Prevention and Intervention in Childhood and Adolescence 14

Special Research Unit 227 — Prevention and Intervention in Childhood and Adolescence

An interdisciplinary project of the University of Bielefeld

conducted by *Prof. Dr. Günter Albrecht, Prof. Dr. Michael Brambring, Prof. Dr. Detlev Frehsee, Prof. Dr. Wilhelm Heitmeyer, Dr. Alois Herlth, Prof. Dr. Klaus Hurrelmann, Prof. Dr. Hans-Uwe Otto, Prof. Dr. Helmut Skowronek*

Language acquisition problems and reading disorders: Aspects of diagnosis and intervention

Edited by
Hannelore Grimm and Helmut Skowronek

W DE G

Walter de Gruyter · Berlin · New York 1993

Prof. Dr. *Hannelore Grimm*,
Department of Psychology, University of Bielefeld, Bielefeld, Germany

Prof. Dr. *Helmut Skowronek*,
Department of Psychology, University of Bielefeld, Bielefeld, Germany

With 18 figures and 49 tables

Library of Congress Cataloging-in-Publication Data

Language acquisition problems and reading disorders : aspects of diagnosis and intervention / edited by Hannelore Grimm and Helmut Skowronek.
p. cm. — (Prevention and intervention in childhood and adolescence ; 14)
Includes bibliographical references.
ISBN 3-11-014120-5 (acid-free paper)
1. Language disorders in children — Congresses. 2. Dyslexia — Congresses. I. Grimm, Hannelore. II. Skowronek, Helmut. III. Series.
RJ496.L35L348 1993
618.92'855 — dc 20 93-27052
CIP

Die Deutsche Bibliothek — Cataloging-in-Publication Data

Language acquisition problems and reading disorders : aspects of diagnosis and intervention / ed. by Hannelore Grimm and Helmut Skowronek. — Berlin ; New York : de Gruyter, 1993
(Prevention and intervention in childhood and adolescence ; 14)
ISBN 3-11-014120-5
NE: Grimm, Hannelore [Hrsg.]; GT

⊗ Printed on acid-free paper which falls within the guidelines of the ANSI to ensure permanence and durability.

Printing: WB-Druck GmbH, Rieden am Forggensee. Binding: Lüderitz & Bauer GmbH, Berlin.
Cover Design: Hansbernd Lindemann, Berlin. Photo: Helmut von Berg, Berlin.

Preface

In October 1991 an international symposium "Language acquisition problems and dyslexia: Aspects of diagnosis and intervention" was held in Bielefeld, Germany. Researchers from Austria, Canada, Germany, the Netherlands, Norway, the United Kingdom, and the USA presented the current state of research in the areas of specific language impairment (SLI) and reading disorders (RD), discussed productive directions for future research into the relationship between language impairments and reading disabilities, and crystallized out the most urgent problems which still need resolving, despite the massive progress research has made in both fields in recent years.

That this meeting of researchers in the fields of developmental language disorders and reading disorders was arranged in Germany was a result of the growing awareness of the two editors of this volume that there was a link between our research interests, and of our intention to work in cooperation with each other. When we started to discuss our research questions and problems we soon recognized that knowledge and experience in the one research field was combined with relative ignorance in the other field. This gave rise to two ideas. First, that other researchers very probably shared our fate of knowing a lot about reading disorders but only little about specific language impairment or vice versa. The second idea consequently was to bring together the most outstanding researchers in both fields so that they might inform each other and discuss mutual interests and problems. The result is documented in eleven articles, each with a comprehensive commentary (with one exception due to organizational difficulties).

It would not be reasonable to attempt to summarize the detailed information presented in each article. Instead we would like to merely name four issues which appear especially important and worthy of more scrutiny: (a) The forging of explicit links between underlying language deficits and problems in learning to read. It has not been well understood what aspects of preschool language impairment are related to which subsequent reading disorders. It seems clear, however, that the causes of reading difficulties cannot be attributed to deficits in phonological processing alone. There also appears to be a connection between early syntax deficits and later problems in reading comprehension. (b) If there is a connection between oral language disorders and reading problems then future studies need to clarify the common causes underlying both deficits. Obviously, problems of visual perception and memory cannot be the right candidates. But what is the situation with digit-span problems and speed of verbal item identification, for example? (c) The third issue concerns the question of individual differences. In both fields, that of SLI and of RD, it is a truism that there are great differences between children. What is the exact nature of these differences and which factors are responsible? We need to find out highly specified subgroups in order to grasp the existing relationships between patterns of language disorders and reading problems. The argument is that different children may experience problems in learning to read for different reasons. (d) Such knowledge is not only of great theoretical interest but undoubtedly will have an important impact on the development of remediation techniques. We need more studies which directly confront treatment and its effectiveness. After all, it is our primary aim to help these impaired children as effectively as possible.

Finally, we would like to thank the German Research Council for the grant making possible this conference which was held within the framework of the Special Research Unit 227 "Prevention and Intervention in Childhood and Adolescence" and took place at an idyllic spot within the Teutoburger Forest near the historical site where in 9 B.C. Varus' legions were defeated by Hermann, the head of the Cheruscans. We also wish to express our thanks to all contributors. In particular, we would like to thank E. Wolter, who took care of the text processing, mounted tables and figures and made the book camera-ready for the publishers.

Hannelore Grimm
Helmut Skowronek

Bielefeld, April 1993

Contents

Part 1
Deficits in children with specific language impairment (developmental dysphasia)

Part 2
Disorders of written language (developmental dyslexia)

Contributors

Aram, Dorothy M., Emerson College, Division of Communicative Disorders, 168 Beacon Street, Boston, Massachusetts 02116, U.S.A.

Beck, Isabel, Learning Research and Development Center, 3939 O'Hara Street, Pittsburgh, Pennsylvania 15260, U.S.A.

Catts, Hugh W., Department of Speech, Language and Hearing, University of Kansas, Lawrence, Kansas 66044, U.S.A.

Connell, Phil J., Department of Speech and Hearing Sciences, Indiana University, Bloomington, Indiana 47405, U.S.A.

Deutsch, Werner, Institut für Psychologie der Technischen Universität Braunschweig, Spielmannstr. 19, 38106 Braunschweig, Germany

Ehri, Linnea C., The Graduate School and University Center of the City University of New York, 33 West 42 Street, New York, New York 10036-8099, U.S.A.

Ellis, Nick, Department of Psychology, University College of North Wales, Bangor, Gwynedd, LL57 2DG, U.K.

Ellis Weismer, Susan, Department of Communicative Disorders and Waisman Center on Mental Retardation and Human Development, University of Wisconsin-Madison, Madison, Wisconsin 53706, U.S.A.

Franks, Steven L., Department of Linguistics/Slavic Languages and Literatures, Indiana University, Bloomington, Indiana 47405, U.S.A.

Georgi, Mara C., Learning Research and Development Center, University of Pittsburgh, 3939 O'Hara Street, Pittsburgh, Pennsylvania 15260, U.S.A.

Grimm, Hannelore, Abteilung für Psychologie, Universität Bielefeld, Postfach 100131, 33501 Bielefeld, Germany

Jansen, Heiner, Abteilung für Psychologie, Universität Bielefeld, Postfach 100131, 33501 Bielefeld, Germany

Mannhaupt, Gerd, Abteilung für Psychologie, Universität Bielefeld, Postfach 100131, 33501 Bielefeld, Germany

Marx, Harald, Abteilung für Psychologie, Universität Bielefeld, Postfach 100131, 33501 Bielefeld, Germany

Menyuk, Paula, School of Education, Boston University, 605 Commonwealth Avenue, Boston, Massachusetts 02215, U.S.A.

Näslund, Jan Carol, University of New Mexico, College of Education, Department of Educational Foundations, Albuquerque, New Mexico 87131-1266, U.S.A

Naremore, Rita C., Department of Speech and Hearing Sciences, Indiana University, Bloomington, Indiana 47405, U.S.A.

Perfetti, Charles A., Learning Research and Development Center, University of Pittsburgh, 3939 O'Hara Street, Pittsburgh, Pennsylvania 15260, U.S.A.

Rice, Mabel L., Child Language Program, The University of Kansas, 1082 Robert Dole Human Development Center, Lawrence, Kansas 66045, U.S.A.

Scheerer-Neumann, Gerheid, Am Gottesberg 59, 33619 Bielefeld, Germany

Schneider, Wolfgang, Institut für Psychologie, Universität Würzburg, Wittelsbacherplatz 1, 97074 Würzburg, Germany

Shatz, Marilyn, Department of Psychology, Human Performance Center, University of Michigan, 330 Packard Road, Ann Arbor, Michigan 48104-1346, U.S.A.

Skowronek, Helmut, Abteilung für Psychologie, Universität Bielefeld, Postfach 100131, 33501 Bielefeld, Germany

Stanovich, Keith E., Ontario Institute for Studies in Education, 252 Bloor St. West, Toronto, Ontario, Canada M5S 1V6

Stone, C. Addison, Department of Communication Sciences and Disorders, 2299 Sheridan Rd., Northwestern University, Evanston, Illinois 60208-3560, U.S.A.

Weinert, Sabine, Abteilung für Psychologie, Universität Bielefeld, Postfach 100131, 33501 Bielefeld, Germany

Wimmer, Heinz, Institut für Psychologie, Universität Salzburg, Hellbrunnerstr. 34, 5020 Salzburg, Austria

Part 1:

Deficits in children with specific language impairment (developmental dysphasia)

Metalinguistic difficulties in children with specific language impairment: Implications for diagnosis and intervention

Paula Menyuk

Recent research with children who show no marked delay in any other aspect of development than language has led to the generation of several hypotheses to account for the delay (Menyuk 1993). These children have been labelled in various ways but specifically language impaired (SLI) or dysphasic are now the labels most frequently applied. Although it is very likely that children so labelled have a malfunctioning central nervous system, there are still many questions about why their difficulties, apparently, lie solely in their language behavior. The more obvious explanations for language delay, such as cognitive retardation or motoric problems, do not fit the case, nor does impoverished or different input (Grimm 1987). However, there are some indications that mothers' patterns of communication interaction with their SLI children possibly underestimate these children's language comprehension and cognitive abilities (Grimm/Weinert 1993). Why this might lead to the particular language difficulties these children are said to have is unclear. In fact, what the cause or causes are for specific language impairment have yet to be clearly determined.

The various explanations that have been offered appear to fall into two categories; non-obvious cognitive differences of a general kind, and non-obvious cognitive differences that are special to language. In this paper I will briefly review some of the data in each of these categories of explanation and see what conclusions might be reached tentatively as to which one seems most explanatory. I will then speculate that metalinguistic difficulties, a class of cognitive difficulties specific to language, are the cause of these children's language acquisition problems, and indicate the reasons for suggesting that such difficulties might best account for these children's language behavior. Finally, the implications of these conclusions for diagnosis and intervention with these children will be touched upon. First, it is necessary to discuss what appear to be some of the general characteristics of these children's language behavior so that there is some understanding of which children are being discussed.

General characteristics of SLI children's language behavior

Children without apparent cognitive and motor problems who have difficulty in acquiring language at the same pace as normally developing children appear to fall into at least three groups. There are those who are simply slow in development, those who primarily exhibit language production difficulties, and those who have both language comprehension and production problems of varying kinds and amounts. The first group's language behavior might be accounted for by the fact that, although they are by definition not retarded, they are also at the slow end of the continuum of development in all aspects of development, and, therefore, should not be categorized as SLI (specifically language impaired) children at all. This hypothesis was put forth by Lynn Snyder (1987) and seems to be a highly reasonable one. If this were the case, then studies of so-called SLI children who are very young (2 to 3 years) would provide us with very questionable data. We could not be sure whether or not they were very slow normal or SLI children.

Children who fall into the second group are those who achieve normal, near normal, and even way above normal scores on tests of language comprehension but are more than one standard deviation below the norm on tests of language production. Given their normal language comprehension these children may be dyspraxic or dysphasic. That is, they may have problems with motor planning or with motor movements which lead to a general clumsiness and particulary poor articulation of speech. Such articulation requires highly complex motor movements. This group of SLI children appears to be a small one but it is difficult to determine where the cut off point is between them and children who fall into the next group.

The final group contains children with both comprehension and production problems who are not simply generally slow in language development. That is, they are delayed in development but also follow patterns of language development not observed in normally developing children (Fletcher 1991), acquire linguistic structures never used by normally developing children (Grimm/Weinert 1990; Menyuk 1983), and go about the task of language acquisition in ways that are different from that of normally developing children (Grimm this volume; Grimm/Weinert 1991; Menyuk 1991). There has been a great deal of argumentation about this position of difference rather than just delay. As stated initially, there has also been a great deal of argumentation about whether these children have a general cognitive problem or only one that is concerned with the process of language acquisition. Obviously the two types of argumentation are related. Evidence supportive of both delay and difference has been found in studies of these children, and these data will be discussed next. It is possible that studies that have come up with opposing data on this issue have really dealt with different groups (group 1 and 3 described above).

Research into all aspects of language behavior has been carried out with SLI children. Their acquisition and use of morphophonological, lexical, semantactic and discourse rules have been examined, as well as their cognitive abilities in non-linguistic domains. These aspects of language behavior and behavior in general are dealt with in some detail by other papers in this volume. Here, only a few examples of studies that deal with the issue of whether the behavior observed can be described as a delay or a difference in development will be discussed. The findings of these studies will then be used to explore whether these children's language behavior might best be explained by a general or specifically linguistic problem, that is, metalinguistic difficulties.

Phonological analysis of the spontaneous speech produced by SLI children as compared to their normally developing age peers indicates that both delay and differences can be found. Schwartz/Leonard/Folger/Wilcox (1980) found that the same phonological processes are used by both groups of children during the word acquisition period. For example, such processes as weak syllable deletion (bella for umbrella) and stopping of consonants (tip for ship) are found in the speech of both groups of children. The only difference is that these processes appear later and last longer in SLI children. On the other hand Stoel-Gammon (1991) has found that, in at least one group of SLI children, unique phonological realizations are mapped onto an age appropriate lexicon. These might be dyspraxic children. In another group there is delay in lexical acquisition, and many speech sound targets are collapsed into a few. These children may be either delayed in development or SLI. In another study of older language disordered children (5 years) it was found that some were still mapping unique phonological realizations onto lexical items. For some children lexical usage was age appropriate, and for others it was not (Menyuk 1983). The first group, who used an age appropriate lexicon, might also be dyspraxic or Group 2 children. The second group might be SLI children. Examples of some unique realizations were substitution of /m/ for /d/ or a glottal /h/ for all stops. These substitutions do not appear in the phonology of normally developing children.

The bound morphemes of English are said to cause particular difficulties for SLI children, although modals such as "do" and "can" are also late acquisitions for these children. The question addressed by a number of researchers is whether or not SLI children are particularly slow in the acquisition of certain morphemes as compared to others and therefore show a different as well as delayed pattern of development. Leonard (1989) suggests that the pattern is different as well as delayed in young children acquiring the morphological system, and Menyuk/Looney (1972) found that certain grammatical morphemes are still missing from the language production of children who are 5 years of age. Examples of such morphemes are the stridents as plural markers, contracted copula (as in "bats" and "he's nice") and third person singular. On the other hand, Lahey et al. (in press) have found that the morphological markers produced by SLI and normally developing children, during the period of 1 up to 4 MLU, were quite similar with one outstanding exception. The contracted copula was omitted by significantly more SLI children at all MLU levels.

The findings of many studies of the semantactic development of SLI children indicate that they are not only delayed in the comprehension and production of semantactic structures, but also that they plateau in this development when certain critical stages are reached (Menyuk 1978). For example they have difficulty in expanding simple SVO sentences at about age 3 to 6, and then have difficulty in expanding sentences by conjunction and embedding when they are 9 plus years. They also more frequently produce these structures with errors (Johnston/Kamhi 1984) and, as stated previously, produce structures not produced by their normally developing peers (Fletcher 1991; Grimm 1987). Some of these structures are errors of ordering in combination with morphophonological errors (for example, from Fletcher 1991 "my mum was take me a picture" for "my mum took a picture of me", and "here they got eyes to me" for "here they gave me eyes", or "here they are looking at me"). Semantactic development appears to be one aspect of language acquisition where few claims have been made that SLI children are simply delayed. It may be that consistent morphophonological differences, such as those found with the contractible copula, are more a function of semantactic than morphophonological differences. Problems with this form might be similar to problems with modals such as "can" and "do", that is, difficulties in verb phrase expansion. It has also been suggested that many of these children's morphophonological problems are due to their difficulties in marking agreement between the noun phrase and verb phrase in sentences (Clahsen 1992).

Behaviors such as overextension of lexical items during the lexical acquisition period have been found in the language samples of both normally developing and SLI children (Chapman et al. 1983). Again, such overextensions, like morphophonological processes, begin later and continue longer in the speech of SLI children. However, differences as well as delays have been found in the lexical behavior of older SLI children (German 1982). Some older SLI children appear to have a smaller vocabulary than their normally developing age peers whereas others appear to have a retrieval problem. The latter do a great deal of substitution and reformulation of lexical items in their spontaneous speech. They also exhibit delay and circumlocutions ("it's to dig with" for "shovel") in the confrontation naming behavior. Finally plateaus in lexical development, like plateaus in semantactic development, may occur in SLI children, although there are few data to support this notion. For example, there is an indication that SLI children plateau in their ability to name colors and letters rapidly (Chesnick et al. in preparation; Menyuk 1993). SLI children have particular difficulty with metaphoric language (Nippold/Fey 1983).

Little research on SLI children's speech act development has been carried out but more on their discourse processing. The data collected thus far on speech act development indicate, again, both delays and differences. The functions of the speech of young normally developing and SLI children appear to be similar (Leonard et al. 1982). Both groups demand and name, but SLI children name less than their peers. However, a plateau in the development of indirect requests occurs, and SLI children of 6 to 9 years are about 2 years behind their normally developing peers in this ability (Prinz/Ferrier 1983). Speech act development is a function of conjoined lexical and semantactic development, as well as the development of intentions, and, therefore, it may be difficult to parcel out whether the plateau in speech act development in these children is due to delays in the development of pragmatic rules or differences in knowledge of the semantactic structures needed to carry out speech acts. Findings on the difficulties that these children have in discourse suggest that for some the latter is the primary problem.

When examining these children's development of discourse knowledge, conversational interaction and narrative recall have been studied, but only in older SLI children. Once again, both delays and differences have been found but what is most interesting in these findings are data which suggest that the comprehension abilities of the SLI children in the study have a marked effect on their discourse behavior. For example, there were children within an older SLI population (approximately 9 to 14 years) who showed more turn errors, interrupted more and interacted less than others within this population. The children who exhibited these behaviors more frequently were those with reduced receptive skills. These children's patterns of recall of stories has been found to be both similar (Graybeal 1981) and different (Johnston 1982) from their normally developing peers. That is, it has been found that although some SLI children recall fewer propositions they do recall most aspects of the story's grammar in the right order. It has also been found that some SLI children show temporal inversions and transformations in their recall, and their patterns of recall and story construction are atypical of children of their age. These differences may be related to their language comprehenion abilities. Those who show differences in sequence of recall may be those with comprehension difficulties.

In summary, there are data which support the conclusion that language development in SLI children is delayed but follows the same pattern of development as that of normally developing children. There are also data which support the conclusion that patterns of language development are different in these children. Most of the data that points to similarities between the two groups of children are data obtained when these children are at the beginning stages of language development, and the data on differences are concerned with development at later stages. Therefore, one might hypothesize that these children are delayed initially, and then become different as they mature. This appears to be an incorrect conclusion because some of these children are still similar to their normally developing peers even at later ages while others are not. It was stated initially that there might be at least three groups of children in this population; slow, and therefore late developing children, children who have output problems, and children who have both input and output problems. The data obtained on these children's development of the various aspects of language lend some support to this possibility. A summary of findings and conjectures concerning patterns of development in aspects of language is presented in Table 1. The statements concerning Group 2, children with output problems, is largely conjecture.

If there are differences among these children in their patterns of language behavior and development, there might also be different explanations to account for their behavior and patterns of development. Dyspraxic children's behavior might be simply explained by constraints on either their planning of output or their output programming of planned units of language. The behavior of children who are slow in development might be explained by a general slowness in developing categories and relations of all kinds, not

Tab. 1: Rough summary of findings on patterns of language development in three groups of language impaired children

		Groups of Children	
Aspect of Language	Group I	Group II Output Problems	Group III Input and Output Problems
Phonology	Delayed	Plateau/Unique Realizations in Production Perception Normal	Delay/Unique Realizations Perception?
Morphology	Delayed	Unique Realizations Comprehension Normal?	Particular Difficulties with Certain Free and Bound Morphemes
Semantax	Delayed	Comprehension Normal Production Delay/Plateau	Delay/Plateau/Difference in Comprehension/Production
Lexicon	Delayed	Age Appropriate	Delayed and Different in Retrieval Time/Type
Pragmatics	Delayed	Comprehension Normal Production Labored	Difficulties in Turntaking Indirect Speech Acts/ Connected Discourse

just linguistic ones. There are some data which indicate that children within this population have difficulties in the rate at which they process visual as well as auditory information (Johnston/Weismer 1983; Tallal et al. 1981). Differences in the rate at which information of all kinds can be processed obviously could lead to a slowing down of the rate at which different aspects of language are acquired, and thus account for the behavior and development of the delayed children. However, just stating that they are slow is not an explanation. One needs to determine why they are slow. In addition, the children who would not be accounted for by simply calling upon differences in rate of information processing are the third group of children, those who exhibit differences in development. For them some alternate explanation must be provided. It will be argued below that metalinguistic difficulties, due to differing sources for each group, can account for the behavior and development of children in Group 1 and 3. The argument, not so by the way, will be in support of the modularity principle for acquisition of some aspects of language.

Role of metalinguistic processing in normal development

Before discussing the role of metalinguistic difficulties in non-normal development it is necessary to talk about the role of metalinguistic processing in normal development. In an outstandingly clear summary of the varying positions held by theoreticians concerning the explanations for language development, Hirsh-Pasek/Golinkoff (in press) refer to the "outside-in" and the "inside-out" theorists. They further subdivide the "outside-in" theorists into "social-interactionists" and "cognitivists". In both types of explanation, the child constructs the grammar of the language. The social interactionists emphasize the importance of the communication interactions between child and caregiver in which the caregiver *makes clear* how the categories and relations in the environment are marked by the language. The cognitivists suggest that the child starts with a rich conceptual base of categories and relations, and looks for associations between these and the categories and relations marked in language. Then by a general process of pattern recognition they develop the grammar of the language.

The "inside-out" theorists are those who support the modularity principle either totally or partially. For them language learning is separate and different from other kinds of learning. This implies (although certainly not stated by Hirsh-Pasek/Golinkoff) that the underlying hardware for at least some aspects of language learning is probably also separate and different from that of other kinds of learning. From this point of view the grammar of the language is discovered, not constructed. There are also two schools of "inside-out" theorists. The first school suggests that the child looks for proofs for innate ideas about the categories and relations in language that are not specific to a particular language. Thus, the child comes with a set of hypotheses about the nature of language or a so-called core grammar. The second group is concerned with the linguistic "mechanisms" (perhaps other possible words are "cues" and "strategies") the child uses to learn language and only language.

Although the above discussion is probably very familiar to researchers in child language development, there is a reason for reviewing it. It is useful to think about these views in a discussion of explanations for the language behavior and development of SLI children. It is also useful in discussing the role of metalinguistic processing in language development, and metalinguistic difficulties in specific language impairment. We started out by reviewing some facts about SLI children. Their language difficulties cannot be easily explained by either group of "outside-in" theorists, the social interactionists and the cognitivists. The position of the first group of "inside-out" theorists of a richly endowed child is, for the most part, untestable. The position of the second group of "inside-out" theorists, that there are mechanisms used by the child to discover the grammar of the language, seems most germane to the discussion. What is meant by the position is certainly open to interpretation. One possible interpretation is that the child comes prepared to use certain kinds of information, let's call them surface structure cues, to categories and relations in the language, and then must have some means or strategy for storing the units and relations for further use. It is this further use, or the ability to retrieve or be aware of the units and relations, that could be termed metalinguistic ability.

The term metalinguistic abilities can be used by different researchers in differing ways. One view is that these abilities are a product of advanced cognitive development (Karmiloff-Smith 1986). When children reach the concrete operation period (approximately 8 years), the child is then said to be able to take a reflective stance about language; that is, view it as an object in its own right apart from its use, and be aware of the categories and relations in the language. Another view is that this reflective stance begins at a very early stage of language development, and continues throughout the entire developmental period (Menyuk 1991). Further, metalinguistic abilities are necessary for the acquisition of all aspects of language, and change in nature as knowledge of the language changes. Figure 1 describes changes in metalinguistic ability with time. The figure attempts to capture the notion that metalinguistic abilities are not simply the ability to assume a reflective stance but involve other competences that are necessary for first *discovering* and then *storing* the categories and relations in language. A necessary first

---

I DISCOVERY OF CUES

II STORAGE OF INFORMATION

III REFLECTION OR AWARENESS

IV JUDGEMENT/COMPARISON

V AUTOMATICITY IN USE/EXPLANATION

Fig. 1: Stages in development of metalinguistic ability

stage is being able to judge what are important cues. The child must then become aware of what the cues are and be able to judge whether or not the data fits the cues. Finally, the child must be able to automatically process these cues.

Some of the evidence in support of this position has been discussed elsewhere (Menyuk 1991). Here some of that evidence and additional evidence will be briefly summarized. At the very beginning of language development, during the first two years of life, a number of behaviors are manifested which can be viewed as being able to judge what are important cues, storing units, and taking a reflective stance. During the first year of life there is evidence that infants are sensitive to cues that correspond to clausal units first, then phrasal units and then word units (Hirsh-Pasek 1989). Prosodic cues probably play the most important role in this behavior. A very convincing argument has been presented that the transition from expression of meaning through paralinguistic means (prosody, facial expression and gesture) to expression of meaning by linguistic means requires a reflective stance. Bloom/Capatides (1987) found that the more frequently infants expressed affect the later were their first words. The more time the infants spent in neutral affect, the younger their age when first words appeared. The researchers suggest that this is due to the fact that word use requires this reflective stance.

Manifestations of lexical and semantactic judgement abilities continue throughout the second year of life when the basic relations and categories in the language are being acquired. Two examples of this are young children's introduction of phonemic distinctions which don't exist in their language to disambiguate words (Leopold 1939), and their ablity to judge which panel of a split screen depicts an appropriate actor, action, object relation (Hirsh-Pasek et al. 1985). These two behaviors suggest, respectively, the ability to judge that different phonological sequences mark different words in the language, and that order of words in a sequence mark different relations among these words.

During the third and fourth year of life detection of semantactic and morphophonological error and correction of such errors is manifested. One can observe judgement of errors in ordering of animate actor, action and inanimate object (Gleitman/Gleitman/Shipley 1972) and correction in terms of semantic relations. Children alternate between the use of correct and incorrect forms, and self correct (Menyuk 1964). They also respond to requests for clarification by addressing all aspects of their utterances (Stokes

1976). They are aware that they should respond to such requests and attempt to be intelligible. They also alter the semantax of their utterances and thus indicate that they judge that ambiguity may lie in the structure of their utterances.

Over these years and the following years of life children excercise these abilities of judgement and correction with increasingly complex structures, and over pieces of discourse. Children develop notions of appropriate sequence in stories of their culture when they are 4 years of age, and are able to detect incorrect sequences and sudden shifts in topic at this age. They are able to judge and correct non-grammatical and anomalous sentences that first contain simple SVO structures at ages 3 to 5 (for example, "I see a leaves" and "The nail hit the hammer") and then sentences that contain embedded structures at ages 6 to 7 (for example, "I know what is he doing" and "He broke his leg because he went to the hospital"). They also can judge paraphrase (for example, "I sent a valentine to every girl" and "I sent every girl a valentine") and can detect ambiguity (for example, "Do you want the lion to chase you or the tiger?") when they are about 10 years of age (Flood/Menyuk 1983). At around 6 or 7 years of age children are able to provide explanations for the judgements that they are able to make. Table 2 provides some examples of the changes that occur in linguistic meta-ablities with time.

We have described evidence for metalinguistic abilities and for changes in metalinguistic abilities with time, but the role of metalinguistic abilities in the language acquisition process has not been described. The view espoused here is that it is necessary for the child to be aware of the categories and relations in language before they can be used automatically. In turn, automatic use of the categories and relations in language is necessary for acquisition of additional structures because only automatic processing leaves space and time for additional information to be dealt with (Siegler 1991). The application of metalinguistic abilities to the language acquisition process and the sequence of development from unconscious judgement and use to awareness and, finally, automaticity is described in Figure 2.

Tab. 2: Some evidence of metalinguistic processing over first several years of life

Age	Behavior
First Year	Sensitivity to Clausal, Phrase and Word Units Shift in Speech Discrimination to Native L Categories Shift from Paralinguistic to Linguistic Expression
Second Year	Judgment of Depiction of Correct SVO Relations Use of Speech Sound Contrasts to Disambiguate Speech Sound Avoidance
Third and 4th Year	Judgment of Correct and Incorrect SVO Relations Correction of Incorrect SVO Relations Selfcorrection of Errors of All Aspects Variable Response to Request for Clarification Increase Intelligibility Alter Linguistic Units and Relations
Fourth to 8th Year	Judgment of Topic Maintenance and Sequence in Stories Detection of Anomaly, Non-grammaticality and Explanation Judgment of Paraphrase and Ambiguity and Explanation

TIME I	TIME II	TIME III
Processing Strategies Set I	Processing Strategies Set II	Processing Strategies Set III
Intuitive Knowledge Rules Set I	Intuitive Knowledge Rules Set II	Intuitive Knowledge Rules Set III
	Conscious Knowledge Rules Set I	Conscious Knowledge Rules Set II
		Automatic Processing Rules Set I

Fig. 2: Development of automaticity

Role of metalinguistic difficulties in the language development of SLI children

Specifically language impaired children are, presumably, only slow in developing linguistic categories and relations, not non-linguistic ones. However, as stated, there are data which indicate that SLI children are slower in their rate of response and can process smaller amounts of data than their age matched peers in both the linguistic and non-linguistic domain. The children who have provided these data may, however, be Group 1 children, the over-all slow developers, who show delay in language development initially and continue to develop at a much slower rate than their peers of any age, but show no differences in patterns of development. These children exhibit delays in both comprehension and production of language. They have both metalinguistic difficulties and general metaprocessing difficulties which retard their development, but are not so severe that they can be categorized as retarded.

Group 2 are children who have language production problems and who may be what we have called dyspraxic. They are not children who have general metaprocessing or metalinguistic difficulties but only constraints on their language output. There are data which indicate that these children are in families where speech and language problems are quite frequent and, therefore, a genetic component to their difficulty is suspected. These families also evidence more frequent incidence of dyslexia (Lewis/Ekelman/Aram 1989). Children who fall into Group 3 are children with both language comprehension and production difficulties. They are the ones who show differences in their patterns of development and language behavior, and their difficulties are metalinguistic ones, not general metaprocessing difficulties.

A brief review of the findings with these children in different aspects of the language indicate the following differences:

1. At the phonological level they develop speech sound representations in words that are markedly different in features than target speech sounds.
2. At the morphophonological level they have long lasting difficulty with certain morphemes, particularly those that are morphosyntactic, and may show plateaus in this development.
3. At the lexical level they have great difficulty in word retrieval and confrontation naming and frequently substitute a lexical item with words such as "that" and "this" or a descriptive phrase.
4. At the semantactic level they have long lasting difficulty at each stage

where further development is marked by first expansion of phrase and then expansion of clause. They distort the sequence in which these phrases and clauses should be expanded, and frequently commit errors of marking.
5. At the pragmatic level they have difficulty with consistent appropriate responding in conversation and in recall of sequences in narratives.

The explanations that have been presented previously to account for the above findings are the reduced rate at which SLI children can process speech information, and the fact that they can only process limited amounts of information within a given time frame. Both types of explanation, it has been argued (Menyuk 1991), could be subsumed under an explanation of difficulties in metalinguizing. Automaticity in processing of information speeds up the rate at which that information is processed, but automaticity first requires conscious awareness of the structure of the information. When processing of some part of the information becomes automatic then *additional* information can be processed in immediate memory. The explanation, as stated previously, could be appropriate for both language delayed children and SLI or dysphasic children. The difference between the two groups in patterns of development and behavior could be explained by the particular difficulties the SLI children have in language comprehension. Such difficulties lead not only to slowed down development but also distorted development.

A study (Menyuk et al. 1991) was recently carried out in which children labelled as SLI, using established criteria of 1 or more years below the mean on tests of language production, and 6 months or more below the mean on language comprehension, were asked to engage in varying metalinguistic tasks. Included in the population were children considered to be at risk for later reading difficulties because of early language difficulties or very low birth weight. The children ranged in age from 4 - 5½ years at the beginning of the study and were 7 - 8½ years at its end. In the area of phonology they were asked to segment morphemes into syllables and speech sound segments. In the area of semantax they were given an oral Cloze task, asked to judge and correct grammatical and non-grammatical sentences (non-grammatical morphophonologically and structurally), and answer questions about simple and complex sentences). Their confrontation naming and their lexical recall abilities in non-cued and cued situations was examined. Their discourse ability was examined by asking them to recall a story. A comparison of their metalinguistic abilities and those of normally developing and at risk children was carried out. Using cluster analyses of the scores obtained on the intake measures, it was found that some SLI and some at risk children clustered together in these ablities but that, although some at risk children performed significantly more poorly than their normally developing age peers, they did significantly better than did the SLI children. Thus, the population seemed to divide itself into the normally developing group, a group performing significantly more poorly than the normally developing children but significantly better than the SLI group, and the SLI group.

To examine the children's development of metaprocessing skills in the three groups the children's scores on tasks were also grouped in terms of the aspect of language being examined; that is, phonology, semantax, lexicon and discourse. Their raw scores (number correct) for each aspect were converted to standard scores (a mean of 0 and a standard deviation of 1). The children were tested three times over a three year period, shortly after the study began, then approximately midway in the duration of the study, and then near its end. A comparison of the metalinguistic skills of the three language ability groups in all the areas showed that the SLI group was most different in pattern of development of semantax and phonology (Chesnick et al. in preparation). Further, children who were normally developing were significantly better at these tasks than children who were slow in development at all three times of testing. These latter children, in turn, were significantly better at these tasks than SLI children at all times. These findings are shown in Figure 3.

A great deal of data has been collected by a number of researchers that provides evidence that both delayed and SLI children have difficulty in bringing to conscious awareness the categories and relations that exist in every aspect of language. Every time these children are tested or are asked to engage in an experiment, conscious awareness of differing units of language is required (Menyuk et al. 1991). Therefore, most of the language performance data reported in the literature, not based on spontaneous speech samples, probably reflect this difficulty in metalinguizing. However, the above statement is a logical conclusion, and the explanation provided for the patterns of language development and the language behavior of the three groups of language disordered children is largely a theoretical one. Much more research is needed before the theory can be evaluated. Some suggestions for such research are described below.

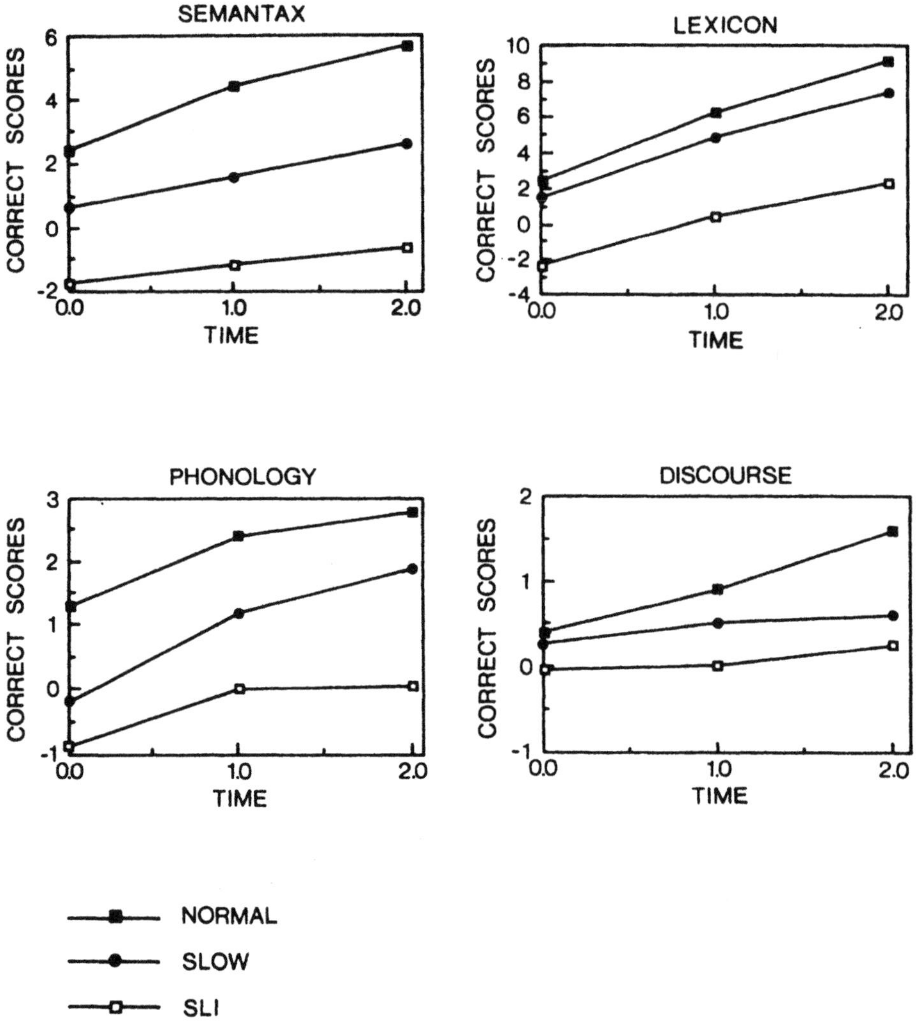

Fig. 3: Metalinguistic performance of the three groups of children

Implications for diagnosis and intervention

We need to know a great deal more about the language development and metalinguistic abilities of SLI children before very clear statements can be made about the implications of what has been said for diagnosis and intervention. However, research designed to gain a better understanding of these children's difficulties is, in fact, a form of diagnosis. In like fashion, a better diagnosis of these children's difficulties would provide a better plan of what needs to be taken into consideration when planning intervention. Therefore, the suggestion that more research is needed is in reality a call for better diagnoses of these children's problems, and, therefore, better bases for the interventions to be carried out with them.

If the above theory is correct, then one should think about research with these children in terms of three areas of development, metaprocessing in non-linguistic domains, patterns of development of spontaneous speech, and metalinguistic abilities. The theory should predict differences in patterns of development and behavior among the three groups of children in all three types of development. Group 1 children should show slowed development in all three areas. Group 2 children should show markedly slow patterns of development only in spontaneous speech with, perhaps, particular difficulty in realization of target speech sounds. Group 3 children should show delay and difference in the development of spontaneous speech, and in the development of their metalinguistic abilities but not in metacognitive abilities.

Despite the fact that intervention should be based on proven difficulties we are currently engaged in a study examining under which conditions these children's metaprocessing of the various units of language at different levels might be improved.[1] We are also examining whether or not improvement in their metaprocessing of these units speeds up and corrects their acquisition of these units. If we find that this is the case, then we will have substantive evidence that our theory is possibly correct. If this is not the case, then we will have to rethink the matter.

Note

[1]This research is supported in part from a grant from N.I.D.C.D. Improving language processing in impaired children (DC00537).

References

Bloom, L. & Capatides, J. (1987). Expression of affect and the emergence of language. Child Development, 58, 1513-1522.

Chapman, K., Leonard, L., Rowan, L., & Weiss, A. (1983). Inappropriate word extensions in the speech of young language disordered children. Journal of Speech and Hearing Disorders, 48, 55-61.

Chesnick, M., Menyuk, P., D'Agostino, R., & Belanger, A. (in preparation). Development of metalinguistic skills in children of varying language ability.

Clahsen, H. (1992). The acquisition of inflectional morphology: A comparison of English and German. Paper presented to the Applied Linguistic Program, Boston University, Boston, MA.

Fletcher, P. (1991). Evidence from syntax for language impairment. In J. Miller (Ed.), Research on child language disorders: A decade of progress. 169-188. Austin, TX: Pro-Ed.

Flood, J. & Menyuk, P. (1983). The development of metalinguistic awareness and its relation to reading. Journal of Applied Developmental Psychology, 4, 65-80.

German, D. (1982). Word-finding substitutions in children with learning disabilities. Language, Speech, and Hearing Services in Schools, 13, 223-230.

Gleitman, L., Gleitman, H., & Shipley, E. (1972). The emergence of the child as grammarian. Cognition, 1, 137-164.

Graybeal, C. (1981). Memory for stories in language impaired children. Applied Psycholinguistics, 2, 269-283.

Grimm, H. (1987). Developmental dysphasia: New theoretical perspectives and empirical results. The German Journal of Psychology, 11, 8-22.

Grimm, H. & Weinert, S. (1990). Is the syntax development of dysphasic children deviant and why? New findings to an old question. Journal of Speech and Hearing Research, 33, 220-228.

Grimm, H. & Weinert, S. (1991). Conditions of normal language acquisition viewed from the analysis of causes of disordered language development. Paper given at Biennial Meeting of the Society for Research in Child Development, Seattle, Washington.

Grimm, H. & Weinert, S. (1993). Patterns of interaction and communication in language development disorders. In G. Blanken, J. Dittmann, H. Grimm, J.C. Marshall, & C.-W. Wallesch (Eds.), Linguistic disorders and pathologies. An international handbook. 697-711. Berlin: de Gruyter.

Hirsh-Pasek, K. (1989). Infants' perception of fluent speech: Implications for language development. Paper given at Biennial Meeting of Society for Research in Child Development, Kansas City, MO.

Hirsh-Pasek, K. & Golinkoff, R.M. (in press). Skeletal supports for grammatical learning: What infants bring to the language learning task. In C.K. Rovee-Collier (Ed.), Advances in infancy research, Vol. 10. Norwood, N.J.: Ablex.

Hirsh-Pasek, K., Golinkoff, R., Beaubien, F., Fletcher, A., & Cauley, K. (1985). In the beginning: One word speakers comprehend word order. Paper given at 10th Annual Boston University Language Development Conference, Boston, MA.

Johnston, J. (1982). Narratives: A new look at communication problems in older language disordered children. Language, Speech and Hearing Services in Schools, 13, 144-156.

Johnston, J. & Kamhi, A. (1984). Syntactic and semantic aspects of utterances of language impaired children: The same can be less. Merrill-Palmer Quarterly, 30, 65-86.

Johnston, J. & Weismer, S. (1983). Mental rotation abilities in language disordered children. Journal of Speech and Hearing Research, 26, 397-403.

Karmiloff-Smith, A. (1986). From meta-processes to conscious access: Evidence from children's metalinguistic and repair data. Cognition, 23, 95-147.

Lahey, M., Liebergott, J., Chesnick, M., Menyuk, P., & Adams, J. (in press). Variability in the use of grammatical morphemes: Implications for understanding language impairment. Applied Psycholinguistics.

Leopold, W. (1939). Speech development of a bilingual child: A linguist's record: Vol. 1. Evanston, IL.: Northwestern University Press.

Leonard, L. (1989). Language learnability and specific language impairment in children. Applied Psycholinguistics, 10, 179-202.

Leonard, L., Camarata, S., Rowan, L., & Chapman, K. (1982). The communicative functions of lexical usage by language impaired children. Applied Psycholinguistics, 3, 109-125.

Lewis, B., Ekelman, B., & Aram, D. (1989). A familial study of severe phonological disorders. Journal of Speech and Hearing Research, 32, 713-724.

Menyuk, P. (1964). Alternation of rules in children's grammar. Journal of Verbal Learning and Verbal Behavior, 3, 480-488.

Menyuk, P. (1978). Linguistic problems in children with developmental dysphasia. In M. Wyke (Ed.), Developmental dysphasia. 135-158. London: Academic Press.

Menyuk, P. (1983). The role of context in misarticulations. In G. Yeni-Komshian, J. Kavanaugh, & C. Ferguson (Eds.), Child phonology, Vol. I. 211-228. New York: Academic Press.

Menyuk, P. (1991). Metalinguistic abilities and language disorder. In J. Miller (Ed.), Research on child language disorders: A decade of progress. 387-397. Austin, TX.: Pro-Ed.

Menyuk, P. (1993). Children with specific language impairment (developmental dysphasia): Linguistic aspects. In G. Blanken, J. Dittmann, H. Grimm, J. Marshall, & C. Wallesch (Eds.), Linguistic disorders and pathologies: An international handbook. 606-625. Berlin: de Gruyter.

Menyuk, P., Chesnick, M., Liebergott, J., Korngold, B., D'Agostino, R., & Belanger, A. (1991). Predicting reading problems in at risk children. Journal of Speech and Hearing Research, 34, 893-901.

Menyuk, P. & Looney, P. (1972). Relationships among components of the grammar in language disorder. Journal of Speech and Hearing Research, 15, 395-406.

Nippold, M. & Fey, S. (1983). Metaphoric understanding in preadolescents having a history of language acquisition difficulties. Language, Speech, and Hearing Services in Schools, 14, 171-180.

Prinz, P. & Ferrier, L. (1983). Can you give me that one? The comprehension production and judgement of directives in language impaired children. Journal of Speech and Hearing Disorders, 48, 44-54.

Schwartz, R., Leonard, L., Folger, M., & Wilcox, M. (1980). Early phonological behavior in normal speaking and language disordered children. Journal of Speech and Hearing Disorders, 45, 357-377.

Siegler, R. (1991). Children's thinking. Second Edition. Englewood Cliffs, N.J.: Prentice-Hall.

Snyder, L. (1987). Defining language disordered children: Disordered or just "low verbal" normal? Proceedings of Symposium on Research in Child Language Disorders, 3, 197-209. U. of Wisconsin, Madison.

Stoel-Gammon, C. (1991). Issues in phonological development and disorders. In J. Miller (Ed.), Research on child language disorders: A decade of progress. 255-266. Austin, TX: Pro-Ed.

Stokes, W. (1976). Children's replies to requests for clarification: An opportunity for hypothesis testing. Paper given at 3rd Annual Boston University Conference on Language Development.

Tallal, P., Stark, R., Kallman, C., & Mellits, D. (1981). A reexamination of some nonverbal perceptual abilities of language impaired and normal children as a function of age and sensory modality. Journal of Speech and Hearing Research, 24, 351-357.

Syntax and morphological difficulties in German-speaking children with specific language impairment: Implications for diagnosis and intervention

Hannelore Grimm

Prototypical definition

German is a highly inflected language including mobility of verbs and other constituents and is thus especially appropriate for the investigation of syntax problems and morphological difficulties in dysphasic or specific language impaired (SLI) children. In the following, these two terms will be used interchangeably.

In order to ensure agreement on what kind of children we are talking about, I shall first give a sort of prototypical definition. This definition applies for all children we examined - even if not quite perfectly in every case.

As shown in Table 1, SLI children are characterized by a late and slow

Tab. 1: Specific language impairment: Main characteristics

- late and slow development of language
- normal overall developmental progress
- adequate hearing ability
- no evident profound neurological damage
- no profound emotional and behavioral problems
- normal home background

Three discrepancies typically shown:

* severe deficits in language abilities
  - normal nonverbal test intelligence

* Severe problems in language production
  - better abilities in language comprehension

* Severe deficits in learning the morpho-syntactic aspects of language
  - better learning of the semantic/pragmatic aspect

development of language. They exhibit delays of one year or more in language production but are less retarded in language comprehension. This language deficit exists in spite of a normal overall developmental progress and adequate hearing ability. The children also show no evident profound neurological damage. However, the new sophisticated scanning devices for documenting neurological status were not used (see Miller 1991 for discussion of this point). Further, there is a normal home background and an absence of profound emotional and behavioral problems.

In particular, the children typically show the following three discrepancies: First, in spite of having severe deficits in language abilities, they perform within a normal range in nonverbal intelligence tests; second, their language production ability is more disturbed than their comprehension ability; and third, the morpho-syntactic aspects of their language are more disturbed than the semantic and pragmatic aspects.

To avoid any misunderstanding, it should be pointed out that the discrepancy between language skills and test intelligence cannot mean that the dysphasic children are completely normally intelligent children, who - for some inexplicable reason - are only unable to acquire language normally. Thus, the mother of a boy enrolled in my longitudinal study repeatedly pointed out - and she was quite irate about it - that she could not understand why psychologists classified her son as having an above-average intelligence, whereas he could not speak well, had a poor memory and could not read or write properly (Grimm 1987; 1988). This mother addressed two important aspects: First, that the intelligence diagnosis is based solely on nonverbal tasks. This restriction, however, is made neither in common psychometric theories nor in subjective theories of intelligence. Second, it should be emphasized that all intelligence tests can only have a restricted ecological validity. What is measured only represents one part of the whole range of intelligent behavior. Thus, one cannot predict directly from the performance in an intelligence test the level of performance in other cognitive tasks.

In Table 2 all past and present studies done in my lab with dysphasic children are listed. Up till now, we have examined in total 170 SLI-children between the ages of 3;9 to 12;7 years. We have observational data, test data, and experimental data either from a longitudinal study, from a follow-up study or from crosssectional studies. This data base should be broad enough to be able to characterize some of the children's language problems and to formulate tentative causal explanations for these problems.

Tab. 2: *Research Projects*

Study	Topic	Number of Subjects	Age	Design	Data
Grimm (e.g. 1983; 1986a, b; 1987)	General language development; syntax acquisition	8 SLI 8 NL	3;9-4;8[1] 2;1-2;11	longitudinal; follow-up	natural observation; test data
Grimm 1988; 1989	general language development	90 SLI	4;3-12;7	cross-sectional	test data
Weinert/Grimm et al., 1989	text processing	16 SLI 16 NL	6;6-8;6 6;10-7;7	cross-sectional	experimental; test data
Grimm 1991a	language and cognition	8 SLI 16 NL	3;9-4;8 2;1-4;8	cross-sectional	natural observation
Weinert 1991	syntactic rule learning	24 SLI 42 NL	5;5-8;5 5;1-6;7	cross-sectional	experimental; test-data
Grimm, running project (Research Grant No. Gr 588/10-1, Gr 588/10-2)	syntax, metalinguistics and memory	24 SLI 24 NL	5;0-8;0 5;0-8;0	cross-sectional	experimental; test-data

[1]age at timepoint t1; mean age at timepoint t5; 7;3

Syntax

Typical word order problems

As a particular description of syntax, I want to start with the sentence patterns used by the 8 dysphasic preschoolers in my longitudinal study over the period of one year (Grimm 1986a, 1987). At the beginning of the study, the children were between 3;9 and 4;8 years old (see Table 3). Their spontaneous speech was characterized by very simple sentences comprising only one or two other elements in addition to the verb, whereby obligatory elements were often left out. The average number of words per utterance (MLU) lay between 3.22 and 4.41 with a mean of 3.81.

Tab. 3: Samples of normal and specifically language impaired children (SLI)

	SLI children N = 8	normal children N = 8
age[a]	4;2 (3;9 - 4;8)	2;6 (2;1 - 2;11)
sex	6 m; 2 f	6 m; 2 f
IQ[b] (non-verbal-S.O.N.)	113 (SD = 22)	116 (SD = 9)
stammering	all	none

[a] means with range
[b] means with standard deviation

No relationship between sentence complexity and the distinctness of the children's articulatory problems was found; the child with almost unintelligible speech had the second highest MLU of 4.10; and the child with the lowest MLU of 3.22 had the least problem with articulation. Therefore, the conclusion appears justified that these children's syntax problems cannot be traced back to phonological difficulties only. Neither could phonological difficulties explain why these dysphasic children produce such idiosyncratic sentences that do not belong to the typical developmental errors. Examples of such sentences are given in Table 4. It is important to stress that such sentences seem to be typical for German SLI children, for not only did we find them in the children in our study but also Clahsen (1988) found them in other German-speaking dysphasic children.

Tab. 4: Examples of incorrect sentences with the verbal part or subject in final position (from Grimm 1987; 1988)

Examples	Standard German
Ich heute gehen raus (I today go out)*	Ich gehe heute raus (I go today out)*
Ein Dach da lege hin (A roof there lay down)	(Ich) lege da ein Dach hin (I) lay there a roof down
Eine Brust ich sehn hab (A breast I seen have)	Ich habe eine Brust gesehen (I have a breast seen)
Ich das guck an will (I that look at will)	Ich will das angucken (I will that at look)
Weg ist sie (Gone is she)	Sie ist weg (She is gone)

*Word for word translations

These sentences can be characterized syntactically in the following way: The main verb, or the auxiliary or modal verb plus the main verb are incorrectly placed at the end of the sentence; furthermore, prefixes and verbs, as well as subjects, are placed in a wrong word order. These sentences are extremely incorrect in Standard German and are produced neither by adults nor by normally developing children. Thus, the MLU-matched control children in our longitudinal study (see Table 3) produced no comparably wrong sentences, and in a more extensive study with 115 normal language children in age groups between 2;7 and 5;11 years I found among the 13.000 analyzed utterances not one sentence with the typical dysphasic form (Grimm 1973).

That this specific word ordering problem cannot be interpreted as being purely a problem of dealing with syntactic and morphological complexities is made clear by the fact that in an elicited imitation task the children changed the word order in even very simple sentences in accordance with their incorrect ordering, placing verb or subject at the end of the sentence (see Grimm/Weinert 1990).

The following impressive figures demonstrate that this incorrect word order was predominant in the spontaneous speech of the 8 SLI children in the longitudinal project: In 69% of the sentences produced by the SLI children with an average age of 4;2 years at timepoint 1, either the verbal part or the subject was placed at the end of the sentence. And in 75% of these cases this word order was incorrect so that an average of 53% of all sentences produced may be characterized as typically dysphasic.

Figure 1 shows that there was, however, great variability among the children: At the first timepoint, four of the eight dysphasic children produced 90 to 100% idiosyncratic sentence patterns out of all sentences with verb and subject in final position. The other four children produced between 50% and 75%. In comparison, the percentages for the MLU-matched controls lay between under 10 and 80.

However, it is important to observe that the incorrect sentences produced by the younger controls are typical for children in this developmental stage and thus differ decidedly from the dysphasic sentences. The important qualitative difference lies in the fact that the sentences with wrong word order produced by the younger controls were morphologically simple and short. In contrast, the incorrect sentences produced by the SLI children were not simply incomplete but significantly longer and morphologically more complex. This important qualitative difference is clearly indicated by the following figures: The incomplete sentences with verb or subject in final position produced by the control children contained on average only 2.90 constituents as compared to the other sentence patterns which contained an average number of 4.02 constituents. In contrast to this significant difference, the typically dysphasic sentences with verb or subject in final position on average displayed the same number of constituents as other sentence patterns (3.74 versus 3.81).

When one follows the history of these sentences over time, one can clearly recognize that at timepoint 2, after 4 months, the controls still formed only very few sentences with wrong word order, that is, with verb or subject in final position. Here again, the different status of these sentences is made clear: The end positioning of the verb is indeed characteristic for normal children in their early language development; however, as soon as the children acquire morphological rules, they also start using different sentence patterns and stop using wrong final verb sentences. In contrast, the developmental change in the dysphasic children is far more heterogeneous. Only the children 1 and 8 made such rapid progress that at timepoint 2 they were producing only few idiosyncratic patterns. However, even after a whole year the three children 5, 6, and 7 had failed to reduce the proportion of

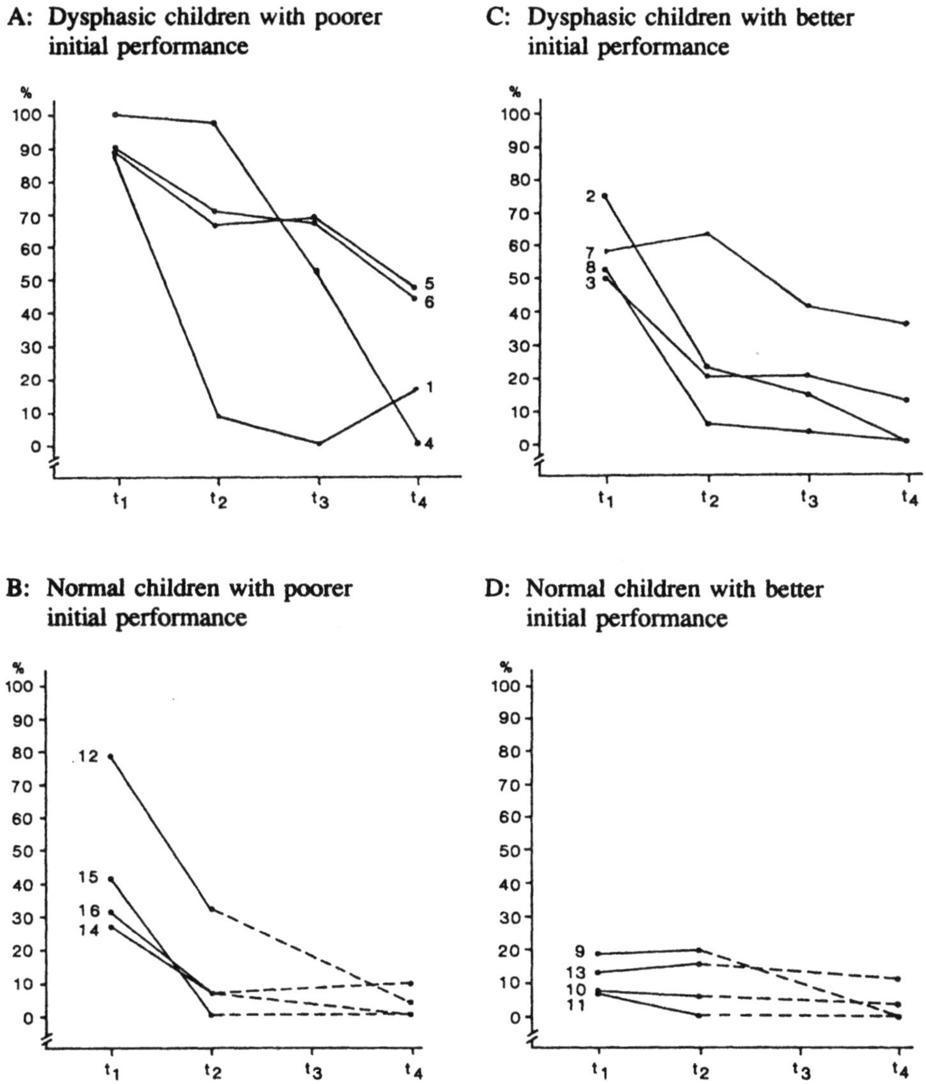

Fig. 1: Decrease in incorrect sentences during the course of one year (t1-t4)

incorrect sentences to a "normal level". This supports to a high degree the supposition that we are here dealing with specific sentences indicating that there is something linguistically special to master for the SLI children. This particular problem could be interpreted as being a permutation problem since the children encounter difficulties in separating units that are semantically linked and in placing them in different and variable syntactic positions. And this permutation problem might be best explained by the assumption that the dysphasic children's underlying representations of phrases and clauses are different from the representations of normally developing children. Limitations of processing when actually producing these utterances do not seem to provide sufficient explanation.

Delay or deviancy?

It is interesting that there is considerable controversy in the literature whether SLI children produce qualitatively special utterances or not. For instance, Leonard (1979; Leonard/Sabbadini/Leonard/Volterra 1987), who studied American- and Italian-speaking SLI children, did not report any such word ordering problems, and concluded that the syntax development of SLI children is simply delayed and not deviant. Accordingly, Miller (1991, 6) stated in a recent review: "At the sentence level, language-matched disordered speakers acquire the major grammatical categories and the rules for combination in the same order as normal children". Fletcher (1991), however, noticed special formulation problems in his SLI group which he characterized as "intuitively more serious than the omission of a grammatical element such as determiner, an auxiliary, or an inflection" (177). He quotes, among others, the following examples (178):
"my mum was take me a picture"
"here they got eyes to me"
"he put webs"
"what's that is"
"that's how long".
To my ears - and these are German ears - these sentences do sound relatively wrong, but not nearly as wrong as the incorrect sentences of our dysphasic children. This may be due to the fact that German is one of the languages requiring numerous permutations and that missing permutations are therefore especially conspicuous, so that the dysphasic utterances really do sound "all over the place", as one mother put it.

In order to understand better the language problems the dysphasic children have, it certainly is not sufficient to describe the deficits cross-sectionally only or to isolate one aspect and examine it longitudinally. We obviously need extensive longitudinal data which optimally should range from the emergence of the language disorder at preschool age right up to adolescence. Unfortunately, I can only offer data from a longitudinal study over one year with a follow-up after 2 years.

Table 5 shows the pattern change of 4 indicators of spontaneous speech over 1 year. Four points are remarkable (see Grimm 1986a):
First, the mean complexity of the verbal part is a highly valid measure or index of productive language development. Main verbs, auxiliaries and modals as well as adverbs were credited 1 point; missing obligatory verbs received 0 points. This index differentiates very clearly between the dysphasic children and the controls: Starting from the corresponding initial level at t1, a significant difference in favor of the younger children is already perceptible after four months. These children then only omit very few verbs and increasingly use modal verbs and auxiliaries. Even after one year, the much older dysphasic children have not reached this developmental level, thus showing a delay of more than 2 years.

Second, there is a distinct relationship between the developmental change in average verb complexity and the production of different sentence patterns. In the younger normal language children it is especially apparent that the increase in average verb complexity is correlated with a decrease of cor-

Tab. 5: Spontaneous speech variables in SLI and normal children during the course of one year (from Grimm 1986a)

Variables	Subjects	t1[1]	t2	t3	t4
CV	SLI	1.00 (0.08)[2]	1.05 (0.08)	1.10 (0.11)	1.11 (0.13)
	normal	1.04 (0.11)	1.26 (0.17)	---	1.36 (0.16)
SV	SLI	69.0 (18.6)	53.1 (27.6)	34.4 (20.1)	31.7 (14.3)
	normal	42.0 (13.2)	23.9 (8.7)	---	18.5 (6.7)
SVW	SLI	75.3 (19.1)	44.7 (34.3)	33.4 (27.7)	19.4 (20.0)
	normal	28.0 (23.6)	10.7 (11.2)	---	3.6 (4.6)
CORP	SLI	30.5 (9.0)	32.5 (8.7)	30.3 (6.7)	38.4 (12.4)
	normal	34.6 (5.9)	39.3 (7.0)	---	44.9 (8.9)

CV = Mean complexity of the verbal part
SV = percentage of sentences with verb or subject in final position
SVW = percentage of wrong SV sentences
CORP = percentage of corpus sentences of all utterances produced

[1] Mean age at t1 of the SLI children: 4;4 years; mean age of the controls: 2;6 years; the timepoints were 4 months apart
[2] Mean with standard deviation

rect as well as incorrect sentences with verb or subject in final position. They increasingly produce more other sentence patterns with different word orderings. Also up to 70% of the sentences the dysphasic children produce at timepoint 4 have neither subject nor verb in final position. However, these sentence patterns are less variable than those of the controls: As also well-documented in the literature, the sentences are simple, without expansion of the nominal phrase or the verb phrase and are not coordinated or embedded. Additionally, the sentences show many syntactic and morphological errors. I will return to the morphological problems later on.

Third, looking at the standard deviations, one can confirm that the SLI children are more heterogeneous in their syntactic development than the normal children.

Fourth, when comparing the number of corpus sentences, the two groups again do not differ significantly at the first timepoint. This may be interpreted that the SLI children try just as hard as the younger controls to use their verbal means productively. Thereby it is important to stress that corpus sentences are defined as those correct or incorrect utterances which are linguistically analyzable in that they are neither unintelligible, nor ambiguous, nor incomplete in that they contain neither subject nor predicate. They also represent more than simple denominations or social formulas such as "Hi". Interestingly, the increase in corpus sentences over one year is lower in the dysphasic children than in the normal controls. At timepoint 4, when they were on average 3;6 years old, the controls produced approximately 14% more corpus sentences than the SLI children at timepoint 1, when these were on average 4;2 years old. This allows the conclusion that in general the language of the dysphasics remains more fragmentary. In interaction with their mothers they are often content with language fragments and avoid forming sentences. This avoiding tendency is in accordance with the impression given that the production process is often so arduous as if the children had to generate their sentences anew each time, even though these are structurally similar (see also Grimm 1983).

Methodological excursion: The Heidelberg Language Development Test

Before I start on further results, it will be necessary to briefly introduce the Heidelberg Language Development Test (Grimm/Schöler 1991, 1st ed.

1978; Grimm/Schöler 1985), which we have applied to all children in our samples.

Table 6 gives an overview of the six language components that are operationalized by 13 subtests. I do not intend to go into greater detail but only want to give some information about the different subtests:
1. **Comprehension** is measured by an object manipulation task: the child hears 17 sentences of differing complexity and shows what he/she has understood by the use of toy objects.

Tab. 6: Heidelberg Language Development Test (Grimm & Schöler 1991; first published 1978) (from Grimm 1988)

I Sentence Structure	1. Comprehension	Ex: The dog bites the bear who catches the cat.
	2. Imitation	Ex: The tiny mouse is chased by the lion
	3. Production	Ex: Sun - cold
II Text	1. Delayed free recall of a story (134 words)	
III Metalinguistics	1. Correction of semantically inconsistent sentences	Ex: The child laughs in sheer grief.
IV Morphological Structure	1. Plural-singular formation	Ex: Kölz → Kölzer
	2. Transformation of verbs	Ex: falen → Faler, Falerin, Falerei
	3. Transformation of nouns	Ex: Tacken → tackig, tackiger, am tackigsten
V Wort Meaning	1. Classification 2. Word Completion	Ex: basket, bag, bucket → pocket, sack etc.
VI Interactive Meaning	1. Flexibility in naming 2. Relationship between verbal and nonverbal information 3. Encoding and recoding of meaning	

2. The **Imitation** task consists of 12 sentences, also of differing complexity, that have to be repeated immediately after being heard.
3. **Production** means that 10 syntactically and semantically correct sentences have to be formed from given words.
4. The story used in the subtest **Text memory** refers to an event that is not part of a child's everyday experience. All elements are, however, familiar to the children.
5. The **Metalinguistic** task consists of 9 items and is self-explanatory.
6., 7., 8. The **Morphological** tasks consist of 18, 4 and 6 items respectively. In each case, artificial words are presented in order to find out which morphological rules have been acquired.

In order to give an impression of the complexity of the German morphological rule system, the different possibilities for forming plurals are briefly explained. Since the subtest "Plural-singular formation" differentiates best between groups, I will restrict myself to this subtest in the discussion of the test data.

As Table 7 shows, there are 8 morphological markers (see e.g. Clahsen/Rothweiler/Woest 1991). However, it would be completely mistaken to assume that the child's only task is to learn which markers go with which determined nouns. There is only one reliable rule, namely that nouns with -e go with marker -n. All other relations are highly arbitrary. Accordingly, Clahsen et al. (1991) recommend that the rules should be understood as more or less strong tendencies. Comparing the German examples with the English translations, it becomes clear that the arbitrary plural system is bound to a similarly arbitrary article system, which does not help to make things easier.
9. In the **Classification** task, appropriate objects on picture cards have to be chosen to match six different categories such as animals or food.
10. With the **Word Completion** task, the referential aspect of meaning is assessed. Each of the 14 items consists of three words defining a semantic space, and the children have to find out the appropriate fourth word. In the example given, 'tray' for instance would only be partly correct and would get 1 point. 0 points would be given for a totally incorrect answer such as 'plastics'.
11., 12., 13. With the following tasks under the label **Interactive Meaning**, pragmatic aspects of language use are measured. In the first task, the children are shown two pictures of persons and are told that their name is, for instance, Kurt Schneider. They then have to say how Kurt Schneider would

Tab. 7: Morphological plural markers in German

Markers	Examples
1. zero marker	der Lehrer - die Lehrer (the teacher - the teachers)
2. modification	die Mutter - die Mütter (the mother - the mothers)
3. -e	das Bein - die Beine (the leg - the legs)
4. -e + modification	die Kuh - die Kühe (the cow - the cows)
5. -er	das Kind - die Kinder (the child - the children)
6. er + modification	der Rand - die Ränder (the edge - the edges)
7. -(e)n	die Straße - die Straßen (the street - the streets) die Frau - die Frauen (the woman - the women)
8. -s	das Auto - die Autos (the car - the cars)

be addressed by different persons, for instance, by his wife, his daughter or a shop assistant. In the next task, sentences that express different emotions such as joy or anger are read aloud to the children. They then have to assign the sentences to appropriate pictures of faces. And finally, in the third task, the children have to express one and the same meaning in different ways. To do this, they must take on the roles of people who show different emotions such as joy or sadness in one and the same situation.

This language development test is that most widely used in German-speaking countries; it appears appropriate for characterizing the language problems displayed by language disordered children.

Follow-up study

Syntactical and morphological difficulties

The 8 dysphasic children of the longitudinal sample were tested at the beginning of the study, then one year later, and again two years later.

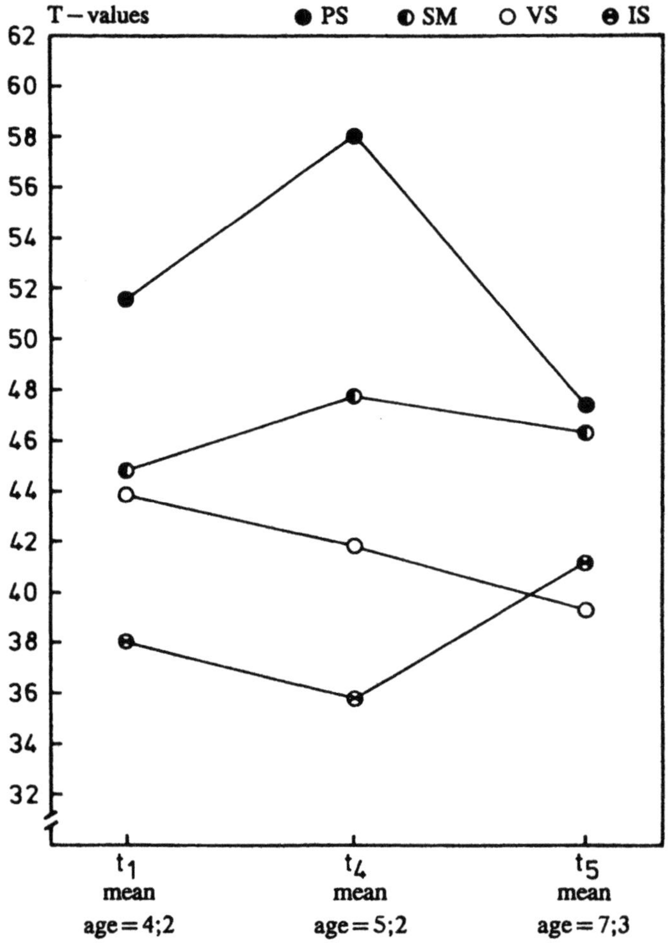

Fig. 2: *Standard values in the comprehension text (VS), the morphology test (PS), the imitation test (IS), and the semantic tests (SM) over a three-years-period (from Grimm 1986a, Grimm/Weinert 1990)*

Some of the data are presented in Figure 2. The T-values of the Comprehension subtest show that initially the children have no serious comprehension problems when compared with the norm group of the same age, at least not at timepoint 1. The normal range of the T-score is 50 plus/minus 10. At school age, at timepoint 5, the children have deteriorated significantly in this aspect. Since there is also a significant decrease in morphological ability (PS), the conclusion appears justified that in formal abilities the gap between dysphasics and their age group increases over time. The test data on semantic abilities, that is the compound data of the subtests 9 and 10, remain within normal range, so that the conclusion is warranted that the eight SLI children do not suffer from a severe semantic deficit. At first sight, the result that the performance in the imitation subtest is, in contrast, significantly better at school age appears surprising. The explanation for this, however, is that the children have learnt to reproduce correctly structurally simple sentences. That they nevertheless show far poorer values than the norm group can be attributed to the fact that they still make many morphological errors.

In the Tables 8a - 8c the reproductions given by a dysphasic child at preschool (age: 5;8 years) and school age (age: 7;4 years) and a normal preschooler (age: 5;8 years) are compared. These reproductions can be considered as representing very typical performances. In the reproductions of the nearly 6-year-old dysphasic child (Table 8a) syntactical and morphological errors abound in every sentence. In those items in which the verb is not in final position the word order is changed during reproduction to comply with the typically incorrect dysphasic sentence construction with verb in final position. In comparison, the reproductions of the age-matched normal child are nearly perfect (cf. Table 8b). Therefore, for comparison purposes, only the 6 most difficult items were chosen in addition to the two training sentences. Finally, Table 8c demonstrates the SLI child's improvement in performance with respect to syntax whereby, however, many morphological errors still occur.

These examples, together with the errors in the subtest "Plural-singular formation" and supplemented by the spontaneous speech data, provide a desolate picture of dysphasic children's morphological skills (see also: Clahsen et al. 1991): They have extreme difficulties with subject-verb agreements and the required agreement within nominal phrases; they confound articles, very often produce nominatives instead of other required cases, fail - as already mentioned - to separate verbs and particles and produce these at different positions in the sentence, use wrong auxiliary and

Tab. 8a: Imitation of grammatical structures[1] *- SLI-child (age: 5;8)*

Presentation	Reproduction	
Der Ball rollt den Abhang hinunter.	Der Ball de Abemine runter rollt.	
Die Katze leckt die ganze Schüssel aus.	Die Katze die ganze Schüssel ausleck.	
Der Teppich wird von dem Vater ausgeklopft.	Den Teppich √ n Vater aufgeklopft.	(no passive)
Die kleine Maus wird von dem Löwen gejagt.	Die Maus ihre/irche? Löwen jagt wird.	
Es ist heute morgen kein schönes Wetter.	√ Heute morgen kein schön Wetter is.	
Bevor du spielst, mußt du den Tisch abräumen.	He du spiel √ hen Tisch abräumen muß.	(no temporal subordinate clause)
Es sitzt der kleine Vogel im Gebüsch.	Und √ der kleine Vogel in Gebüsch sitzt.	
Ursula wird von Peter auf dem Rücken getragen.	√ Die Peter jage √ Rücken tragen wird.	
Das Fahrrad wird von dem Omnibus an die Wand geschoben.	Das Fahrrad √.√ Wand geschoben.	(no passive)
Die Tante, die weit weg wohnt, kommt zu Besuch.	Den Tante √ Besuch kommt.	(no relative clause)
Der Schrank, den ich mir gekauft habe, ist schön.	Der Schrank √ gekauft hab, is schön.	(no relative clause)
Vater hat einen Rucksack gekäuft, bevor wir wanderten.	Der Vater √ ein Rucksack √ und dann de wandern.	(no temporal subordinate clause)
Das ist der Mann, dessen Sohn krank ist.	Dere ein Mann, sein Sohn is krank.	(no relative clause)
Die Sonne scheint, nachdem es immer geregnet hatte.	Die Sonne scheint nach immer regne.	

[1]Subtest of the Heidelberg Language Development Test (Grimm & Schöler, 1991; first edition 1978)

—— syntactic error ...... preposition error
- - - morphological error ~~~ articulation error
▬ conjunction error √ missing elements

Tab. 8b: Imitation of grammatical structures[1] *- NL-child (age: 5;8)*

Presentation	Reproduction
Der Ball rollt den Abhang hinunter.	Der Ball rollt den Abhang hinunter.
Die Katze leckt die ganze Schüssel aus.	Die Katze leckt die ganze Schüssel aus.
Das Fahrrad wird von dem Omnibus an die Wand geschoben.	Das Fahrrad wird von den Omnibus an die Wand geschoben.
Die Tante, die weit weg wohnt, kommt zu Besuch.	Die Tante, die weit weg wohnt, kommt zu Besuch.
Der Schrank, den ich mir gekauft habe, ist schön.	Der Schrank, den ich mir gekauft habe, is schön.
Vater hat einen Rucksack gekauft, bevor wir wanderten.	Vater hat einen Rucksack gekauft, bevor wir wanderten.
Das ist der Mann, dessen Sohn krank ist.	Das ist der Mann, dessen Sohn krank ist.
Die Sonne scheint, nachdem es immer geregnet hatte.	Die Sonne scheint, dann nach es immer geregnet hatte.

[1]Subtest of the Heidelberg Language Development Test (Grimm & Schöler, 1991; first edition 1978); Reproductions of the more difficult items only.

- - - morphological error

~~~ articulation error

▬ conjunction error
~~~

Tab. 8c: Imitation of grammatical structures[1] *- SLI-child (age: 7;4)*

Presentation	Reproduction
Der Teppich wird von dem Vater ausgeklopft.	Der √Teppich wird von den Vater abgeklopft.
Die kleine Maus wird von dem Löwen gejagt.	Die √Maus wird von den großen Löwen gejagt.
Es ist heute morgen kein schönes Wetter.	Es ist √morgen kein schönes Wetter.
Bevor du spielst, mußt du den Tisch abräumen.	Vor du spielst, mußt du den Tisch abräumen.
Es sitzt der kleine Vogel im Gebüsch.	Da sitzt ein kleiner Vogel auf'm Gebüsch.
Ursula wird von Peter auf dem Rücken getragen.	-
Das Fahrrad wird von dem Omnibus an die Wand geschoben.	Der Fahrrad √Omnibus an den Wand geschoben. (no passive)
Die Tante, die weit weg wohnt, kommt zu Besuch.	Die Tante, der ganz weit weg wohnt, die kommt zu Besuch.
Der Schrank, den ich mir gekauft habe, ist schön.	Den Schrank, was ich nich? gekauft habe, find ich schön.
Vater hat einen Rucksack gekauft, bevor wir wanderten	Papa hat einen Rucksack gekauft, vor wir gewandert haben.
Das ist der Mann, dessen Sohn krank ist.	Das ist der Mann, wo der Mann den Sohn krank is.
Die Sonne scheint, nachdem es immer geregnet hatte.	Die Sonne scheint, früher es noch geregnet hat.

[1]Subtest of the Heidelberg Language Development Test (Grimm & Schöler, 1991; first edition 1978)

- - - morphological error	..... preposition error
▬ conjunction error	~~~ articulation error
-.-. wrong relative pronoun	√ missing elements

verb inflections or even produce uninflected auxiliaries and verbs, and shorten words and make restricted use of prepositions. Additionally, to return to the subtest "Plural-singular formation", they fail to mark plurals far more often than normal children, whereby this applies even more for artificial words. They overgeneralize predominantly with the marker -n, whereas normal language children also use the markers -e and -s in their overgeneralizations.

According to Clahsen et al. (1991), normally developing children master plural formation by the end of their preschool years. The rate of error in 3 to 4-year-olds is approximately 50%. In dysphasic children, however, plural formation and the morphological rule system in general remains extremely disordered.

As demonstrated by the data already reported and as shown by further results which will be presented later, it appears that the grammatical morphology is extremely slow in development in dysphasic children (see also Schöler 1985). However, the children do not generate idiosyncratic forms as in the syntax, but apparently follow the same sequence as normal children do. We therefore need not postulate different underlying representations for explaining the morphological errors. On account of quantitative limitations only, an on-line processing hypothesis should be sufficient as explanation (see also Menyuk 1993). I cannot go into further detail here, because we have not yet analyzed the morphological errors in sufficient depth. But it seems to me that there is a strong tendency for these children to plateau, so that many of them will never acquire an intact morphological system.

Text processing difficulties

Very probably, insufficient morphological and syntactical resources are responsible for the fact that the SLI children also display extreme difficulties when trying to reconstruct cohesive texts.

The difficulties the children had with the subtest "Text memory" are demonstrated in Tables 9a and 9b, again in typical examples. The SLI child (Table 9a) retold the story incompletely and omitted so many details that the meaning of the story was completely lost. Besides that, she used a simplified and often erroneous syntax and also made many morphological mistakes. When comparing this reproduction with the reproduction of an age-

Tab. 9a: Recall performance in the subtest 'Text memory'[1] *- SLI-child (age: 5;8)*

Story	Reproduction of the story	
Eines Tages sagte ein Sohn zu seinem Vater:		
"Ich werde mich verstecken,	dann hier Sohn hier verstecken	(syntactically incomplete
und du wirst mich nicht finden."	gar nicht finden	and ambiguous)
Der Vater antwortete:		
"Verstecke dich, wo du willst",		
dann ging er ins Haus.		
Der Sohn verzauberte sich in eine Erdnuß.	dann verwandeln hab eine Nuß	(syntactically incomplete
Die Erdnuß wurde von einem Huhn hinuntergeschluckt.	hierche Huhn runterschluck	and ambiguous)
Das Huhn wurde von einer Katze gefressen.	hierche komm dann eine Katze	
Die Katze wurde von einem Hund gefressen.		
Nach kurzer Zeit		
wurde der Hund von einer Schlange gefressen.	eine Schlange und ein Hund	(syntactically incomplete)
Die Schlange wurde in einem Fischnetz gefangen.		
Als der Vater nach seinem Sohn suchte,		
sah er die Schlange in dem Fischnetz.	ihrche Netz abeschneide	(syntactically incomplete)
Er machte die Schlange auf und fand den Hund.		
Dann fand er die Katze, dann das Huhn	ihrche dann Huhn gefunde	(syntactically incomplete)
und in dem Huhn die Erdnuß.		
Er zerbrach die Schale	dann Nuß aufgeschneide	(syntactically incomplete)
und entdeckte seinen Sohn.	dann wiedergefunde das Sohn	(syntactically incomplete)
Der Sohn war so verblüfft,		
daß er nie wieder versuchte,		
seinen Vater hereinzulegen.		

[1]Subtest of the Heidelberg Language Development Test (Grimm & Schöler, 1991, first edition 1978)

___ syntactic error   ~~~ articulation error

\- - - morphological error

Tab. 9b: Recall preformance in the subtest 'Text memory'[1] *- NL-child (age: 5;5)*

Story	Reproduction of the story
Eines Tages sagte ein Sohn zu seinem Vater:	Ein Junge sagt eines Tages zu seinem Vater:
"Ich werde mich verstecken,	"Ich verstecke mich
und du wirst mich nicht finden."	wo du mich nie finden kannst."
Der Vater antwortete:	Und dann sagt der Vater:
"Verstecke dich, wo du willst",	"Versteck dich, wo du willst."
dann ging er ins Haus.	Der Junge ging herein
Der Sohn verzauberte sich in eine Erdnuß.	verwandelte sich als eine Erdnuß
Die Erdnuß wurde von einem Huhn hinuntergeschluckt.	Das Huhn ißt die Erdnuß. (no passive)
Das Huhn wurde von einer Katze gefressen.	Die Katze ißt das Huhn. (no passive)
Die Katze wurde von einem Hund gefressen.	Der Hund ißt/frißt die Katze. (no passive)
Nach kurzer Zeit	Nach einer kurzen Zeit
wurde der Hund von einer Schlange gefressen.	frißt die Schlange den Hund (no passive)
Die Schlange wurde in einem Fischnetz gefangen.	und die Schlange war in einem Fischnetz gefangen.
Als der Vater nach seinem Sohn suchte,	
sah er die Schlange in dem Fischnetz.	Da sah der Vater die Schlange,
Er machte die Schlange auf und fand den Hund.	machte die auf und dann entdeckte er den Hund.
Dann fand er die Katze, dann das Huhn	und dann entdeckte/und dann kam die Katze und dann das Huhn
und in dem Huhn die Erdnuß.	In dem Huhn die Kokos/die Erdnuß
Er zerbrach die Schale	und machte die Schale auf von der Erdnuß
und entdeckte seinen Sohn.	und entdeckte seinen Sohn.
Der Sohn war so verblüfft,	Und sein Sohn versprach ihm
daß er nie wieder versuchte,	
seinen Vater hereinzulegen.	daß ihn nie mehr reinlegt.

[1]Subtest of the Heidelberg Language Development Test (Grimm & Schöler, 1991; first edition 1978)

—— syntactic error

matched normal language child, one becomes really aware of how severe the handicap of the dysphasic children must be.

In an experiment with other text material, the text processing difficulties could be confirmed and were augmented by an interesting aspect (Weinert/Grimm/Delille/Scholten-Zitzewitz 1989). The children - 16 SLI schoolchildren with an average age of 7;7 and 16 age-matched control children - heard a coherent and an incoherent version of a story, the familiar farmer's story (e.g. Thorndyke 1977). The coherent version had a complex hierarchical structure, whereas in the incoherent version the aims of the two main actions were omitted and the other elements were ordered in a simple temporal "and then" fashion.

Figure 3 shows firstly that the normal children reproduced significantly more propositions than the SLI children. Even more interesting is the second finding that the normal children reproduced significantly more propositions of the coherent version than of the incoherent one. This means that the inherent structure facilitated their recall performance. Or in other words: The children were able to use the inherent structure for their recall. In contrast, the SLI children failed to make use of this structural information, which is demonstrated by the fact that their performance was equal for both versions. A possible explanation for this could be that on account of their syntactic problems, the dysphasic children also have problems in forming hierarchical representations of texts. It appears plausible to assume that insufficient underlying representations of sentences are related to insufficient underlying representations of texts. Whether morphological difficulties bear a share of the responsibility for these structural problems is difficult to say. The fact is that the SLI children not only recalled far fewer propositions, but also made very numerous morphological errors.

Interindividual differences

Changes in developmental patterns

Up to now the dysphasic or SLI children have been dealt with as if they formed a homogeneous group. Now this is certainly not the case; developmental dysphasia, or specific language impairment, is not a unitary construct. Therefore it is important to disclose the interindividual differences concealed behind mean values. Thus, as previously mentioned, the 8 chil-

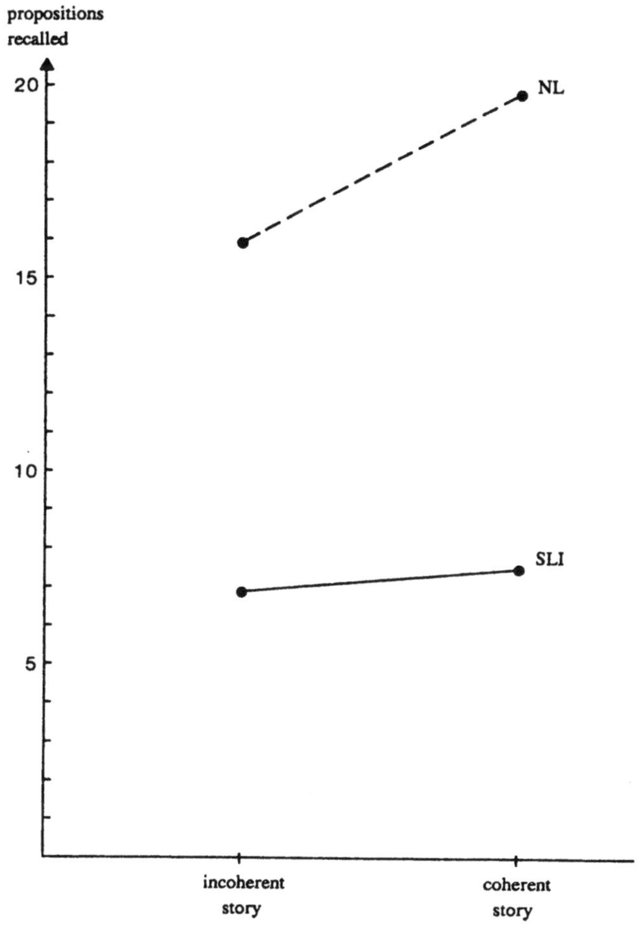

Fig. 3: *Mean number of propositions recalled by specifically language impaired (SLI) and normal-language (NL) children (from Weinert/Grimm et al. 1989)*

dren in the longitudinal study formed 2 groups, since at the first investigation time the one group showed more syntactical word ordering errors than the other. Interestingly enough, the same grouping could be formed on the basis of the subtests of the Heidelberg Language Development Test. This grouping concurrence clearly supports the view that the portion of sentences with wrong word order is a sensitive measure for quantifying language performance.

Three years later, the only difference in the grouping was that child 3, who had been in the better group, changed to the poorer group. One may therefore conclude that the development is stable in the sense that the children within the two different groups displayed similar changes in their language ability.

These changes can be briefly summarized in two points (more extensively in Grimm 1986a; on account of missing data for t5, child 6 is omitted):
(1) After three years all children in the poorer group had lower T-values in all subtests than the children in the better group. The poorer children's performance was clearly below average not only in the syntactic and morphological subtests but in all subtests; the average T-value in the Word Completion task was, for example, under point 10. This suggests that we are dealing with children suffering from a cumulative language deficit. The difference in performance between these children and the age-matched norm group increased enormously over three years.

In clear contrast, after three years the language problems in the better group were limited primarily to syntax. Besides rather minor morphological inaccuracies in the Imitation task, only the performance of child 2 in the subtest "Plural-singular formation" with a T-value of 42 lay on the borderline to below-averageness. In comparison, the poorer group had an average T-value of 14 in this morphological task.

At this point it seems necessary to refer again in general to the developmental change in morphology. As already shown in Figure 2, when the dysphasic children were tested at timepoint 1, the average T-value in the subtest Plural-singular performance reached over 50; the range, however, was rather wide, namely between 31 and 90. In comparison to the MLU-matched younger children, the dysphasic children were moreover more advanced morphologically in spontaneous speech. In fact, my argument was that the combination of wrong word ordering and more advanced morphological marking is characteristic for the typical dysphasic sentence pattern during the earlier stages of language learning. After one year the children achieved in comparison with their age group even above average values in the subtest "Plural-singular formation". This good performance could, however, as seen previously, only be retained in the better group. The other children of the poorer group apparently made no considerable further progress and two years later showed a highly significant worse performance than their norm group.

These developmental patterns clearly demonstrate the importance of studying language disorders in longitudinal designs. The most important point is that we may come to completely different assumptions about the nature of the dysphasic disorder, depending on which slices of time the same children were examined at. If we had examined the children at preschool age only we would have found that they show a rather normal or even above average morphological performance and we would probably have concluded that the morphological component does not belong to SLI children's serious problem areas. However, if we had examined the children at school age only we would have concluded that in addition to their syntactic problems they - and I am here referring to the poorer group - would at least have had equally large problems with the morphology from the beginning. In both cases we would therefore have made false assumptions.

(2) Over the time, a regression to the mean in language comprehension can be established: In the 3 year follow-up, the children in the better group showed less increase in performance than the children in the poorer group. The rank correlation between the T-values in the subtest "Comprehension" at timepoint 1 and the difference in the T-values between the first and the last timepoint (t5) is correspondingly significantly negative -.64. A tentative interpretation of this could be that the capacity for change in syntax is limited in these SLI children. Since the children in the better group at school age showed predominantly syntactical problems, the assumption is that the syntactical component is resistant to change after a certain developmental level has been reached. This would mean that after the children have acquired simpler structural forms, a stagnation effect sets in, so that a further and complete mastering of the syntactical rule system is handicapped or even prevented.

Predictive validity

In closing the discussion of the longitudinal study, the significant results on the predictive validity of the four measures "Mean complexity of the verbal part", "Comprehension", "Imitation" and "Plural-singular formation" are summarized in Table 10.

Rank correlations have been computed between the last three measures at timepoint 1 and the raw scores obtained in the subtests of the Heidelberg Language Development Test at timepoint 5, the two subtests "Transformation of verbs" and "Relationship between verbal and nonverbal information" being not included. The first measure "Mean complexity of the verbal part"

Tab. 10: Correlations between language performances at t1 and t5 (from Grimm 1986a)

timepoint 1	timepoint 5	Correlation (Spearman)
Comprehension	Plural-singular formation/ Transformation of nouns	.85, p=.00
Comprehension	Text memory	.68, p=.03
Imitation	Plural-singular formation/ Transformation of nouns	.57, p=.07
Imitation	Word meaning	.57, p=.07
Plural-singular formation	Comprehension/Imitation	.59, p=.06
Plural-singular formation	Text memory	.75, p=.02
Plural-singular formation	Sentence production/ Metalinguistics	.63, p=.05
Mean complexity of the verbal part	Comprehension	.64, p=.06

was only correlated to three measures, "Comprehension", "Imitation" and "Plural-singular formation". Four results seem to be especially salient: First, besides the significant relationship between "Imitation" and "Word Meaning" (cf. Table 6) there are no further significant relations between the syntactic-morphological abilities at timepoint 1 and semantic and pragmatic abilities (components V and VI in Table 6) at timepoint 5. Second, remarkably close relationships could be established between the two subtests "Comprehension" and "Plural-singular formation" and the subtest "Text memory". At the first investigation timepoint, when the children were between 3;9 and 4;8 years old, none of the 8 children were able to reproduce the story text. Three years later, those children with better comprehension and better morphological ability were to reproduce the same story far better than the other children. Third, the grade of elaboration in the verbal part is closely related to the later ability to process syntactic structures; and this syntactic processing ability measured at timepoint 1 is again very highly correlated with the later acquisition of the morphological rule system.

Thus, as already elaborated above, the SLI children with comparatively better syntactic abilities in the earlier stages of their language development are much better prepared to acquire the complex morphology of German than the SLI children with poorer syntactic abilities. This is corroborated by the significant correlation between the subtest "Imitation" at timepoint 1 and the two morphological subtests "Plural-singular formation" and "Transformation of nouns" at timepoint 5. In this context it should be reminded that the third morphological subtest "Transformation of verbs" was not administered at timepoint 5. Fourth, the significant relationship between "Plural-singular formation" and the later ability to produce and correct sentences seems to be mediated by a metalinguistic demand required by all three tasks.

Subgrouping by cluster analysis

Figure 4 shows a five-cluster-solution that may be understood as an initial attempt to develop a typology of specific language impairment.

90 SLI children between 4 and 13 years were tested with the Heidelberg Language Development Test. Most of them had been diagnosed by speech therapists. The sample was composed of 75 boys and 15 girls; this gender distribution is typical in that always considerably more boys than girls show language disorders. The nonverbal IQ was calculated on the basis of either the Wechsler Scales, the Snijder-Oomen, or the CPM; only 8 children scored slightly lower than 85 (Table 11).

Tab. 11: Sample of 90 SLI children (from Grimm 1989)

age	gender		non-verbal	social class	
	m	f	IQ	middle/upper	lower
4-6 yrs.	15	4	109.2(17.9)[1]	10	6
7-9 yrs.	46	6	106.4(16.5)	21	14
10-13 yrs.	14	5	107.9(14.0)	9	10
in sum	75	15	105.3(16.1)	40[2]	30[2]

[1] mean with standard deviation
[2] some data are missing

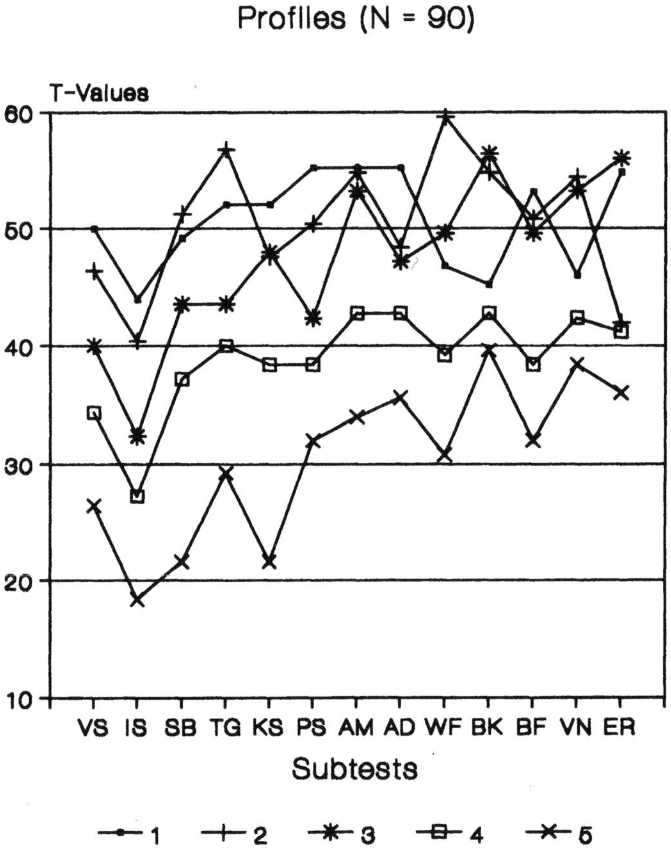

Cluster 1: N=10; Cluster 2: N=9; Cluster 3: N=27; Cluster 4: N=27; Cluster 5: N=17

Sentence structure:	VS, IS, SB
Text memory:	TG
Metalinguistic ability:	KS
Morphological structure:	PS, AM, AD
Word meaning:	WF, BK
Interactive meaning:	BF, VN, ER

Fig. 4: 5-Cluster Solution

The standardized test data (T-values) were submitted to cluster analysis using Ward's method and to multiple discriminant analysis. I cannot go into greater theoretical or statistical detail here, but only want to draw attention to four main observations (Grimm 1988, 1989):
(1) In comparing the 5 profiles, one can ascertain that the children in the clusters differ on the one hand in the general performance level reached and on the other in which language components were disordered. The variance with respect to which components of language are disturbed is supported by the results of the discriminant analysis, since the groups are best differentiated by different subtests.
(2) Even if the profiles are asynchronous, it is common for all profiles that the sentence structure is reliably the most disordered component.
(3) Although the 5 clusters represent the best cluster solution, these clusters are not all internally homogeneous. In fact, clusters 1, 2, and 4 turn out to be rather heterogeneous: Thus the mean profiles correlate rather strongly with each other, whereas the correlations of the individual profiles with the mean group profiles show only middle values. It is important to point out this methodical aspect, since the results of cluster analyses are often trusted blindly. Actually, the interpretation of clustering results is somewhat subjective and needs to be checked by other methods.
(4) I have tried to establish the relationships between the variables of age, social status and of neurological status and the five clusters. Because some data are missing, I can only present the following results with due caution: In the better clusters 1 and 2, the children are on average younger (mean ages: 7;5 and 6;9 years) than in the poorer clusters (mean ages: 9;10, 7;10 and 8;2 years). Of the children with an IQ of 115 and higher, 52% are in the better clusters 1 and 2 and only 22% are in the worst clusters 4 and 5; in contrast, 65% of the children with an IQ of 100 or lower are in the worst clusters 4 and 5 and only 9% are in the better clusters 1 and 2. It seems that the children with poorer performances in the language development test are also those who are weaker in the nonverbal test performance. Whether these children are not merely coincidentally also those belonging to the lower social class is difficult to answer, since the relevant data of 11 children in cluster 5 are missing. The data for cluster 4 are, however, complete. And these 27 children are distributed equally over the upper, middle and lower social class. It seems premature, however, to conclude that social class is not an important variable since alone 90% of the children in cluster 1 and 2 belong to the middle and upper class so that only 10% belong to the lower class. This distribution could lead to the interpretation that the language disorders of the children in the poorer clusters are far more socially determined than the language disorders of the children in the better

clusters, whereby the differentiation in "better" and "poorer" refers to the total performance level.

Finally, it is interesting that the groups can also be differentiated according to neurological status. However, it must be stressed here that the children were examined according to traditional methods (as for example the method used by Touwen (1982)). The highest percentage of children with positive outcome were found in cluster 3, which had always had an intermediate position in the other variables. Not one of the children in cluster 5 showed positive neurological results. When one combines this with the fact that the children of cluster 5 had on average a relatively low nonverbal IQ, one could conclude that the children's low language performance level represents a general learning deficiency.

We urgently need more studies which describe in detail the substantial variance with respect to which components of language are disturbed and to what degree, which developmental changes the language components experience, which relationships between different language profiles and other nonverbal variables exist, and how these relations change throughout the developmental course. As Miller (1991, 5) correctly remarks, "the concept of changing profiles of language disorder complicates the problem of characterizing disordered language performance." This performance "may look different at different points in time as a result of continued development, adaption, or intervention."

Implications for diagnosis and intervention

The critical diagnostic question is to determine which manifestations of early behavior lead to later language disorders. We haven't found a satisfactory answer to this question yet, so that it is almost impossible to diagnose a child as being dysphasic under the age of three. One reason seems to be that children may manifest different language development milestones at widely different ages and yet develop language normally. In order to find out which unattained milestones are predictive for later language disorders we need careful and long-term follow-up studies. Thus, for example, as many as half of the 24-month-old toddlers identified as language delayed on the grounds of their failure to speak more than 50 words or to combine words into short phrases continue to show expressive language delay at age 3 (see for example: Fischel/Whitehurst/Caulfield/De Baryshe 1989; Rescorla/Escarce/Hadicke-Wiley 1991). However, we are completely ignorant about the ultimate prognosis. Will these children catch up on their language delay in the years following, or will they continue their career as language disordered children? In the latter possibility, we will very probably have to do with children showing problems in many areas. There is now a substantial body of research demonstrating that language impairment in preschool years is strongly related to later academic difficulties and behavioral maladjustment. Thus, for example, Silva/McGee/Williams (1983) found that 60% of the children who had been diagnosed as language delayed at age three had distinct difficulties at school at age seven (see also Grimm in press). Comparable results were achieved by Stevenson (1987), who stated succinctly "it is clear that language processing disabilities lie at the core of the most children's reading problems" (14).

On account of their difficulty in deriving the relevant information from spoken and written language and on account of additional problems experienced in mathematics, the SLI children can develop generalized intellectual and also motivational problems which Stanovich (1986, 113) characterized as "academic learned helplessness". It is obvious that the more serious the children's language problems are, the more pronounced this helplessness will be, and this has also been empirically proven (see for example Howlin/ Rutter 1987).

Taking an optimistic view, early screening would reliably spot those under-three-year-olds exhibiting a language delay with negative prognosis; these children would then receive therapy and so a negative academic career would be avoided. This is a view with many unknown quantities.

With regard to the screening, I should like to argue that it cannot suffice merely to assess attained verbal abilities such as size of vocabulary, number of word combinations, or the comprehension of verbal instructions. Rather, we need to include further abilities or performances which we know differentiate well and reliably between normal language and language impaired children.

In my longitudinal study I have shown that the 8 dysphasic children differed from the 8 normal control children with respect to how often and in which way they openly process their mother's language input (e.g. Grimm 1986a,b, 1987; summarized e.g. in Grimm 1991b, Grimm/Weinert 1993). All children were observed in semi-structured interaction situations with their mothers, and an on-line analysis was made of the way in which the children openly processed their mother's speech. All the children's utterances that were formally related to the immediately preceding maternal utterances were registered. Then, in a second step, these formally related utterances were coded according to two main strategies of language processing (see e.g. Grimm 1984, 43-44, Grimm 1987, 16):

(1) Elementaristic strategy: The child picks out one single word or phrase from the immediately preceding maternal utterance.

Example: Mother: "The ball lies here"
Child: "Ball".

(2) Gestalt-like/holistic strategy comprising two substrategies:

(a) The child imitates the whole sentence/more than one phrase.

Example: Mother: "Here we can build one again"
Child: "Here can build one".

(b) The child transforms the mother's preceding utterance.

Example: Mother: "Where is the devil?"
Child: "Here is the devil."

The first interesting result is that during the one-hour interaction situation on average 14% of the utterances produced by the younger controls were formally related to the maternal utterances. In contrast, only 7% of the SLI children's utterances were formally related to the maternal utterances. That this quantitative difference cannot be explained by different quantities of maternal utterances formally related to the children's utterances is clearly proven by the fact that both groups of mothers on average produced 24% of formally related utterances. These data might be taken as evidence that on the one hand almost every fourth utterance the mothers directed towards their children was teaching-oriented. On the other hand, the younger normal controls were more learning-oriented than the dysphasic children. That is, in the dyads with the language disordered children one could observe much teaching but little learning.

Even more interesting than the quantitative difference between the two groups of children is the qualitative finding that compared to the SLI children the normal language children significantly more often made use of the gestalt-like strategy of processing larger speech units from their mother's input, while at times adding to or reworking elements of the units in an active and constructive way. As Table 12 shows, the SLI children restricted themselves mainly to the elementaristic processing of their mother's input. Interestingly, one year later this difference still existed when the SLI children were on average 5;2 years old and the normal controls were on average 3;6 years old (for details see Grimm 1987).

Tab. 12: Children's language processing strategies (absolute numbers: means and standard deviations

	SLI children	normal children	U-test (Mann-Whitney, two-tailed)
Elementaristic strategy: Child picks out a single word/phrase	30.25 (16.48)	38.75 (18.55)	ns
Gestalt-like strategy: a) Child picks out more than one phrase	2.25 (1.91)	10.88 (7.86)	p<.01
b) Transformation of mother's sentence	4.75 (2.31)	13.75 (11.17)	p<.01
Total	37.25 (16.69)	63.38 (22.30)	p<.05

Comparisons between normal and dysphasic children: ns: not significant (p>.10)

It is a very important finding that the SLI children under study processed incoming language in a different way. If it is correct that different acquisition mechanisms underly and are responsible for different processing strategies (e.g. Bates/Bretherton/Snyder 1988), then the most important task is to find out the mechanisms leading to the deficient use of the gestalt-like strategy in SLI children. As one line of research it seems promising to look for memory restrictions. The short-term memory could be regarded as the bottleneck of information processing because of its limited capacity. Therefore, structural and/or procedural deficits in short-term memory might cause problems in the registration, processing and storing of input, thus leading to a deficient individual data base for language learning. Thus, the theoretical argument could be the following: On account of their short-term memory restrictions, the SLI children are prevented from memorizing longer speech units that may form the basis for the inductive acquisition of formal linguistic regularities. The induction of linguistic rules (e.g. of word classes and word order rules) ensues by means of a distribution analysis. For this, the normal language learner has stored longer speech units. These units serve as models for the implicit comparing processes by which the learner can discover covarying characteristics. Since the SLI children very seldom adopt longer speech units and far more often adopt only single words from the input language, the consequence is that they must have greater difficulties with the inductive process of rule learning. Single words can be regarded as a deficient data base that does not allow distribution analyses to be performed successfully.

This explanatory hypothesis could alternatively be interpreted in the sense that the gestalt-like processing of language input helps the normal language learner to crack the code at least at the earlier stages of language learning. Similar arguments have been forwarded by Peters (1983) and Shatz (1987) for primary language acquisition and by Wong-Fillmore (1979) for secondary language learning.

A second, though not necessarily independent explanatory hypothesis could be that it is difficult for the SLI children to process language in a gestalt-like manner because they have severe problems in exploiting the rhythmic-prosodic structure of incoming speech. It is argued that incoming speech is clearly structured by prosodic features such as pauses, intonation patterns and stress. This is especially true for the speech directed to small children, as demonstrated in the Motherese research (e.g. Ferguson/Snow 1977). The child is thus supported in her/his parsing task, so that (s)he can easily recognize coherent units.

That these two explanatory hypotheses point in the right direction is supported by the following empirical findings: First, it is a replicated and robust result that SLI children show severe deficits in memory tasks. In our lab we could ascertain that the examined SLI children, aged 4;0 to 8;0 years, reliably showed severe deficits in digit and word-span tests (e.g. Grimm 1986a; Weinert 1991). However, the SLI children do not only have significantly greater problems than age-matched children to reproduce disconnected item lists, they also have considerable problems in reproducing natural language material immediately. Already Menyuk/Looney (1972, 278) suspected therefore that the limits on immediate memory "do not allow time for storage of the complete phrase or sentence and a deeper analysis than that required to derive meaning-bearing elements. Therefore these children come up with the simple forms of rules that are reflected in their repetitions."

Second, it is a common observation that language impaired children are very poor in dealing with rhythm. They often have problems in moving rhythmically, clapping their hands rhythmically, imitating melodies and singing songs. This was also observed by the mothers in my longitudinal study. In addition, there is also experimental support. In a study by Kracke

(1975), dysphasic children - who, however, were also receptively very disordered - had to decide whether two rhythmic sequences were the same or different, and she discovered that the dysphasics tried laboriously to remember the patterns by repeating the individual stimuli. Thereby they achieved far poorer results than normal language and deaf control children who were able to use the inherent structural organisation of the patterns for their comparisons in a holistic way. Especially interesting is a further study by Weinert (1991, 1992), who taught normal language and dysphasic children sentences of an artificial or miniature language, which were presented either with or without prosodic cues to the underlying phrase structure. She found out, among other results, that the dysphasic children had far more difficulties than the other children in using the rhythmic-prosodic cues when trying to acquire the miniature language. Most interestingly, only those dysphasic children who showed better rhythmic abilities as indicated by a rhythm discrimination task were also able to learn more than 6 prosodically enriched sentences and to induce at least some of the formal sentence rules.

Third, Connell (1987) found that for SLI children an imitation teaching procedure was far more effective than a modeling-teaching procedure with regard to the acquisition of a non-English, invented language rule. Both procedures are characterized in the following way (Connell 1987, 105): "Imitation teaching is a procedure in which a learner is taught to repeat the language behavior of a model with the expectation that, in the process, the learner will acquire some aspect of the language spoken by the model. ... Modeling teaching is a procedure that is similar to imitation teaching with the exception that the learner is only required to observe the language of the model rather than make an overt response."

From the very probable relationships between gestalt-like language processing, memory abilites, and rhythmic abilities (see also Grimm/Weinert 1991), we can thus deduce as an important consequence for a screening instrument that it should include the assessment of the children's capability to actively adopt larger parts of the input language as well as the assessment of their memory and rhythmic abilities.

For purposes of intervention it seems correspondingly appropriate to suggest that therapists use gestalt-like language processing strategies in their language teaching programs. One of these strategies can certainly be the imitation of preceding utterances. As Connell has pointed out, the use of this strategy could be "the first step of language-teaching programs that teach language rules" (Connell 1987, 111). Certainly, far more research is needed. It is especially necessary to establish whether, and in which way, SLI children can also be taught to employ the rhythmic-prosodic cues and improve their memory performance for their arduous language acquisition task.

References

Bates, E., Bretherton, J., & Snyder, L. (1988). From first words to grammar. Individual differences and dissociable mechanisms. Cambridge: Cambridge University Press.

Clahsen, H. (1988). Normale und gestörte Kindersprache. Linguistische Untersuchungen zum Erwerb von Syntax und Morphologie. Amsterdam: Benjamins.

Clahsen, H., Rothweiler, M., & Woest, A. (1991). Lexikalische Ebenen und morphologische Entwicklung: Eine Untersuchung zum Erwerb des deutschen Pluralsystems im Rahmen der lexikalischen Morphologie. In M. Rothweiler (Ed.), Spracherwerb und Grammatik. 105-126. Opladen: Westdeutscher Verlag.

Connell, P.J. (1987). An effect of modeling and imitation teaching procedures on children with and without specific language impairment. Journal of Speech and Hearing Research, 30, 105-113.

Ferguson, C.A. & Snow, C. (Eds.) (1977). Talking to children: Language input and acquisition. Cambridge: Cambridge University Press.

Fischel, J., Whitehurst, G., Caulfield, M., & De Baryshe, L. (1989). Language growth in children with expressive language delay. Pediatrics, 82, 218-227.

Fletcher, P. (1991). Evidence from syntax for language impairment. In J.F. Miller (Ed.), Research on child language disorders: A decade of progress. 169-187. Austin: Pro-Ed.

Grimm, H. (1973). Strukturanalytische Untersuchung der Kindersprache. Bern: Huber.

Grimm, H. (1983). Kognitions- und interaktionspsychologische Aspekte der Entwicklungsdysphasie. Sprache & Kognition, 3, 169-186.

Grimm, H. (1984). Zur Frage der sprachlichen Wissenskonstruktion. Oder: Erwerben dysphasische Kinder die Sprache anders? In E. Oksaar (Ed.), Spracherwerb, Sprachkontakt, Sprachkonflikt. 30-53. Berlin: Walter de Gruyter.

Grimm, H. (1986a). Entwicklungsdysphasie: Verlaufsanalyse gestörter Sprachentwicklung. In B.Narr & H.Wittje (Eds.), Spracherwerb und Mehrsprachigkeit / Language acquisition and multilingualism. Festschrift für Els Oksaar zum 60. Geburtstag. 93-114. Tübingen: Narr.

Grimm, H. (1986b). Ontogenese der Sprache als Fortsetzung nicht-sprachlichen Handelns. In H.G. Bosshardt (Ed.), Perspektiven auf Sprache. Interdisziplinäre Beiträge zum Gedenken an Hans Hörmann. 166-184. Berlin: de Gruyter.

Grimm, H. (1987). Developmental dysphasia: New theoretical perspectives and empirical results. The German Journal of Psychology, 11 (1), 8-22.

Grimm, H. (1988). Diagnosis of language disordered children: Is developmental dysphasia a unitary construct? Paper given at the University of California, Fresno on 24.3.1988.

Grimm, H. (1989). Entwicklungsdysphasie - kein einheitliches Konstrukt. Heilpädagogische Forschung. Themenheft: Sprachentwicklungsprobleme - Leseprobleme, XV(1), 3-14.

Grimm, H. (1991a). Developmental dysphasia as a case of restricted dialogue. Paper presented at the Symposium "Mutualities in dialogue", Study Group "Dynamics of Dialogue" in the Werner Reimers Foundation, Bad Homburg, Germany, November 13-15.

Grimm, H. (1991b). Kognition - Grammatik - Interaktion: Entwicklungspsychologische Interpretationen der Entwicklungsdysphasie. In M. Grohnfeldt (Ed.), Handbuch der Sprachtherapie, Band 4: Störungen der Grammatik. 83-109. Berlin: Spiess-Verlag.

Grimm, H. (in press). Gestörter Sprachlernprozeß: Ursachen und schulische Folgen. In W. Niemeyer (Ed.), Tagungsband "Kommunikation und Lese-Rechtschreibschwäche". Bochum: Winkler-Verlag.

Grimm, H. & Schöler, H. (1985). Sprachentwicklungsdiagnostik. Was leistet der Heidelberger Sprachentwicklungstest? Göttingen: Hogrefe.

Grimm, H. & Schöler, H. (1991). Heidelberger Sprachentwicklungstest. Braunschweig: Westermann (1st Edition 1978).

Grimm, H. & Weinert, S. (1990). Is the syntax development of dysphasic children deviant and why? New findings to an old question. Journal of Speech and Hearing Research, 33, 220-228.

Grimm, H. & Weinert, S. (1991). Conditions of normal language acquisition viewed from the analysis of causes of disordered language development. Paper given at the Biennial SRCD Meeting, Seattle, April 18-20.

Grimm, H. & Weinert, S. (1993). Patterns of interaction and communication in language development disorders. In G. Blanken, J. Dittmann, H. Grimm, J.C. Marshall, &

C.-W. Wallesch (Eds.), Linguistic disorders and pathologies. An international handbook. 697-711. Berlin: De Gruyter.

Howlin, P. & Rutter, M. (1987). The consequences of language delay for other aspects of development. In W. Yule & M. Rutter (Eds.), Language development and disorders. 271-294. London: MacKeith.

Kracke, I. (1975). Perception of rhythmic sequences by receptive aphasic and deaf children. British Journal of Disorders of Communication, 10, 43-51.

Leonard, L.B. (1979). Language impairment in children. Merrill-Palmer Quarterly, 25, 205-232.

Leonard, L.B., Sabbadini, L., Leonard, J.S., & Volterra, V. (1987). Specific language impairment in children: A cross-linguistic study. Brain and Language, 32, 233-252.

Menyuk, P. (1993). Specific language impairment (developmental dysphasia): Linguistic aspects. In G. Blanken, J. Dittmann, H. Grimm, J.C. Marshall, & C.-W. Wallesch (Eds.), Linguistic disorders and pathologies. An international handbook. 606-625. Berlin: De Gruyter.

Menyuk, P. & Looney, P. (1972). A problem of language disorder: length versus structure. Journal of Speech and Hearing Research, 15, 264-279.

Miller, J.F.(1991). Research on language disorders in children: A progress report. In J.F. Miller (Ed.), Research on child language disorders: A decade of progress. 3-22. Austin: Pro-Ed.

Peters, A.M. (1983). The units of language acquisition. Cambridge: University Press.

Rescorla, L., Escarce, E., & Hadicke-Wiley, M. (1991). Identification of language delay at age 2. Unpubl. Manuscript.

Schöler, H. (1985). Überlegungen zum Erwerb morphologischer Strukturformen bei dysgrammatisch sprechenden Kindern am Beispiel des Pluralmorphems. In I. Füssenich & B. Gläß (Eds.), Dysgrammatismus - Theoretische und praktische Probleme bei der Interdisziplinären Beschreibung gestörter Kindersprache. 165-179. Heidelberg: Schindele.

Shatz, M. (1987). Bootstrapping operations in child language. In K. Nelson & A. Van Kleeck (Eds.), Children's language, Vol. VI. 1-22. Hillsdale, N.J.: Lawrence Erlbaum Associates.

Silva, P., McGee, R., & Williams, S. (1983). Developmental language delay from 3 to 7 years and its significance for low intelligence and reading difficulties at age seven. Developmental Medicine and Child Neurology, 28, 783-793.

Stanovich, K.E. (1986). Cognitive processes and the reading problems of learning-disabled children: Evaluating the assumption of specificity. In J.G. Torgesen & B.Y.L. Wong (Ed.), Psychological and educational perspectives on learning disabilities. 87-131. New York: Orlando: Academic Press.

Stevenson, J. (1987). Language development and delays and the predictors of later reading failure. Paper given at the symposium "Prevention and intervention in childhood and youth", Univ. of Bielefeld.

Thorndyke, P.W. (1977). Cognitive structure in comprehension and memory for narrative discourse. Cognitive Psychology, 9, 77-110.

Touwen, B.C.L. (1982). Die Untersuchung von Kindern mit geringen neurologischen Funktionsstörungen. Stuttgart: Thieme.

Weinert, S. (1991). Spracherwerb und implizites Lernen. Studien zum Erwerb sprachanaloger Regeln bei Erwachsenen, sprachunauffälligen und dysphasisch-sprachgestörten Kindern. Bern: Huber.

Weinert, S. (1992). Deficits in acquiring language structure: The importance of using prosodic cues. Applied Cognitive Psychology, 6, 545-571.

Weinert, S., Grimm, H., Delille, G., & Scholten-Zitzewitz, R. (1989). Was macht sprachgestörten Kindern das Textverstehen so schwer? Heilpädagogische Forschung, Themenheft: Sprachentwicklungsprobleme / Leseprobleme, XV(1), 25-37.

Wong-Fillmore, L.(1979). Individual differences in language ability and language behavior. New York: Academic Press, 203-228.

Commentary on Menyuk and Grimm: How well do we understand specific language impairment?

Marilyn Shatz

Two decades of intensive research into children's language development have taught us that there is considerable variability in the timing and nature of children's language acquisition. Some two-year-olds speak in three-word utterances whereas others use one word at a time. Some children focus on names for things whereas others seem more oriented toward doing social work with their words. With so many individual differences, what, then, distinguishes children who are said to make abnormal progress in language development? One oft-cited view is that language impairment in children is nothing other than language delay. The papers by Paula Menyuk and Hannelore Grimm are provocative in that they question this view. Both provide data to support their claims for deviance rather than delay, and they offer theoretical proposals, albeit very different ones, about the causes of deviance during the course of language acquisition. Their data challenge thinking not only in the field of language disorders, but in the areas of normal language development and linguistic and psycholinguistic theory as well. Yet, despite their major contributions, the inevitable conclusion is that we still have a very long way to go before we understand specific language impairments.

My commentary summarizes the authors' most important points, offers critical appraisal of their theoretical proposals, and makes some suggestions for future research. Following the lead of the papers themselves, I have organized my comments according to a tripartite framework addressing the issues of diagnosis, method, and theory. On the first two, there is much agreement between the two authors, and their work will be considered together. There is more divergence at the explanatory level, and here my comments will be theory- and researcher-specific.

The need for better and more specific diagnoses

Specific language impairment (SLI) is the diagnostic category for instances of child language problems unaccompanied by evidence for general problems of development or specific neurological impairments. However, such a designation depends on the worth of the evidence. If the tests for other kinds of impairments are insensitive, inconclusive, or incomplete, then the diagnosis of "normality" everywhere but in the language system may be inaccurate. Moreover, abnormalities of, say, the perceptual system may not have measurable behavioral consequences in systems other than language early on. That is, deficits in a basic ability may show themselves earliest in the language system even though later they may become manifest elsewhere. For example, it may be difficult to demonstrate general memory deficits in slow language learners at the age of two, although memory undoubtedly affects language learning at that age; older children who show both language deficits and problems with digit span may have had memory problems all along, but they were manifest only in one sphere earlier.

Unsurprisingly, then, early diagnoses of specific language impairment can be inaccurate. Some children so diagnosed may have subtle but pervasive problems that will ultimately affect more than just the language system. Others may have primarily output problems, with difficulties in planning and producing the articulatory units of speech. Still others may be only delayed, making up the tail end of the rate curve for language development. Both Menyuk and Grimm argue that diagnoses should be more specific, separating out children with clear problems of deviance that go beyond articulation difficulties or slow learning.

One reason - mentioned by both authors - why the diagnostic issue is so important is that different kinds of problems undoubtedly require different solutions; with better specified diagnoses, more individualized therapies can be designed for particular problems. However, even the "true" SLI children seem heterogeneous. Menyuk notes that qualitative differences between SLI and normal children can appear in a variety of language areas. Indeed, some children seem to demonstrate broad and pervasive difficulties across many areas of language competence; others seem to have more focused problems. And, as Grimm notes, whereas cluster analyses indicate mean group characteristics of SLI types, individual profiles are only moderately related to such categorizations. Classifying together only and all children who demonstrate non-articulatory deviance may still result in too broad and diverse a grouping to serve as a basis on which to create specific therapies.

The use of the SLI designation for a broad range of cases results, then, in a curious paradox. The designation itself, *specific* language impairment, carries with it the theoretical presupposition that there is an autonomous language system that can be damaged in the absence of damage elsewhere. Accordingly, there should be identifiable syndromes associated with damage to that system that can be accounted for on the basis of the workings of the system alone. However, in practice, SLI cases are defaults - diagnoses of SLI are made not because we can identify uniquely linguistic disorders but because *no other basis of impairment can be found.* The designation of SLI can be misleading to researchers who might believe it labels some clear commonality in symptomatology or underlying causes when, in fact, it labels those cases of which we are most ignorant.

There may be some hope in defining a subpopulation of the children now characterized as SLI who share an underlying language system-specific deficit: early and prolonged syntactic deviance seems to be one common characteristic of some SLI children. However, we are not even sure whether there are one or more kinds of syntactic deviance. Moreover, we need to know whether and how much the potential for syntactic difficulties interacts with the learning of a particular language. Grimm's paper raises the question of whether syndromes of syntactic deviance will be language-particular. Will, for example, all "true" SLI children show at least some difficulties in the acquisition of morphology and the syntax of verbs, or will such problems be a function of the degree of irregularity and arbitrariness of the individual language being learned? The answer to such a question could be critical not only for therapists but for theorists trying to determine the nature of a universal grammar and its possible role in language acquisition.

The value of more comprehensive methods

Menyuk's and Grimm's insights about diagnostic inadequacies are no accident. They are the consequence of comprehensive research methods that have allowed them to see the diversity of disorder in language-impaired children. The authors have shown that comprehensive testing for a range of abilities, both linguistic and non-linguistic, is essential for more accurate diagnoses. The need for intensive longitudinal studies of some children also seems clear, not only to make better diagnoses, but to discover a true picture of the profiles over time of children exhibiting deviance.

In addition to comprehensive testing, deeper probing in more specific areas would be useful. Children who exhibit deviance in a particular aspect of language should have that area thoroughly investigated. There are many paradigms, for example, for assessing verb knowledge. Using them with children who manifest some difficulties with verbs gives fuller descriptions of the deficits and provides a sounder basis for causal theorizing. Menyuk notes it is often difficult to decide how to characterize errors children make. Possibly, deeper probing could help uncover whether a particular error is, say, phonologically or syntactically based.

Identifying children within a language group who share well-described particular problems will allow for future comparative work across languages. Grimm's work on deficits in the syntactic development of German children provides some initial opportunities to examine questions about the universality of deficit types and the influence of particular languages on the nature of language impairment. Just as the cross linguistic investigation of aphasia has produced insights into the nature of language organization and processing (Bates 1992), so the cross linguistic study of early language impairment should provide insights about the capacity for language acquisition.

Cross linguistic research will not be easy. If it is difficult to decide what aspect of the language system to assign a particular error to, consider how difficult it will be to decide whether two errors in two different languages have a common basis. Clearly, this kind of research will involve a bootstrapping operation: how one classifies errors depends in part on the theory of grammar one holds and what theory one holds should depend (at least in part) on how well or elegantly the theory accounts for the cross linguistic data on deficits.

What goes wrong? Accounting for language impairment

Menyuk and Grimm are in agreement that environmental factors alone cannot account for the deficits observed in language impaired children. This is not to say that there is no influence of socio-economic factors. Grimm's data suggest that higher socioeconomic classes suffer less from language impairments; whether they are less vulnerable or have access to better remedial services is unclear. Nonetheless, both authors focus their explanatory accounts on characteristics of the child rather than external factors, although their theoretical paths diverge thereafter.

Menyuk's theory of metalinguistic ability

Using the classificatory terms of Hirsh-Pasek/Golinkoff (in press) Menyuk points out that the existence of SLI children is problematic for theorists of the "outside-in" schools of language acquisition. She proposes that "inside-out" theories are better able to account for those children who have significant language impairments despite having no detectable general cognitive deficits and having caretakers who provide them with adequate linguistic and social stimulation. Note that the terminology of Hirsh-Pasek and Golinkoff commits Menyuk to the notion that language learning is at least partially different from other kinds of learning and hence dependent on mechanisms of acquisition unique to language. General cognitive strategies are "outside-in" devices - clearly, "outside" refers to "outside the language system" not "outside the child."

Menyuk's candidate for a language-unique strategy for learning is metalinguistic ability. However, for her theoretical proposal to be considered explanatory, it will have to be clarified and better-specified. Now, metalinguistic ability is a vague term covering a broad range of behavioral phenomena associated with language acquisition, from discovering the cues revealing of structure, to reflecting on and assessing linguistic data, to using the discovered structures automatically (see p. 11, Fig. 1). But, to say that children discover the appropriate cues to language structure does not tell us HOW they do so. Possibly the perceptual-cognitive capacities involved in such discoveries are indeed unique to language, but Menyuk offers no evidence on that point other than the fact that children diagnosed as SLI do not have as-yet-discoverable general perceptual-cognitive difficulties.

As Menyuk uses the term, metalinguistic ability is not limited to conscious processes. Indeed, it seems little different from the class of behaviors one might call procedures for language learning. Menyuk is undoubtedly correct in arguing that young children are active language learners who at times reflect on their own and others' language. Yet, lumping together all the behaviors Menyuk cites as "metalinguistic" may obscure important differences among them. For example, some children may not be able to reflect on their language, whereas others may have trouble discovering and using the appropriate cues to structure. It is certainly not self-evident that the two kinds of children would suffer the same consequences.

Menyuk also proposes a stage theory of development, as different aspects of language are acquired in separate "rules sets" over time, although all sets pass through the same processing phases toward automaticity (see p. 14, Fig. 2). Recent findings on children's language-learning related behaviors are compatible with Menyuk's idea that some aspects of linguistic knowledge can be at an earlier intuitive level, while others will have reached a higher, conscious one. Normal two-year-olds can spontaneously revise their own syntactic efforts ("That a chimney. That's a chimney,") but do not make meta (that is, self-reflective) comments about syntax, although they do make such comments about phonology or the lexicon ("I call my ball ballie, I do,") (Shatz/Ebeling 1991). Presumably revision requires only intuitive knowledge whereas meta comments require conscious knowledge.

It would be of great interest to know whether SLI children both revise and make meta comments on the same aspects of language that normal children do. If they can revise but not make meta comments, it would suggest that revisions and self-reflective comments are *not* part of a single ability and that self-reflection is necessary for ultimate success at language learning. If they can make meta comments but not revise, it would suggest that some syntax-specific difficulty, *not* a language-general deficit in reflectiveness, is responsible for grammatical misanalysis. In either case, the data would provide a means of clarifying and evaluating Menyuk's proposal of metalinguistic ability as a cause of SLI.

It is important to keep in mind the distinction between traditional metalinguistic tasks that require conscious reflection, and metalinguistic abilities, now defined more broadly as sometimes not requiring reflection, when considering how Menyuk proposes to account for both delay and impairment. Menyuk argues that children who have only a general processing problem of speed should be language delayed but not impaired - they cannot process rule sets through the system as fast as normal children. Therefore, at any given age, they should have less of their knowledge at the conscious level than should normals. Hence, they should do less well on metalinguistic tests, not because they cannot be reflective or have other metalinguistic ability deficits, but because they have less knowledge that has passed to the conscious level for them reflect on. SLI children, however, have a genuine deficit in some (unspecified) comprehension skill that results in distorted, not just delayed development. Menyuk's point seems to be that a specific ability must be impaired for true language impairment to occur - slow processing alone will suffice for delay, as well as poor performance on metalinguistic tasks, but will not result in deviance.

Yet, it is possible that slow processing can result in deviance as well, if new information keeps entering the language-learning system irrespective of the state of analysis of the information already in the system. Imagine a continuously moving conveyor belt with new data pushing information along through the various levels of analysis at a constant rate, irrespective of whether all the analytic work at a particular level has been done. If the rate at which the conveyor belt moves is slow, then, despite slow analytic processes, information would be fully analyzed even though less information per unit time would be processed. However, if a normal-speed conveyor belt were coupled with slow analytic processes, the result would be incompletely processed information. Possibly the difference between delayed and impaired children has to do with the nature of processing time difficulties and not with additional deficits in the impaired children.

In sum, although it too needs to be much better specified, Menyuk's proposal for the stages of processing that linguistic information undergoes may have more explanatory promise than the broad notion of metalinguistic ability that leaves too vague the mechanisms involved in each stage of development.

Grimm's theory of gestalt versus elementaristic strategies

Processing abilities also play an important role in Grimm's account of possible causes of SLI. Grimm proposes that normal children take in and store together larger segments of speech (gestalt processing), whereas SLI children seem able to deal only with words or short phrases (elementaristic processing). Consequently, Grimm argues, SLI children do not have the input available in pieces large enough to accomplish adequate distributional analyses of structural characteristics. Grimm suggests that deficits in the ability to use rhythmic and prosodic cues to speech segmentation are a possible cause for elementaristic processing.

There is much to be said for Grimm's proposal. For one, she has impressive data showing differences between normal and dysphasic children in rhythmic abilities. For another, her proposal allows her to be neutral on the question of whether the children's problems are due to mechanisms unique to language or language learning. Indeed, rhythmicity is the sort of ability where, without the capacity itself being unique to the language system, a deficit in it could have early and obvious consequences for language development.

Still, there are some troubling gaps in the explanatory account. Perhaps the most glaring is that there is no well-specified route from the general explanatory constructs to the specific syntactic and morphological deficits that Grimm's German dysphasic children exhibit. For example, how does elementaristic processing push the children toward the (incorrect) verb-final solution to word order? Why should elementaristic processing be especially problematic for a relatively arbitrary morphological system like German plurals, where there are few general rules to uncover? Answering questions like these will necessitate more precise linguistic descriptions of the children's productions. Do the children have distorted or incorrect grammars that consistently generate their errorful utterances, or is their behavior more chaotic than that? If they have consistent grammars, can the grammars be accounted for by applying normal analytic procedures to an inadquate data base or are the analytic procedures themselves impaired? That is, is it necessary to postulate deficits beyond the segmentation system to account for the specifics of deviance? Since we have little idea what "normal" analytic procedures are, the task of accounting for specific distortions, necessary though it be, is formidable indeed.

Towards an adequate explanation of language impairment

Despite their theoretical differences, both Grimm and Menyuk suggest major processing deficiencies of some sort as the bases for language impairments. One of the most intriquing questions that emerge from their work is the issue of whether deviance in either speed of processing or segmentation of input can account for deviance in structural organization. There are ways to construe both theoretical approaches such that a general deficit could lead to misanalysis of structure - without there being any deficiencies in the analytic procedures themselves that operate on stored information. If all misanalyses of structure could be traced either to difficulties in the speed of processing or the segmentation of input, then the problems of diagnosis and treatment of language impairments would be greatly simplified. The work by Menyuk and Grimm have helped us see what further must be done in order to assess whether such accounts of language impairment will suffice.

Acknowledgement

This paper was prepared while the author was a visiting scholar at the Institute for Human Development, University of California, Berkeley.

References

Bates, E. (1992). Cross linguistic studies of language breakdown in aphasia. Plenary address presented at the Cognitive Society Conference, July, 1992.

Hirsh-Pasek, K. & Golinkoff, R.M. (in press). Skeletal supports for grammatical learning: What infants bring to the language learning task. In C.K. Rovee-Collier (Ed.), Advances in infancy research. Vol. 10. Norwood, NJ: Ablex.

Shatz, M. & Ebeling, K. (1991). Patterns of language learning-related behaviours: evidence for self-help in acquiring grammar. Journal of Child Language, 18, 295-313.

Perceptual and cognitive deficits in children with specific language impairment: Implications for diagnosis and intervention

Susan Ellis Weismer

Introductory remarks

The mechanisms underlying language acquisition and language disorders remain a mystery. The interrelationships between perceptual/cognitive processes and language skills have been investigated by researchers who view language within the larger framework of information processing capabilities or conceptual development. How findings of associations between processing limitations and language functioning are interpreted rest on one's conception of specific language impairment (SLI) and views regarding causality. A thought-provoking debate on this topic among a number of researchers in the area of child language disorders was recently published (Aram 1991; Dale/Cole 1991; Johnston 1991b; Kamhi 1991; Leonard 1991a, b; Tomblin 1991). Consideration of these complex issues is outside the scope of the present discussion. However, I would concur with researchers such as Johnston (in press) and Dale/Cole (1991) who propose that we move away from medical models focused on primary causal conditions. Instead, we may be better served by psycholinguistic or educational models which take into account the type of resources and constraints that SLI children bring to the task of language learning.

I will begin by selectively reviewing evidence for perceptual and cognitive deficits in SLI children, focusing on areas of inquiry that seem particularly relevant to the discussion of clinical implications. Recent comprehensive reviews of this research have been provided by Johnston (1988), Kamhi (in press), Leonard (1987), and Tallal (1988). In the second half of the paper, I will address assessment and intervention implications of these findings.

Perceptual abilities

Evidence of perceptual deficits in SLI

The nature of perceptual abilities in children with specific language impairments has been most extensively investigated by Paula Tallal and her colleagues. These researchers have used an experimental paradigm known as the Repetition Test (Tallal/Piercy 1973a, b) which investigates discrimination, sequencing, rate processing, and serial memory for speech and nonspeech stimuli. Numerous studies by Tallal and associates have demonstrated temporal processing deficits in SLI children across tasks employing verbal and nonverbal auditory stimuli (Johnston/Stark/Mellits/Tallal 1981; Tallal/Piercy 1973a, 1973b; 1974; Tallal/Stark/Kallman/Mellits 1980, 1981; Tallal/Stark/Mellits 1985a, b). Findings of impaired perceptual processing in language impaired children have also been reported for visual, tactile, and cross-modal stimuli (Tallal et al. 1981; Tallal et al. 1985b). Results indicate that the amount of time SLI children require for sensory information processing is orders of magnitude greater than that of normal language (NL) children, but that there is no significant difference between SLI and NL children on tasks of temporal integration when stimuli are presented more slowly (cf. Tallal 1988).

Elliott/Hammer (1988) compared auditory discrimination skills of school-age children with language learning problems and those with normal language abilities in a three-year longitudinal study. They administered a set of fine-grained auditory discrimination tasks designed to determine the smallest acoustic differences (i.e. "just noticeable differences" or JNDs) that could be discriminated. Language impaired children demonstrated poorer auditory discrimination skills (i.e. larger JNDs) than NL children across the three-year span.

Relation between perceptual functioning and language skills

In addition to documenting the existence of auditory perceptual deficits in SLI children, attempts have been made to more directly examine the relationship between these children's perceptual functioning and their language skills. Tallal and associates have found that SLI children have specific difficulty processing brief, rapidly sequenced speech signals (Tallal/Stark 1981) and that the speech production errors made by language impaired children follow the same pattern as speech perception (Tallal et al. 1980). Further, Tallal et al. (1985a,b) have reported that the degree of nonverbal temporal perceptual impairment is highly predictive of receptive language deficits in SLI children (with correlations of .85) and that a combination of perceptual and motor variables classified 98% of the subjects correctly as normally developing or SLI (however, see Elliott/ Hammer/Scholl 1990 regarding criticism of the experimental design/statistical analyses employed in this study). Elliott/Hammer/Scholl (1989) found that fine-grained measures of auditory discrimination correctly classified 79% of the younger group of subjects (6-7 year-olds) in their study and 64% of the older group (8-11 year-olds).

Recently, Curtiss/Tallal (1991) have reported findings from a large-scale longitudinal investigation examining various outcomes of preschool language impairment. One aspect of this study addressed the relationship between nonlinguistic sequential processing abilities and language acquisition. Performance on temporal processing tasks was compared to receptive and expressive language scores obtained from the CYCLE (Curtiss/Yamada 1988). Items on the CYCLE were divided into two distinct clusters designated as +sequentially-cued or -sequentially-cued: +sequentially-cued items consisted of semantically reversible SVO sentences in which word order uniquely cued grammatical and thematic role; whereas -sequentially-cued items included negative, attributive or stative sentences in which roles and relations were signalled by key grammatical formatives. SLI subjects' performance on the language items was significantly poorer on the +sequentially-cued cluster than the -sequentially-cued cluster whereas performance of the age-matched controls was not significantly different on the two clusters. For the SLI children, a modest but significant correlation was found between performance on the nonverbal sequencing task and the +sequentially-cued cluster for year 2 (.49) and year 3 (.39). Based on these findings, Curtiss and Tallal propose that a nonlinguistic sequential impairment may underlie SLI children's difficulty in processing linguistic structures in which sequential order of linguistic elements uniquely cues grammatical or semantic information.

Summary and interpretation

Numerous studies have found that compared to their agemates, SLI children demonstrate auditory perceptual deficits affecting linguistic and nonlinguistic processing of rapidly presented information. Whether these deficits are unique to auditory processing or extend to other modalities is a matter of continuing debate (cf. Elliott et al. 1990; Tallal 1990). Elliott views language impaired children's perceptual processing problems as auditory in nature. Tallal and associates argue that the deficit is more fundamental in character and contend that there is evidence of a "neural timing" deficit (Tallal 1988). (It should be noted, however, that Tallal's own findings have indicated some conflicting evidence concerning the presence of visual processing deficits in SLI, e.g. Tallal/Piercy 1973b). There are clearly differences across investigations in the tasks and type of perceptual processing skills tapped, but the overall findings of auditory processing limitations are consistent. Also, there is agreement that performance on perceptual processing tasks helps us distinguish between NL children and those with language difficulties. Further, particular types of temporal processing deficits (i.e. sequential impairments) have been shown to be related to specific language difficulties.

How shall we view these associations between perceptual processing deficits and specific language impairment? Various researchers have challenged causal interpretations (cf. Kamhi in press; Leonard 1987). To begin with, such claims have been criticized on theoretical grounds. Research in this area has focused on serial, bottom-up processing while ignoring the contribution of contextual factors, knowledge states, prior experience, and other conceptual processes in perception and memory (cf. Bohannon/Warren-Leubecker 1988). Furthermore, it is not clear what role temporal perceptual abilities play in language development. Theoretical accounts of language acquisition hypothesizing the nature of the relation between rapid auditory processing skills and language learning are lacking. The exception to this is Leonard's (1989) attempt to relate SLI children's difficulties with morphological development to the acoustic properties of these forms based on Pinker's (1984) Learnability Theory.

Another area of concern with a perceptual deficit explanation of SLI centers on the particular paradigm that has been used and what it taps, given that the bulk of the evidence for this view comes from performance on the Repetition Test employed by Tallal and associates. Normally developing children younger than 4½ years cannot successfully perform these tasks (Tallal 1976). Since NL children of that age have developed relatively sophisticated language skills (Lahey 1988), researchers have questioned the significance of successful performance for language learning (Kamhi in press). In addition, Tomblin/Quinn's (1983) finding that NL children's performance on the Repetition Test improved with a modest amount of experience has been viewed as refuting the notion that poor performance on these tasks reflects a limitation in fundamental temporal resolution capability. Finally, research with populations other than SLI children has provided counterevidence to causal claims. Ludlow/Cudahy/Bassick/Brown (1983) found that hyperactive boys without identified language or learning problems performed poorly on rapid auditory processing measures. Thus, auditory perceptual deficits seem to fall short as the explanation for language impairment. Nevertheless, these findings can provide important information about the type of pertinent processing limitations that many SLI children possess as they attempt to learn language.

Cognitive abilities

Children with SLI, in order to be classified as such, must perform within normal range on standardized measures of nonverbal intelligence. However, research findings based on a variety of experimental tasks have documented particular cognitive deficits in a number of areas. Various researchers have discussed this apparent paradox (Johnston 1982; Kamhi/Minor/Mauer 1990; Leonard 1987). Explanations that have been offered focus on the fact that nonverbal intelligence measures tap only a selected area of cognitive skills, with many of the items assessing visual perception of static figures and designs which is a relative area of strength for these children (Johnston 1982). Other aspects of cognitive functioning seem to be more problematic for language impaired children. I will review pertinent investigations, dividing them according to those which focus on symbolic skills versus nonsymbolic cognitive functioning.

Symbolic skills

It has been hypothesized that language impaired children have a general representational deficit rather than a selective language impairment, such that they have a limited ability to create and deploy symbols (Morehead 1972; Morehead/Ingram 1973). The areas of nonverbal symbol use that have been investigated most in relation to children with specific language impairments are symbolic play and visual imagery.

Symbolic play. When SLI children are compared to age-matched normal language controls, they consistently exhibit less pretend play and less use of advanced play schemes, i.e. those involving symbolic substitution of one object for another or the integration of play behaviors around a theme (Terrell/Schwartz 1983; Udwin/Yule 1983). Various investigations, in particular those by Terrell and colleagues, have reported that language impaired children are not deficient in their symbolic play skills when compared to children with equivalent *expressive* language skills (Terrell/Schwartz 1983, 1988; Terrell/Schwartz/Prelock/Messick 1984). In fact, the SLI children exhibit more mature play than their language-matched peers even though they perform considerably below age expectations. This finding is most likely related to differences in the comprehension levels between the two groups. Bates and colleagues have noted that higher levels of symbolic gesture use are associated with higher language comprehension skills (Bates/Thal/Whitesell et al. 1989). When both *receptive and expressive* language levels were taken into account in establishing linguistic equivalency between groups, Roth/Clark (1987) found that SLI children demonstrated significant deficits in symbolic, adaptive, and integrative play.

Visual imagery. A number of studies have found that language impaired children evidence difficulties in visual imagery skills (de Ajuriaguerra/Jaeggi/Guignard et al. 1976; Johnston/Ramstad 1983). They have been shown to perform significantly more poorly than chronologically age (CA) matched and mental age (MA) matched normal language controls across a range of different tasks (Camarata/Newhoff/Rugg 1981; Johnston/Ellis Weismer 1983; Kamhi 1981; Savich 1984). When groups are matched in terms of mean length of utterance (MLU), language impaired children exhibit better imagery skills than the younger, normal language children (Camarata et al. 1981; Kamhi 1981). This finding has led some researchers to conclude that the degree of difficulty in visual imagery skills displayed by children with specific language impairments is subtle. Studies are not available, however, to indicate how groups matched on receptive language skills would compare in terms of their proficiency on visual imagery tasks.

Nonsymbolic cognitive functioning

Reasoning skills. Investigators have explored the notion that deficits in cognitive processes supporting problem solving and rule formation might underlie difficulties with language learning. Various theories of language acquisition have incorporated constructs such as hypothesis testing or analogical reasoning (Bloomfield 1933/ 1961; Brown/Fraser 1964; MacWhinney 1978; Pinker 1984, 1989). As Johnston (1988) has noted, many language acquisition theories (with the notable exception of connectionist models) claim that children analyze and compare linguistic input and form hypotheses about the underlying organization of language, later re-evaluating these hypotheses in light of new linguistic input. According to this view, evidence that SLI children demonstrate hypothesis testing deficits could be seen as an important factor in their language learning problems. Similarly, deficits in analogical reasoning could be postulated to play a role in language difficulties since it is posited to be a central mechanism in learning processes (Brown 1989; Holyoak 1984). A related cognitive process that has been investigated with respect to language disorders is inference construction. Investigations have focused on the role of inferential operations in the comprehension and retention of meaningful information, particularly connected discourse (Bransford/Franks 1971; Kintsch/Van Dijk 1978; Paris/Lindauer 1976).

Investigations of SLI children's hypothesis testing skills have produced conflicting results. Two studies by Kamhi and colleagues failed to find significant differences in the performance of SLI and MA-matched normal language controls on hypothesis testing tasks (Kamhi/Catts/Koenig/Lewis 1984; Kamhi/Nelson/Lee/Gholson 1985). However, in both cases this outcome was likely influenced by the use of task items that were too demanding even for the control subjects. Evidence that language impaired children demonstrate limitations in hypothesis testing abilities has been provided by the findings of Hoskins (1979), Nelson/Kamhi/Apel (1987), and Ellis Weismer (1991b).

Research has demonstrated that school-aged children with language disorders and those with language-learning disabilities associated with reading disabilities evidence problems in inferential skills. In studies by Crais/Chapman (1987), Ellis Weismer (1985), and Bishop/Adams (1992), children with language deficits were found to be significantly less adept than age-matched or MA-matched controls in drawing inferences on verbal tasks and on nonverbal (pictorial) tasks.

Recently, the role of analogical reasoning processes in language disorders has been considered by investigators (Kamhi 1988; Kahmi/Gentry/Mauer/Gholson 1990; Nippold/Erskine/Freed 1988). While some differences have been found in the performance of language impaired children compared to normal language children, the evidence for deficits in analogical reasoning is less compelling than for other reasoning skills.

Memory. Investigators have examined the short-term memory skills of children with language impairment in an effort to assess the role that more basic cognitive mechanisms may play in language disorders. Language impaired children have been shown to exhibit deficits on serial memory tasks involving sequences of nonverbal auditory or visual stimuli (Bernstein/Stark 1985; Tallal et al. 1981) and on spatial memory tasks (Wyke/Asso 1979). Investigations of verbal memory in children with language learning difficulties have revealed problems with various components of short-term memory, including use of rehearsal strategies, scanning speed, storage and retrieval (Ceci/Ringstrom/Lea 1981; Kirchner/Klatzky 1985; Sininger/Klatzky/Kirchner 1989). Kirchner/Klatzky (1985) concluded that the verbal rehearsal deficits evidenced by the language impaired children in their study were indicative of limited resource capacity. A subsequent study by Sininger et al. (1989), revealed reduced short-term memory scanning speed in these same language impaired subjects, which is consistent with their limitations in working capacity.

Considering the evidence for short-term memory deficits in children with language impairments, we might ask how these deficits are related to their limitations in reasoning skills. Based on the pattern of results in their study, Nelson et al. (1987) contend that the difficulties in hypothesis testing which the SLI children displayed seemed to relate to deficits in encoding information into short-term memory. Using a modified hypothesis testing task in which the short-term memory requirements were minimized, Ellis Weismer (1991b) found that SLI children still demonstrated significantly more difficulty solving problems than cognitive level controls. This finding is consistent with the results of Ellis Weismer (1985) which indicated that even when language impaired children demonstrated memory for premise information, they were significantly less likely than MA-matched control subjects to generate the appropriate inferences. Although there are, no doubt, links between limitations in SLI children's short-term memory skills and their problem solving abilities, the results of these studies suggest that the reasoning problems which these children exhibit cannot be accounted for solely on the basis of memory difficulties.

Relation to language skills. Some attempt has been made to examine more directly the relation between language impaired children's cognitive abilities and their language skills. Significant, though moderate, correlations have been found between language impaired children's nonlinguistic symbolic abilities and their linguistic skills (Kamhi et al. 1984; Savich 1984; Udwin/Yule 1983). In examining relative performance levels, varying patterns have been reported (cf. Johnston 1988). In some cases verbal abilities and nonverbal symbolic skills have appeared to be equivalent (Terrell/Schwartz

1983), sometimes verbal abilities have been found to be advanced relative to nonverbal symbolic abilities (Roth/Clark 1987), and other times the opposite relationship has been reported (Kamhi 1981; Terrell et al. 1984). Johnston (1988) has contended that these findings are exactly what would be expected based upon a model of two cognitive systems which share the common attribute of symbolism, but differ in other regards. Employing the "local homology" model (Bates/Benigni/Bretherton et al. 1979), Thal/Bates (1988) have argued that language and symbolic play are related only at specific points in time when both draw on similar component processes. In other words, the mechanisms linking language and symbolic play are thought to vary depending upon the developmental stage. Various researchers have proposed that *specific* aspects of language and cognition are temporally associated, but that particular skills may be attained first in either the linguistic or cognitive domain (cf. Kelly/Dale 1989). Few studies have directly investigated the connection between nonsymbolic cognitive skills and language abilities. Nippold et al. (1988) found a significant positive correlation between language impaired children's performance on a verbal analogical reasoning task and two tasks of nonverbal analogical reasoning, but reasoning abilities were not compared to other language skills. No significant correlations were found between SLI children's scores on language measures and their hypothesis testing abilities (Ellis Weismer 1991b) or inferential skills (Bishop/ Adams 1992).

Summary and interpretation

Research has supported the contention that SLI children exhibit representational deficits that extend beyond their problems with linguistic representation. Investigations of symbolic play and visual imagery indicate that children with language impairments evidence limitations in their use of nonverbal symbols as well as verbal symbols when compared to their normally developing peers on the basis of CA, MA or a combination of receptive and expressive language levels. Further, associations between SLI children's symbolic abilities and their language skills have been found. Deficits in nonsymbolic cognitive processes have also been implicated in language disorders. SLI children have been shown to demonstrate short-term memory difficulties on verbal and nonverbal tasks and a lack of proficiency in certain types of reasoning skills. Considering the pattern of results across studies, it appears that in many cases language impaired children exhibit *inefficiency* in various aspects of cognitive processing rather than displaying an inability to perform the task or showing qualitatively different patterns of performance. That is, SLI children can use imagistic strategies, construct inferences, use rehearsal strategies, generate hypotheses and so forth. Compared to their NL peers, however, they are less likely to spontaneously and reliably apply available strategies for processing information. Capacity limitations in SLI children (cf. Johnston 1991a; Johnston/Smith 1989) may be a reflection of factors such as reduced processing speed or deficiencies in attention allocation leading to less efficient strategy use across both verbal and nonverbal domains.

The role of cognitive limitations in SLI children's problems with language learning remains controversial (Johnston 1988; Leonard 1987; Tallal 1988). There are a number of issues to consider in weighing this evidence. It can be argued that SLI children's poorer performance on these cognitive tasks may be a reflection of the language disorder itself. Although explicit demands for language use can be minimized, subjects may well be using language internally to aid their performance on many of the "nonverbal" tasks (cf. Johnston 1991a). Findings of cognitive deficits in certain studies (e.g. Johnston/Ellis Weismer 1983; Wyke/Asso 1979), however, cannot be explained on the basis of SLI children's lack of facility with verbal mediation (refer to discussions of this point by Johnston 1988, 1991a). In another sense though, this claim (that cognitive deficits are a reflection of the language impairment) appears to be true. Several researchers have argued that the nature of the relationship between cognition and language varies as a function of developmental level and the particular features of language or cognition under investigation (Johnston 1985; Thal/Bates 1988). In as much as language serves as a "tool for thought" at later stages of development (Johnston 1991a, in press), we would expect problem solving skills to be integrally related to language abilities and a search for unidirectional influences would be remiss.

Concern with cognitive research in SLI might also be directed at the type of experimental tasks that have been employed and the nature of the cognitive processes they measure. For example, Johnston (1988) has pointed out that explicit, conscious hypothesis testing abilities tapped by concept formation and discrimination learning tasks may well be qualitatively different than the type of implicit hypothesis testing posited to occur in language learning. In attempting to investigate cognitive skills that are hypothesized to be related to language learning, researchers have often drawn on established theoretical frameworks and borrowed experimental paradigms from the field of psychology (such as Hypothesis theory as applied to children's problem solving, cf. Gholson 1980). Admittedly this approach may not be ideal, but Johnston (1991b) notes the challenge of trying to operationalize constructs that have been implicated in language learning problems in order to devise new experimental paradigms to assess these mental processes.

A final factor that complicates the interpretation of this line of research pertains to the comparison groups against which the performance of the SLI children is judged. Several researchers have recently noted the difficulty in obtaining an MA-matched control group in investigations involving language impaired children (Ellis Weismer 1991b; Montgomery/Scudder/Moore 1990; Nippold et al. 1988). Even when there is no statistically significant difference between cognitive levels of language impaired children and MA-matched controls, language impaired children often tend to perform slightly below average as a group and somewhat more poorly than the controls. Investigations of SLI children's cognitive skills have used MA-matches in an attempt to demonstrate that specific aspects of cognition are impaired relative to general intellectual functioning levels. We may need to consider more carefully our procedures for establishing cognitive equivalency between the groups in order to have more assurance in the conclusions regarding specific processing deficits. Use of language-matched comparison groups in examining SLI children's cognitive skills is also problematic. To begin with, studies employing such designs usually equate subjects on the basis of a single index of language across various domains (syntax, semantics, pragmatics) and processes (comprehension and production). When SLI subjects' performance on a reasoning task is found to be similar to younger, language-matched controls it is difficult to know how this should be interpreted. One might conclude that this finding points to the role of language skills in completing the task, i.e. that language impaired children demonstrate reasoning skills that are equivalent to children with the same level of language abilities. Alternately, the similar performance could be related to other areas of processing limitations (such as poor short-term memory rehearsal strategies) that are not the focus of the investigation, but which combine with deficiencies in reasoning skills to make the SLI subjects perform much like the less mature NL controls.

Implications for diagnosis and intervention

Assessment

Findings of perceptual and cognitive processing impairments in SLI children may have potential ramifications in several areas of assessment, including:

identifying children with SLI, predicting language functioning outcomes, and assessing varying linguistic performance under different task demands. As reviewed previously, attempts have been made to relate impaired perceptual processing directly to language functioning and to classify children on the basis of their performance on perceptual tasks as NL or SLI. Tallal (1988, 1991) has suggested that temporal perceptual/motor deficits may be a "marker variable" for language impairment. It may well be important to document perceptual deficits in order to define populations on the basis of such inclusionary criteria for heuristic or research purposes. However, for practical, clinical purposes there are more straightforward means of directly assessing oral language disorders; therefore, the potential clinical significance of assessing perceptual functioning in children with SLI may lie in its predictive value.

There is evidence that a substantial proportion of children with early language impairment continue to exhibit deficits during the school-age period and that they are particularly at risk for problems in reading and writing (Aram/Ekelman/Nation 1984; Aram/Nation 1980; Stark/Bernstein/Condino et al. 1984; Tallal 1988). The importance of this link is acknowledged by the very topics that are being jointly addressed at this conference, namely specific language impairment and dyslexia (see discussions of this issue by Ellis Weismer 1993; Kamhi/Catts/Mauer et al. 1988; Maxwell/Wallach 1984; Tallal 1988). It would be extremely useful if performance on perceptual processing measures could help us predict which SLI children are likely to have continued problems. Results of the San Diego longitudinal study indicate that there is a high incidence of subsequent reading problems in children with early language impairment (cf. Tallal 1988). Investigations by Tallal and colleagues have reported that reading impaired children with decoding (phonics) deficits who have concomitant oral language disorders exhibit patterns of temporal perceptual/motor deficits similar to those of SLI children (Tallal 1980a, b). Those reading impaired children who do not demonstrate oral language disorders or problems learning phonics rules, however, do not exhibit temporal processing deficits (Tallal/Stark 1982). Thus, Tallal has speculated that a common neurological deficit may underlie developmental language disorders and reading disabilities, such that temporal processing impairments may disrupt phoneme perception and production leading to delayed language acquisition and subsequently to reading difficulties. In addition to potential uses to predict SLI children who are most at risk for later written language difficulties, there is at least a possibility that performance on perceptual processing tasks might provide more specific insights into the nature of particular language learning difficulties that SLI children are likely to encounter. With further investigations such as the one reported by Curtiss/Tallal (1991), we may be able to establish patterns of specific associations between linguistic processing and certain perceptual processing deficits (such as sequential impairments), thereby projecting which aspects of the language are vulnerable in the face of these perceptual impairments. At the moment, of course, these potential clinical implications are highly speculative.

With respect to cognitive abilities, most of the clinical applications pertaining to assessment have focused on the area of representational or symbolic skills. Bolstered by findings of specific associations between symbolic play/ gestures and language skills at particular points in normal development (cf. Kennedy/Sheridan/Radlinski/Beeghly 1991; Thal/Bates 1988), assessment efforts have centered on play as an index of symbolic functioning. Formalized means of evaluating these skills have been developed (e.g. the Symbolic Play Test, Lowe/Costello 1976), as well as informal observational checklists. In current clinical practice, some measure of play skills is often included in evaluations of young children suspected of having delayed language development as an indication of their "readiness" for language learning.

Recently, there has been increasing interest in a group of young children referred to in the literature as "late talkers" or "specifically expressively language delayed" (SELD) (Paul/Spangle Looney/Dahm 1991; Rescorla 1989; Thal/Bates 1988; Thal/Tobias/Morrison 1991). Rescorla (1989) has reported that only about half of the children who are identified as late talkers at age two will experience a developmental spurt and catch up to their peers by age three. Thus, a substantial number of these children will have persistent problems. Thal and colleagues have investigated the relationship between language and symbolic gesture in late talkers (Thal/Bates 1988; Thal et al. 1991). The diagnostic significance of this research lies in the attempt to subtype children with language learning difficulties and distinguish between late talkers who will catch up versus those who will be language impaired. The Thal et al. (1991) investigation involved a one-year follow-up study of the relation between symbolic gestures and linguistic skills in ten children who exhibited delayed onset of early lexical production. Four of the ten children who were truly language impaired at follow-up had shown comprehension deficits in addition to significantly poorer performance on all of the gesture tasks at the first visit than the late talkers who caught up. These investigators conclude that gesture production in familiar scripts provides important prognostic information in concert with vocabulary comprehension measures, and suggest that such assessment procedures might be developed to predict continued language learning problems in toddlers as early as 18 months.

Let's turn our attention now to assessment implications of the research on nonsymbolic cognitive functioning in children with SLI. Within the educational literature, the importance of problem solving skills to school success has long been recognized (cf. Brandt 1988; Caine/Caine 1991). Therefore, language impaired children who have concomitant limitations in reasoning skills would seem to be particularly at risk. For instance, deficits in higher-order linguistic and reasoning skills can be expected to negatively impact upon text comprehension abilities and especially on "reading to learn" (Chall 1983) which normally develops at about the fourth grade level (cf. Roth/Spekman 1989). In their text, Larson/McKinley (1987) have suggested assessment procedures for school-age children and adolescents which include evaluation of critical thinking and problem solving abilities.

Evidence of memory and attention deficits in SLI children prompts more concern with "on-line" processing of linguistic information and invites assessment of linguistic performance under different task demands. Tallal (1991) addresses this point in discussing results from the San Diego longitudinal study. She has noted that individual children alternately evidenced mastery or lack of mastery of the same linguistic rules under varied task-processing constraints. The determining variable was not whether the task required comprehension or production of linguistic structures per se, but rather performance appeared to be dependent upon nonlinguistic task demands (e.g. the extent to which information had to be held in memory, the need to select among competing alternatives). Similarly, researchers such as Fletcher (1991) and Johnston (in press) have argued that clinical assessments should include a focus on language performance in addition to linguistic knowledge. As Johnston (in press, 26) notes, successful language use depends not only on knowledge of the language system, but also on the ability to utilize this knowledge reliably and economically. This may mean broadening the scope of our evaluation tools in order to assess the process of language learning as well as the product. In other words, this implies that we consider: a) developing measures that provide information about on-line linguistic processing; b) devising indices that allow us to evaluate the degree and type of trade-offs in linguistic complexity/accuracy under various communicative task requirements; and c) assessing learning potential (such as the type of dynamic assessment techniques suggested by Olswang/Bain 1991).

Intervention

Researchers who have investigated perceptual/cognitive skills in SLI children have typically refrained from making claims about the relevance of their findings for intervention. However, Tallal (1988) includes in her review chapter a detailed discussion of intervention approaches stemming from the literature on central auditory processing (CAP) disorders in children (cf. Katz 1983; Lasky/Cox 1983; Sloan 1986). Varying criteria have been employed in identifying children with CAP disorders, including definitions which would include many children with SLI. This area of investigation has been criticized on a number of grounds (cf. Kamhi in press; Kamhi/Beasley 1985; Rees 1981). Yet, there are various published CAP treatment approaches (Katz 1983; Lindamood/Lindamood 1975) and proponents of these methods. There is scant empirical evidence, however, of the effectiveness of these approaches.

In terms of higher cognitive abilities, Butler (1984) has proposed both assessment and intervention procedures for school-age children with language learning difficulties based on an information processing model. Within this framework, it is suggested that remediation tasks be analyzed in terms of stimulus characteristics, processing characteristics, and information load and that these variables then be manipulated during treatment to facilitate the child's information processing strategies. According to the approach suggested by Butler, direct instruction and practice would be provided in areas such as self-monitoring procedures, use of mnemonic devices, and recall strategies such as active rehearsal. In a text by Wallach/Miller (1988), language intervention principles and techniques are proposed that derive from an information processing framework which incorporates emphasis on various cognitive and metacognitive abilities, including inference construction.

Similarly, strategy-based or "learning strategy" intervention models have been developed in the last ten years. Many of the strategy-based intervention programs are modeled after Feuerstein's Instrumental Enrichment Program (1980) which focuses on cognitive/problem solving skills. Language intervention methods based on the learning strategies approach (designed for school-age children and adolescents) have been described by Buttrill/Niizawa/Biemer et al. (1989), Larson/McKinley (1987), and others. These approaches emphasize the teaching of generalizable strategies to facilitate language learning and language-based academic skills. They include instruction aimed at improving critical thinking and problem solving, listening skills, and metacognitive abilities. Although clinical reports of the success of such cognitive-based language intervention programs are promising, we lack experimental documentation of the effectiveness of these approaches.

Intervention approaches that attempt to directly modify auditory perceptual skills or higher level cognitive abilities are apparently based, at some level, on the assumption that these processing deficits underlie language disorders. Given the controversy regarding the nature of the relationship between nonlinguistic processing deficits exhibited by SLI children and their language impairment, there is an alternate tack that might be taken. We could consider the characteristics of the children who are the focus of our programming efforts and then specially adapt training techniques given what we know about how they process information (cf. Ellis Weismer 1991a). Ellis Weismer/Dollaghan (1989) have proposed an intervention approach which is geared toward providing optimal input or exposure conditions to facilitate language learning by modifying linguistic and nonlinguistic input during training to fit SLI children's processing constraints. Within this framework, linguistic input would be presented in a manner that is posited to reduce processing demands and allow the SLI child to allocate more cognitive resources to the target form.

For example, in an attempt to mitigate auditory processing constraints evidenced by children with SLI, various modifications of the linguistic input have been suggested, including: reduced rate of speech, increased pause length, exaggerated vocal stress, and use of nonauditory cues (such as visual symbols or manual signing) paired with oral language input (see Ellis Weismer 1988; Johnston 1988; Lahey 1988). It is assumed that these modifications may facilitate segmentation of the speech signal and/or heighten the perceptual saliency of the target, thereby reducing processing demands such that the child is able to allocate more attention to the discovery of the linguistic rule. Although several intervention studies have included certain of these linguistic input modifications in their treatment procedures (Constable 1986; Culatta/Horn 1982), there are only a few investigations that have attempted to directly assess the impact of such manipulations on language impaired children's linguistic performance (e.g.Campbell/McNeil 1985; Ellis Weismer/Digney/Krueger/Ricke 1990; McCroskey/Thompson 1973). Ellis Weismer and colleagues (1990) investigated NL and SLI children's ability to learn novel lexical items that were taught under linguistic input conditions which varied with respect to a) rate of speech, b) vocal stress, and c) use of gestures accompanying spoken language. Differential patterns of results were observed for the two groups, with SLI children evidencing greater response to the input manipulations than the NL children. For the SLI group, slowed rates of speech and use of visual cues (gestures) each resulted in improved comprehension and production of the target lexemes. Those lexical targets that had received emphatic stress during training were more often produced correctly than those without emphatic stress; however, no stress effect was found for comprehension.

My colleagues and I are continuing to examine the effects of prosodic manipulations of linguistic input on language learning by children with specific language impairment (see Ellis Weismer in press for literature review and theoretical discussion). Hopefully, this line of research will lead to insights about the ways in which interventionists can optimize the match between SLI children's processing capabilities and the input they receive.

Concluding comments

Future investigations of SLI children's perceptual and cognitive skills might profitably include studies that focus on: a) directly relating specific perceptual or cognitive deficits to particular language problems; b) examining the relation of varying combinations of processing deficits to language functioning, e.g. temporal processing deficits plus limitations in representational skills; c) determining the ability of performance on these tasks to help classify children and to predict language outcomes; and d) consideration of individual subject data as well as group findings.

If we are looking for the cause of specific language impairment, we are likely to be disappointed by this body of research. On the other hand, if we are looking for information that affords us a better understanding of the perceptual and cognitive resources that SLI children can bring to bear on the task of learning language, we are likely to be encouraged by how much knowledge has been gained in the last 15 years. As is the case with beauty, the utility and success of research efforts in this area seem to lie in the eye of the beholder.

References

Aram, D. (1991). Comments on specific language impairment as a clinical category. Language, Speech, and Hearing Services in Schools, 22, 84-87.

Aram, D., Ekelman, B., & Nation, J. (1984). Preschoolers with language disorders: 10 years later. Journal of Speech and Hearing Research, 27, 232-244.

Aram, D. & Nation, J. (1980). Preschool language disorders and subsequent language and academic difficulties. Journal of Communication Disorders, 13, 159-170.

Bates, E., Benigni, L., Bretherton, I., Camaioni, L., & Volterra, V. (1979). The emergence of symbols: Cognition and communication in infancy. New York: Academic Press.

Bates, E., Thal, D., Whitesell, K., Fenson, L., & Oakes, L. (1989). Integrating language and gesture in infancy. Developmental Psychology, 25, 1004-1019.

Bernstein, L. & Stark, R. (1985). Speech perception development in language-impaired children: A four-year follow-up study. Journal of Speech and Hearing Disorders, 50, 21-30.

Bishop, D. & Adams, C. (1992). Comprehension problems in children with specific language: Literal and inferential meaning. Journal of Speech and Hearing Research, 35, 119-129.

Bloomfield, L. (1933/1961). Language. New York: Henry Holt.

Bohannon, J. & Warren-Leubecker, A. (1988). Theoretical approaches to language acquisition. In J. Berko Gleason (Ed.), The development of language (2nd ed.). 167-225. Columbus, OH: Merrill.

Brandt, R. (Ed.) (1988). Teaching thinking throughout the curriculum. Educational Leadership, 45, (7).

Bransford J. & Franks, J. (1971). The abstraction of linguistic ideas. Cognitive Psychology, 2, 331-350.

Brown, A. (1989). Analogical learning and transfer: What develops? In S. Vosniadou & A. Ortony (Eds.), Similarity and analogical reasoning. 369-412. Cambridge, England: Cambridge University Press.

Brown, R. & Fraser, C. (1964). The acquisition of syntax. In U. Bellugi & R. Brown (Eds.), The acquisition of language. 43-79, Monographs of the Society for Research in Child Development, 29, (No. 92).

Butler, K.G. (1984). Language processing: Halfway up the down staircase. In G.P. Wallach & K.G. Butler (Eds.), Language and learning disabilities in school-age children. 60-81. Baltimore: Williams and Wilkins.

Buttrill, J., Niizawa, J., Biemer, C., Takahashi, C., & Hearn, S. (1989). Serving the language learning disabled adolescent: A strategies-based model. Language, Speech, and Hearing Services in Schools, 20, 185-204.

Caine, R. & Caine, G. (Eds.) (1991). Teaching and the human brain. Association for Supervision & Curriculum Development (ASCD) Alexandria, VA.

Camarata, S., Newhoff, M., & Rugg, B. (1981). Perspective taking in normal and language disordered children. Proceedings from the Symposium on Research in Child Language Disorders, 2, 81-88.

Campbell, T. & McNeil, M. (1985). Effects of presentation rate and divided attention on auditory comprehension in children with an acquired language disorder. Journal of Speech and Hearing Research, 28, 513-520.

Ceci, S., Ringstrom, M., & Lea, S. (1981). Do language-learning disabled children have impaired memories? In search of underlying processes. Journal of Learning Disabilities, 14, 159-173.

Chall, J. (1983). Stages of Reading Development. New York: McGraw-Hill.

Constable, C. (1986). The application of scripts in the organization of language intervention contexts. In K. Nelson (Ed.), Event knowledge: Structure and function in development. 205-230. Hillsdale, NJ: Erlbaum.

Crais, E. & Chapman, R. (1987). Story recall and inferencing in language/learning disabled and non-disabled children. Journal of Speech and Hearing Disorders, 52, 50-55.

Culatta, B. & Horn, D. (1982). A program for achieving generalization of grammatical rules to spontaneous discourse. Journal of Speech and Hearing Research, 47, 174-180.

Curtiss, S. & Tallal, P. (1991). On the nature of the impairment in language-impaired children. In J. Miller (Ed.), Research on child language disorders. 189-210. Austin, TX: Pro-Ed.

Curtiss, S. & Yamada, J. (1988). The Curtiss-Yamada Comprehensive Language Evaluation (CYCLE). Unpublished test.

Dale, P. & Cole, K. (1991). What's normal? Specific language impairment in an individual differences perspective. Language, Speech, and Hearing Services in Schools, 22, 80-83.

de Ajuriaguerra, J., Jaeggi, A., Guignard, F., Kocher, F., Manquard, M., Roth, S., & Schmid, E. (1976). The development and prognosis of dysphasia in children. In D. Morehead & A. Morehead (Eds.), Normal and deficient child language. 1345-1385. Baltimore: University Park Press.

Elliott, L. & Hammer, M. (1988). Longitudinal changes in auditory discrimination in normal children and children with language learning problems. Journal of Speech and Hearing Disorders, 53, 467-474.

Elliott, L., Hammer, M., & Scholl, M. (1989). Fine-grained auditory discrimination in normal children and children with language-learning problems. Journal of Speech and Hearing Research, 32, 112-119.

Elliott, L., Hammer, M., & Scholl, M. (1990). Response to Tallal. Journal of Speech and Hearing Research, 33, 619.

Ellis Weismer, S. (1985). Constructive comprehension abilities exhibited by language-disordered children. Journal of Speech and Hearing Research, 28, 175-184.

Ellis Weismer, S. (1988). Specific language learning problems. In D.E. Yoder & R.D. Kent (Eds.), Decision-making in speech-language pathology. 42-43. Philadelphia: B.C. Decker.

Ellis Weismer, S. (1991a). Child language intervention: Research issues on the horizon. In J. Miller (Ed.), Research on child language disorders. 233-241. Austin, TX: Pro-Ed.

Ellis Weismer, S. (1991b). Hypothesis testing abilities of language impaired children. Journal of Speech and Hearing Research, 34, 1329-1338.

Ellis Weismer, S. (1993). Aspects of metalinguistic abilities in developmental dysphasia and dyslexia. In G. Blanken, J. Dittmann, H. Grimm, J. Marshall, & C. Wallesch (Eds.), Linguistic disorders and pathologies: An international handbook. 773-787. New York: de Gruyter.

Ellis Weismer, S. (in press). Effects of prosodic manipulations of linguistic input on specific language impaired children's lexical learning. In R. Chapman (Ed.), Child talk: Processes in language acquisition. Mosby-Yearbook.

Ellis Weismer, S., Digney, K., Krueger, W., & Ricke, C. (1990). Linguistic input manipulations during lexical training. Paper presented at the annual convention of the American Speech-Language-Hearing Association, Seattle, WA.

Ellis Weismer, S. & Dollaghan, C. (1989). Jigsaw: Processing constraints and input modification in language intervention. Miniseminar presented at the annual convention of the American Speech-Language-Hearing Association, St. Louis.

Feuerstein, R. (1980). Instrumental enrichment. Chicago: Scott, Foresman.

Fletcher, P. (1991). Evidence from syntax for language impairment. In J. Miller (Ed.), Research on child language disorders. 169-187. Austin, TX: Pro-Ed.

Gholson, B. (1980). The cognitive-developmental basis of human learning: Studies in hypothesis testing. New York: Academic Press.

Holyoak, K. (1984). Analogical thinking and human intelligence. In R. Sternberg (Ed.), Advances in the psychology of human intelligence (Vol. 2). 199-230. Hillsdale, NJ: Erlbaum.

Hoskins, B. (1979). A study of hypothesis testing behavior in language disordered children. Paper presented at the Annual Convention of the American Speech-Language-Hearing Assoc., Atlanta, GA.

Johnston, J. (1982). The language disordered child. In N. Lass, L. McReynolds, J. Northern, & D. Yoder (Eds.), Speech, Language, and Hearing, Vol. II. 780-801. Philadelphia: W.B. Saunders.

Johnston, J. (1985). Cognitive prerequisites: Evidence from children learning English. In D. Slobin (Ed.), The cross-linguistic study of language acquisition, Vol. 2. 961-1004. Hillsdale, NJ: Erlbaum.

Johnston, J. (1988). Specific language disorders in the child. In N. Lass, L. McReynolds, J. Northern, & D. Yoder (Eds.), Handbook of speech-language pathology and audiology. 685-715. Philadelphia: B. C. Decker, Inc.

Johnston, J. (1991a). Cognitive abilities of language impaired children. Paper presented at the International Symposium on Specific Speech and Language Disorders in Children, Harrogate, England.

Johnston, J. (1991b). The continuing relevance of cause: A reply to Leonard's "Specific language impairment as a clinical category". Language, Speech, and Hearing Services in Schools, 22, 75-79.

Johnston, J. (in press). Definition and diagnosis of language development and disorders. In G. Blanken, J. Dittmann, H. Grimm, J. Marshall, & C. Wallesch (Eds.), Linguistic disorders and pathologies: An international handbook. New York: de Gruyter.

Johnston, J. & Ellis Weismer, S. (1983). Mental rotation abilities in language disordered children. Journal of Speech and Hearing Research, 26, 397-403.

Johnston, J. & Ramstad, V. (1983). Cognitive development in pre-adolescent language impaired children. British Journal of Disorders of Communication, 18, 49-55.

Johnston, J.R. & Smith, L.B. (1989). Dimensional thinking in language impaired children. Journal of Speech and Hearing Research, 32, 33-38.

Johnston, R.B., Stark, R.E., Mellits, E.D., Tallal, P. (1981). Neurological status of language-impaired and normal children. Annals of Neurology, 10, 159-163.

Kamhi, A. (1981). Nonlinguistic symbolic and conceptual abilities of language-impaired and normally developing children. Journal of Speech and Hearing Research, 24, 435-45.

Kamhi, A. (1988). A reconceptualization of generalization and generalization problems. Language, Speech, and Hearing Services in Schools, 19, 304-13.

Kamhi, A. (1991). Specific language impairment as a clinical category--An introduction. Language, Speech, and Hearing Services in Schools, 22, 65.

Kamhi, A. (in press). Specific language impairment: Perceptual and cognitive aspects. In G. Blanken, J. Dittmann, H. Grimm, J. Marshall, & C. Wallesch (Eds.), Linguistic disorders and pathologies: An international handbook. New York: de Gruyter.

Kamhi, A. & Beasley, D. (1985). Central auditory processing disorders: Is it a meaningful construct or a twentieth century unicorn? In J. Singer & R. Hurley (Eds.), Central auditory processing disorders in children. 5-14. Journal of Childhood Communication Disorders, Vol. 9, No. 1.

Kamhi, A., Catts, H., Koenig, L., & Lewis, B. (1984). Hypothesis-testing and nonlinguistic symbolic abilities in language-impaired children. Journal of Speech and Hearing Disorders, 49, 169-76.

Kamhi, A., Catts, H., Mauer, D., Apel, K., & Gentry, B. (1988). Phonological and spatial processing abilities in language and reading-impaired children. Journal of Speech and Hearing Disorders, 53, 316-327.

Kamhi, A., Gentry, B., Mauer, D., & Gholson, B. (1990). Analogical learning and transfer in language-impaired children. Journal of Speech and Hearing Disorders, 55, 140-148.

Kamhi, A., Minor, J., & Mauer, D. (1990). Content analysis and intratest performance profiles on the Colombia and the TONI. Journal of Speech and Hearing Research, 33, 375-379.

Kamhi, A., Nelson, L., Lee, R., & Gholson, B. (1985). The ability of language-disordered children to use and modify hypotheses in discrimination learning. Journal of Applied Psycholinguistics, 6, 435-451.

Katz, J. (1983). Phonemic synthesis. In E.Z. Lasky & J. Katz (Eds.), Central auditory processing disorders: Problems of speech, language and learning. 269-295. Baltimore: University Park Press.

Kelly, C. & Dale, P. (1989). Cognitive skills associated with the onset of multiword utterances. Journal of Speech and Hearing Research, 32, 645-656.

Kennedy, M., Sheridan, M., Radlinski, S., & Beeghly, M. (1991). Play-language relationships in young children with developmental delays: Implications for assessment. Journal of Speech and Hearing Research, 34, 112-122.

Kintsch, W. & Van Dijk, T. (1978). Toward a model of text comprehension and production. Psychological Review, 85, 363-394.

Kirchner, D. & Klatzky, R. (1985). Verbal rehearsal and memory in language disordered children. Journal of Speech and Hearing Research, 28, 556-564.

Lahey, M. (1988). Language disorders and language development. New York: Macmillan.

Larson, V. & McKinley, N. (1987). Communication assessment and intervention strategies for adolescents. Eau Claire, WI: Thinking Publications.

Lasky, E.Z. & Cox, L.C. (1983). Auditory processing and language interaction: Evaluation and intervention strategies. In E.Z. Lasky & J. Katz (Eds.), Central auditory processing disorders: Problems of speech, language and learning. 243-268. Baltimore: University Park Press.

Leonard, L. (1987). Is specific language impairment a useful construct? In S. Rosenberg (Ed.), Advances in applied psycholinguistics, Vol. 1. 1-39. New York: Cambridge University Press.

Leonard, L. (1989). Language learnability and specific language impairment in children. Applied Psycholinguistics, 10, 179-202.

Leonard, L. (1991a). A closer look at explanation in the study of specific language impairment: The author's reply to the commentaries. Language, Speech, and Hearing Services in Schools, 22, 88.

Leonard, L. (1991b). Specific language impairment as a clinical category. Language, Speech, and Hearing Services in Schools, 22, 66-68.

Lindamood, C.H. & Lindamood, P.C. (1975). The A.D.D. program: Auditory discrimination in depth. Allen, T.X.: DLM Teaching Resources.

Lowe, M. & Costello, A. (1976). Symbolic Play Test. Windsor, Berkshire: NFER.

Ludlow, C., Cudahy, E., Bassick, C., & Brown, G. (1983). The auditory processing skills of hyperactive, language impaired and reading disabled boys. In J. Katz & E. Lasky (Eds.), Central auditory processing disorders: Problems of speech, language, and learning. Baltimore: University Park.

MacWhinney, B. (1978). The acquisition of morphophonoloy. Monographs of the Society for Research in Child Development, 43, (No. 1).

McCroskey, R. & Thompson, N. (1973). Comprehension of rate controlled speech by children with specific learning disabilities. Journal of Learning Disabilities, 6, 621-628.

Maxwell, S. & Wallach, G. (1984). The language-learning disabilities connection: Symptoms of early language disability change over time. In G. Wallach & K. Butler (Eds.), Language learning disabilities in school-age children. 15-34. Baltimore: Williams & Wilkins.

Montgomery, J., Scudder, R., & Moore, C. (1990). Language-impaired children's real-time comprehension of spoken language. Applied Psycholinguistics, 11, 273-290.

Morehead, D. (1972). Early grammatical and semantic relations: Some implications for a general representational deficit in linguistically deviant children. Papers and Reports in Child Language Development (#4). Committee on Linguistics, Stanford University.

Morehead, D. & Ingram, D. (1973). The development of base syntax in normal and linguistically deviant children. Journal of Speech and Hearing Research, 16, 330-352.

Nelson, L., Kamhi, A., & Apel, A. (1987). Cognitive strengths and weaknesses in language-impaired children: One more look. Journal of Speech and Hearing Disorders, 52, 36-43.

Nippold, M., Erskine, B., & Freed, D. (1988). Proportional and analogical reasoning in normal and language-impaired children. Journal of Speech and Hearing Disorders, 53, 440-449.

Olswang, L. & Bain, B. (1991). Intervention issues for toddlers with specific language impairments. Topics in Language Disorders, 11, 69-86.

Paris, S. & Lindauer, B. (1976). The role of inference in children's comprehension and memory for sentences. Cognitive Psychology, 8, 217-227.

Paul, R., Spangle Looney S., & Dahm P. (1991). Communication and socialization skills at ages 2 and 3 in "late talking" young children. Journal of Speech and Hearing Research, 34, 858-865.

Pinker, S. (1984). Language learnability and language development. Cambridge: Harvard University Press.

Pinker, S. (1989). Learnability and cognition. Cambridge, MA: The MIT Press.

Rees, N. (1981). Saying more than we know: Is auditory processing disorder a meaningful concept? In R. Keith (Ed.), Central auditory and language disorders in children. 94-120. San Diego: College-Hill Press.

Rescorla, L. (1989). The language development survey: A screening tool for delayed language in toddlers. Journal of Speech and Hearing Disorders, 54, 587-599.

Roth F. & Clark, D. (1987). Symbolic play and social participation abilities of language-impaired and normally developing children. Journal of Speech and Hearing Disorders, 52, 17-29.

Roth, F. & Spekman, N. (1989). Higher-order language processes and reading disabilities. In A. Kamhi & H. Catts (Eds.), Reading disabilities: A developmental language perspective. 159-197. Boston: College-Hill Press.

Savich, P. (1984). Anticipatory imagery ability in normal and language-disabled children. Journal of Speech and Hearing Research, 27, 494-501.

Sininger, Y.S., Klatzky, R.L., & Kirchner, D.M. (1989). Memory scanning speed in language disordered children. Journal of Speech and Hearing Research, 32, 289-306.

Sloan, C. (1986). Treating auditory processing difficulties in children. San Diego: College-Hill Press.

Stark, R., Bernstein, L., Condino, R., Bender, M., Tallal, P., & Catts, H. (1984). Four-year follow-up study of language impaired children. Annals of Dyslexia, 34, 49-68.

Tallal, P. (1976). Rapid auditory processing in normal and disordered language development. Journal of Speech and Hearing Research, 19, 561-571.

Tallal, P. (1980a). Auditory temporal perception, phonics and reading disabilities in children. Brain and Language, 9, 182-198.

Tallal, P. (1980b). Language and reading: Some perceptual prerequisites. Bulletin of the Orton Society, 30, 170-178.

Tallal, P. (1988). Developmental language disorders. In J. Kavanagh & T. Truss, Jr. (Eds.), Learning disabilities: Proceedings of the national conference. 181-272. Parkton, MD: York Press.

Tallal, P. (1990). Fine-grained discrimination deficits in language-learning impaired children are specific neither to the auditory modality nor to speech perception. Journal of Speech and Hearing Research, 33, 616-617.

Tallal, P. (1991). Back to the future: Research on developmental disorders of language. In J. Miller (Ed.), Research on child language disorders. 399-407. Austin, TX: Pro-Ed.

Tallal, P. & Piercy, M. (1973a). Defects of non-verbal auditory perception in children with developmental aphasia. Nature, 241, 468-469.

Tallal, P. & Piercy, M. (1973b). Developmental aphasia: Impaired rate of non-verbal processing as a function of sensory modality. Neuropsychologia, 11, 389-398.

Tallal, P. & Piercy, M. (1974). Developmental aphasia: Rate of auditory processing and selective impairment of consonant perception. Neuropsychologia, 12, 83-93.

Tallal, P. & Stark, R. (1981). Speech acoustic-cue discrimination abilities of normally developing and language-impaired children. Journal of the Acoustical Society of America, 69, 568-574.

Tallal P. & Stark, R. (1982). Perceptual/motor profiles of reading impaired children with or without concomitant oral language deficits. Annals of Dyslexia, 32, 163-176.

Tallal, P., Stark R., Kallman, C., & Mellits, D. (1980). Perceptual constancy for phonemic categories: A developmental study with normal and language impaired children. Applied Psycholinguistics, 1, 49-64.

Tallal, P., Stark, R., Kallman, C., & Mellits, D. (1981). A reexamination of some non-verbal perceptual abilities of language-impaired and normal children as a function of age and sensory modality. Journal of Speech and Hearing Research, 24, 351-357.

Tallal, P., Stark, R., & Mellits, D. (1985a). The relationship between auditory temporal analysis and receptive language development: Evidence from studies of developmental language disorder. Neuropsychologia, 23, 314-322.

Tallal, P., Stark, R., & Mellits, D. (1985b). Identification of language-impaired children on the basis of repaid perception and production skills. Brain and Language, 25, 314-322.

Terrell, B. & Schwartz, R. (1983). Object transformation: The linguistic aspect of symbolic play? Proceedings from the Symposium on Research in Child Language Disorders, 4, 127-136.

Terrell, B. & Schwartz, R. (1988). Object transformations in the play of language-impaired children. Journal of Speech and Hearing Disorders, 53, 459-466.

Terrell, B., Schwartz, R., Prelock, P., & Messick, C. (1984). Symbolic play in normal and language-impaired children. Journal of Speech and Hearing Research, 27, 424-429.

Thal, D. & Bates, E. (1988). Language and gesture in late talkers. Journal of Speech and Hearing Research, 31, 115-123.

Thal, D., Tobias, S., & Morrison, D. (1991). Language and gesture in late talkers: A 1-year follow-up. Journal of Speech and Hearing Research, 34, 604-612.

Tomblin, B. (1991). Examining the cause of specific language impairment. Language, Speech, and Hearing Services in Schools, 22, 69-74.

Tomblin, J.B. & Quinn, M.A. (1983). The contribution of perceptual learning to performance on the repetition task. Journal of Speech and Hearing Research, 26, 369-372.

Udwin, O. & Yule, W. (1983). Imaginative play in language disordered children. British Journal of Disorders of Communication, 18, 197-205.

Wallach, G. & Miller, L. (1988). Language intervention and academic success. Boston: College-Hill Press.

Wyke, M. & Asso, D., (1979). Perception and memory for spatial relations in children with developmental dysphasia. Neuropsychologia, 17, 231-239.

Commentary on Ellis Weismer: How specific is specific language impairment? Some comments by a relative outsider

Werner Deutsch

When more than 30 years ago language acquisition's deep, long sleep suddenly ended, one question became the focus of interest. How is it possible that young children learn their native language so fast and effortlessly? In those days, one answer convinced almost everybody. The human species possesses a genetically determined mechanism that triggers language acquisition, even if the external circumstances were untoward. This assumed mechanism had a built-in program, compatible with all natural languages children may encounter as input. Who was responsible for this conception of language acquisition? It was the prince who kissed awake the sleeping beauty. His name is still on everybody's tongue: Noam Chomsky. His radical critique of behavioristic learning theories and their (non-)applicability to the domain of language has had enduring consequences (Chomsky 1959). Who doubts that language acquisition is based on a biologically given potential? Who would nowadays dare to describe and explain language acquisition exclusively by the repertoire of classical and instrumental conditioning?

The last 30 years have seen serious changes in language acquisition research, too. Susan Ellis Weismer's contribution to this volume is indicative of three of these changes.

1. The formula of incredibly rapid and almost effortless language acquisition became discredited (Klein 1990). Not only do problems and difficulties arise when adolescents or adults try to learn one or more additional languages. Also first language acquisition is a wearisome, laborious enterprise. Some facts! Elementary grammatical structures - as for example syntax and morphology of complex noun phrases - take five or six years until they are mastered by children. The correct - adultlike - use and interpretation of personal pronouns like "he" and "she" is even more protracted, if they serve as reference-maintaining devices across sentences. This is a problem that may cause difficulties even for 10 year old children. Moreover, structures that

are considered as part of a predetermined universal grammar are not at all learned in an error-free manner (cf. Deutsch/Koster/Koster 1986).

What has been mentioned so far are characteristic facts of normal language acquisition. How much more difficult should this process be in children who suffer from developmental deficits! There are good reasons to study those children's language acquisition in some detail, because it opens a window to mechanisms that trigger, stop or prevent children's move from one level of linguistic functioning to the next. However, the study of language dysfunctioning can have an important practical impact too. Is the dysfunctioning only temporary? Does it automatically disappear, even if no intervention from outside takes place? Or is a specific treatment needed to cure the dysfunction?

Ellis Weismer presents a survey of studies involving a group of children who attracted a lot of attention during the last 15 years. To find an appropriate label for this group is a problem itself. In the past, these children were categorized as "developmental agrammatics" or "developmental dysphasics". Many contemporary scholars avoid either of the two expressions and instead prefer the term "Specific Language Impairment" (SLI). Unfortunately, Ellis Weismer does not discuss the terminological issue, but this volume also contains a paper by Hannelore Grimm that completely fills the gap. What is the meaning of SLI? Without going into details, it can be said that SLI applies to children who suffer from specific linguistic deficits - especially, but not exclusively in the domain of syntax and morphology. These deficits seldom appear in normally developing children. SLI children do have (nonverbal) mental abilities that are neither better nor worse than those of their age mates. The present SLI research shows some standard procedures of which Ellis Weismer's survey provides an excellent overview. Taking the risk of reducing and simplifying matters, SLI research proceeds as follows:

1. Take a sample of SLI children.
2. Find a control group of the same chronological, mental, or language age.
3. Administer the same experimental tasks or psychological tests to both groups.
4. Examine whether group differences yield statistical significance.

Ellis Weismer's survey is confined to two domains. She reports on a large number of studies contrasting the performances of SLI children and control groups in perceptual and cognitive tasks. Let us first consider some methodological issues before refering to the findings. Ellis Weismer takes for granted that her readers are familiar with the criteria according to which children are classified as suffering from SLI. The naive reader, however, may ask how SLI-groups are selected. Are they special research samples or do they consist of children who are currently seen by speech therapists? What about the relative proportion of boys and girls in those samples? In general, male persons are more vulnerable to speech- or language disorders compared to females. Does this well-documented fact also hold true for SLI and is it taken into account when subjects for SLI-studies are selected? In one respect, all reported studies are homogeneous. They consist of subjects speaking English as their first (and only?) language. This restriction has advantages since it increases the comparability of the reported studies. But it raises new questions, too. Is it possible to set up criteria for SLI that are valid across languages? Or are SLI criteria dependent on the specific characteristics of the different languages? If the core of SLI consists of morphological and syntactic deficits, one may wonder how structural differences among languages - for example morphologically rich vs. poor languages - could have an impact upon incidental rates for SLI.

In a second respect also, the studies mentioned are homogenous. Ellis Weismer reports on group differences only, although at the very end of her paper she makes a plea for "consideration of individual subject data as well as group findings". Studies with individual subject data are completely missing from her survey, if I have read it correctly. How can this obvious asymmetry be explained? Many researchers attach much more value to group studies than to single (or multiple) case studies. Recently, Danziger (1990) showed that this attitude has a long tradition in psychology. In the beginnings of (experimental) psychology, single subject studies were quite common and published in the leading journals. Later this sort of study was often looked upon as providing idiosyncratic or anecdotal evidence only. Nowadays group studies are associated with the term "nomothetic", whereas case studies fall under the category "idiographic". Lamiell (1992) demonstrated that such classification is not in accordance with the original meaning of "nomothetic" and "idiographic", as suggested by the philosopher Windelband (1894/1904). Aggregate data such as "group findings" do not automatically fit the category "nomothetic", because this notion implies that statements are valid for *all individuals* and not for an *average individual.* SLI-research could certainly benefit from more single-case studies. These studies, however, cannot replace group studies and vice versa. Bridging between the two data sources is a difficult but not impossible task, as Clara and William Stern (1907) clearly showed at the beginning of this century for normal language acquisition (cf. also Deutsch in press).

2. Thirty years ago the ideal speaker/hearer was a fixstar in the sky of psycholinguistics. In the meantime, hardly anybody talks of this star anymore. It has been replaced by the average (normal or impaired, adult or developing) speaker/hearer. Ellis Weismer's survey is indicative of this change, too. The shift is connected to another one. While former psycholinguistic studies were mostly concerned with linguistic competence, many contemporary studies focus on linguistic performance. The question is then, how linguistic knowledge is put to use under varying perceptual, cognitive and motivational conditions. SLI is considered as a problem of linguistic performance.

The term SLI - specific language impairment - is already symptomatic. It leaves open what the nature of the language deficit is, since no specific reference is made to phonological, morphological, syntactic, semantic and pragmatic components of linguistic knowledge. The term "impairment" is relatively vague too. It implies that something does not function as it should or perhaps could. And "specific" means that linguistic performance is not completely disturbed, but only certain aspects of it. Ellis Weismer's topic - perceptual and cognitive deficits in SLI children - would have sounded a bit strange 30 years ago, when the pure linguistic knowledge received so much attention, whereas perceptual and cognitive conditions influencing language use and language learning were considered as 2nd order issues. The shift from competence to performance - the plural 'performances' would be a more appropriate phrasing - made it possible for the relationship between perception, cognition and language use to become a serious research topic.

The present survey convincingly shows that indeed perceptual and cognitive deficits exist in SLI children. These children - on the average - have difficulties in processing sequential information. Control groups - on the average - yield better results in constructing analogies and building inferences than SLI children. No doubt, there is a long list of contrasting group differences. This list will certainly become even longer in the near and more distant future. Is there any study in which the group difference went into the unexpected direction? According to Ellis Weismer's survey, there seems to be no exception to the rule that SLI children never show better average performances than children from control groups. Ellis Weismer does a good job in her discussions of the patterns of unidirectional and zero differences in SLI and control children. It is a masterpiece of diplomacy, because she does not try to construct a single framework for interpretation but instead favors weighing conflicting results. Special emphasis is given to the "Auditory Processing Deficit"-Hypothesis, put forward by Paula Tallal and her coworkers. Although this hypothesis may not serve as the only explanation for the origin of SLI, it certainly deserves special attention. Tallal's hypothesis has been a constant and provocative stimulant for the entire field of SLI research.

3. Contemporary language acquisition research has two sides - a theoretical and a practical one. Without a comprehensive knowledge of normal acquisition processes it is impossible to recognize and classify disorders and deficits. Also, the treatment of developmental dysfunctions requires an orientation toward normal acquisition in order to be effective and realistic. The fully developed adult native speaker certainly does not provide a good point of departure for psychological interventions. Developing children provide the appropriate standards for diagnostic procedures and clinical interventions.

Ellis Weismer pays a lot of attention to the practical side of SLI in the last third of her survey. She makes clear that research and application are far from being closely interconnected. The gap is difficult to bridge. One reason has been mentioned before. While SLI research mainly focusses on contrasting groups, clinical work is usually centered around single cases. Generalisations in either direction - cases to groups and from groups to cases - are problematic. However, the situation is not yet hopeless, as Ellis Weismer points out for the area of diagnosis as well as for intervention. Diagnostic procedures could be improved, if the SLI-assessment included the consideration of perceptual and cognitive deficits. Ellis Weismer argues against the idea to base SLI-classification primarily on non-linguistic criteria. On the contrary, the joint consideration of linguistic, perceptual and cognitive deficits may help to identify children at risk, before they run into serious problems, especially in the area of learning to read and write. As far as intervention is concerned, the implications of perceptual and cognitive deficits in SLI children are unclear. But Ellis Weismer shows a way to improve the situation. She reports on a study by herself and colleagues which examined differential learning effects in SLI and control children. When learning new lexical items SLI-children benefit from facilitating input conditions, as for example reduced speed and exaggerated accentuation patterns. For normal children, however, similar improvements were not obtained. It would be interesting to extend these studies to other areas of learning, especially to the morpho-syntactic domain.

Finally, I would like to close my comments with a short metacomment, revealing my own bias. In the SLI-research that Ellis Weismer includes in her survey the language development of normal children is only used for contrastive purposes. For comparisons, observational data play a minor role and longitudinal studies are not as common as in language acquisition studies with normal children. In this research area, which is at the center of my own work, attempts are made to capture the processes of change from prelinguistic stages up to relatively stable target stages. The focus is on intraindividual changes, although there is much evidence pointing to variations between subjects in their respective intraindividual changes. Sometimes the boundaries between normal and subnormal developments blur. SLI-research - as presented by Ellis Weismer - follows a different path. It states deficits and seeks for possible explanations of how they came about and why they persist. This research overlooks how children individually experience their deficits. The lack is not at all surprising. In search for significant group differences, the individual subjects dissolve into group means. Nonetheless, Ellis Weismer's well-documented survey provides enough food for thought - even for a relative outsider.

References

Chomsky, N. (1959). Review of B.F. Skinner "Verbal Behavior". Language, 35, 26-58.

Danziger, K. (1990). Constructing the subject: Historical origins of psychological research. New York: Cambridge University Press.

Deutsch, W. (in press). Auf vier Wegen zu William Stern. In K. Pawlik & M. Amelang (Hrsg.), Enzyklopädie der Psychologie, Band 1 (Grundlagen und Methoden). Göttingen: Hogrefe.

Deutsch, W., Koster, C., & Koster, J. (1986). What can we learn from children's errors in understanding anaphora? Linguistics, 24, 203-225.

Klein, W. (1990). A theory of language acquisition is not so easy. Studies in Second Language Aquisition, 12, 219-231.

Lamiell, J.T. (1992). What did Windelband mean by nomothetic? Paper presented at the 100th Annual Convention of the American Psychological Association, Washington, D.C., August 1992.

Stern, C. & Stern, W. (1907). Die Kindersprache. Leipzig: Barth.

Windelband, W. (1894/1904). Geschichte und Naturwissenschaft. Strassburg: Heitz.

Social consequences of specific language impairment

Mabel L. Rice

Investigations of children with specific language impairment have focused on possible capacity limitations of these children, and rightfully so. As we study their linguistic systems, their phonology, morphology, lexical inventories, syntactic abilities, and their reading abilities, we enhance our understanding of the fundamental properties of their intellectual functioning and the particular linguistic problems they manifest. In so doing we increase our knowledge of human cognitive systems and possible dissociations, and enhance our ability to design effective intervention procedures.

In this chapter, I will shift the emphasis somewhat, away from the possible inherent limitations of SLI children into consideration of the social/cultural impact of their impaired ability to communicate, and the implications of those consequences for our interpretive models. I will report on a set of findings that were inspired by observations we made in a clinical setting. These findings led to a reconsideration of our assumptions about the relationship between children's language skills and social interactions, and the formulation of a Social Consequences Account of language impairment. In this paper, I will lay out this model, the evidence that led to its formulation, predictions generated by the account, and some implications for diagnosis and intervention.

Social Consequences Account

Let us begin with a preview of the Social Consequences Account. The basic notion is that youngsters with communication limitations are vulnerable to a negative social spiral, starting in the preschool years. This spiral would play out like this: To begin with, some children lack flexibility with language, or intelligibility with speech, that is essential for entry into and maintenance of social discourse with their peers. Because they lack the expected, conventionalized, and socially adjusted uses of language, they are more likely to be ignored, rebuffed, or excluded from peer interactions. Furthermore, they recognize this problem, although probably not on a conscious level, and develop compensatory strategies, such as a greater reliance on adults if adults are available and receptive to their overtures, or a shortening of responses if their speech is unintelligible. These compensatory adjustments, in turn, lead to the probability that these children will be regarded as socially immature, cognitively limited, and from a limited home environment. These biases, then, can constrain the academic options of SLI children.

Background

SLI children have limited discourse skills. Language-impaired children have been described as poor communicators, relative to their normal peers (e.g., Fey 1986). On a number of pragmatic measures, such as clarification responses and the use of cohesive discourse devices, language-impaired children perform below their age peers, on a level more like younger language-matched peers (Lahey 1988). These children are often seen as being less responsive and less able to maintain a conversation with their peers. To the extent that their discourse skills are limited, children with language impairment would be at-risk for social interactions with their peers.

The role of language in social interactions. Children's social status is affected by their communication abilities. By the time of elementary school, children's conversational competencies are associated with their social status. Low-status children are less likely to initiate conversations with their peers (Garnica 1981) and are less sought after as conversational partners (Cooper/Marquis/Ayers-Lopez 1982).

The relationship between peer status and communication ability is formed during the preschool years. Hazen/Black (1989) tie peer status to initiations and responses. They document that liked children were more inclined to clearly direct their initiations to specific listeners, to speak to more than one interaction partner, to respond contingently to others, and to acknowledge others. In a follow-up study, Black/Hazen (1990) explored the interactions of acquainted and unacquainted preschoolers. They report that when entering the play of children they did not know, disliked children were less responsive to peers and more likely to make irrelevant comments than were liked children. With acquainted peers, disliked children were not only less responsive and produced more irrelevant statements than liked children, they were also less likely to clearly direct their communication to specific peers. The authors concluded that responsiveness and contribution to coherent conversation is important to both the establishment and maintenance of social status, whereas failure to socially direct communications may be more related to the maintenance of social status.

To the extent that social acceptance is facilitated by conversational skills, preschool children with limited communication ability would be at-risk. If they are unable to initiate conversational turns, or to respond appropriately to initiations by their peers, they would be less likely to move into the mainstream groupings of their playmates.

Language use as a cultural phenomenon. Theorists who regard the child as a member of a cultural group have long recognized the role of language in children's socialization. Foremost among them is Vygotsky (1978), who viewed language as a conventionalized, socially determined interactive system. Within his model, the association of language and culture is very intimate, wherein cultural knowledge determines the course of language development and, conversely, communicative interactions enculturate a child. Hymes (1972) has bridged the disciplines of anthropology and linguistics with his definition of the full range of linguistic competencies as that of "communicative competence." This concept emphasizes the wide scope of underlying knowledge needed for mastery of linguistic rules and how to use those rules in social contexts. Hymes called for ethnographic studies of culturally-situated language use, which has inspired a number of cross-cultural studies of children's language acquisition.

Observations of children learning language in diverse settings reveal that children become sensitive to cultural conventions revealed in language, including such basics as relative status (e.g., whom one can talk to and how to do so), how to resolve disputes, gender roles, expressions of affection, indications of respect, and even attitudes about children's ability to learn to talk (cf. Ervin-Tripp/Gordon 1986; Heath 1989; Saville-Troike 1982; Schieffelin/Ochs 1986). Language acts as a signal for cultural distinctions that children "pick up." In turn, language users reveal their social position by virtue of their choice of linguistic forms and interactive styles. For example, preschool children are sensitive to registers indicative of relative status. They know that doctors can be bossy to nurses, delivering many directives, but nurses must be more polite in their requests of doctors (Anderson 1977).

In short, children absorb social and cultural distinctions as they are learning to use language appropriately. They are sensitive to differences in how other children communicate, as well as to the style of interactions appropriate for different settings. Intrinsic to this enculturation is awareness of culturally defined ways of grouping people. Children form clusters of liked and less-liked peers, and they recognize individual differences in behavior and demeanor. Their verbal interactions are played out in the web of these culturally-absorbed expectations about the behavior of others.

Evidence for the Social Consequences Account

Language Acquisition Preschool. The setting in which data were collected is the Language Acquisition Preschool (LAP) at the University of Kansas. LAP was designed to teach language in a naturalistic, mainstreamed setting. Mainstreaming refers to a least-restrictive environment, in which handicapped children receive intervention with their normally developing peers. Such integrated settings have been developed in response to conclusions drawn from the normative literature, suggesting that children use language as a way to express their ideas and social needs, in a naturalistic setting. Another impetus has been the passage of U.S. Public Law 99-457, which mandates such mainstreamed settings for preschool intervention programs.

Three groups of children, approximately equal in number, are enrolled: normally developing children, children learning English as a second language (ESL), and children with specific language impairment (SLI). The children are all between 3 and 5 years of age.

The SLI children meet several criteria, which can be summarized as speech and/or language skills significantly below the expectations for their chronological age, combined with normal or above performance on a nonverbal test of intelligence, normal social functioning, and no evidence of perceptual or neurological problems. These children are ones with a "hidden handicap." To a casual observer of the group, they cannot be identified on the basis of how they look or how they behave. They come from all socioeconomic groups. With these youngsters, therefore, we have an opportunity to investigate the effects of speech and/or language impairment on social interactions, without the complications introduced by clinically significant social or intellectual or sensory deficits, racial differences, or major socioeconomic differentiation.

The ESL children meet the following criteria: recent arrivals to the U.S., who demonstrate normal language development in their native language, who are just introduced to English, and who are as close to 3 years of age as possible. Most of these children are in the families of middle-class graduate students or faculty at the University. Therefore, the ESL children are less proficient than the SLI children at the outset, although they often catch up with and sometimes exceed the SLI children. They also differ from the SLI children in that they have a history of successful communication development.

Several features of LAP are relevant for the following discussion. The curriculum is a modification of the High Scope cognitive/social approach (Hohmann/Bonet/Weikart 1978). Throughout the daily activities there is encouragement of child-directed learning, with many opportunities for children to interact verbally with each other and the teachers. Language development is emphasized throughout the curriculum; there is no special "language time", nor is individual therapy provided for the SLI or ESL children (although each SLI child has an Individual Education Plan, with explicit remediation goals); all special instruction is tailored to a child's moment-to-moment interests in the context of the classroom activities.

One activity of each day is play-center time, which is a 40-min period when children can choose their own activity, among four options: art activities, books and puzzles, blocks and toy vehicles, or dramatic play. The theme for dramatic play changes from day to day. Some of the children's favorites are: visit to a fast food restaurant; visit to the veterinarian (when they take their stuffed animals for a check-up); bathe the babies (dollies); and outdoor camping. During the play-center time children can wander from activity to activity, talk to whomever they choose, or play quietly by themselves. It is during this time that individual therapy activities are negotiated with the SLI children, and any other children who chose to participate in the interactions.

Summative evaluation over 3 years documents the effectiveness of the curriculum (Bunce/Rice/Wilcox 1990). A sample of 14 SLI children who were enrolled in the program during that time, for an average of 3 semesters, demonstrated significant gains in vocabulary, receptive and expressive language, and in articulation. Their mean scores on standardized tests increased from an initial level of one or more standard deviations below the normative mean, to performance within the normal range. In comparison, the normal models' scores improved somewhat, but not at a level of statistical significance. Thus, the rate of improvement was actually higher for the SLI children than for the normal controls. Improvement was also evident in the SLI children's mean length of utterance, which increased from an entry level average within Brown's (1973) Stage 2 (2.25) to an exit level of late Stage 5 (> 4.0). These improvements are thought to be related to the children's therapy goals, 88% of which were achieved or showing improvement.

Overall, the general descriptors of LAP are that it provides a least-restrictive environment for intervention with 3- to 5-year-old SLI children, in a mainstreamed, naturalistic, child-centered setting. A special feature is that SLI children are not singled out for individual language therapy, but instead are interacted with in targeted ways in the midst of the general classroom activities.

Peer interactions. In this naturalistic mix of young children with varying levels of communicative competence, it soon became apparent that there were interesting things happening in the patterns of social interactions. We devised a means of measuring social interactions, with an on-line data recording system, the Social Interactive Coding System (SICS), that did not require videotaping and the consequent time-consuming transcript analysis procedures. We were interested in obtaining clinically relevant information in a timely fashion. The targeted interactive skill was that of initiations and responses, cross-coded according to the person the children were interacting with. Initiation is defined as a verbal attempt to begin an interaction with another person. Responses can be verbal or nonverbal. In effect, the coding captures who is talking to whom, and who initiated the interaction (Rice/Sell/Hadley 1990).

Initiations and responses are conversational moves that are sensitive to the interface of verbal and social abilities (cf. Black/Hazen 1990; Fey 1986; Hazen/Black 1989). In order to initiate successfully, a child must have a good sense of when to approach another child, be able to negotiate joint attention, and find an appropriate way to talk about something. Successful initiations are associated with social success, whereas a disproportionately high number of responses are associated with a passive social role.

Children's social interactions were observed during play-center time, when the children have relatively free choice of activities and interactants. The results of two studies (Hadley/Rice 1991; Rice/Sell/Hadley 1991) revealed that the social interactions of the LAP children were significantly influenced by the children's facility with communication. Insofar as the findings are presented in detail elswhere (Hadley/Rice 1991; Rice et al. 1991) only the key findings relevant to this discussion will be summarized here. It is important to note that extensive observational samples were collected from multiple SLI children in the naturalistic LAP setting. In Rice et al. (1991), 26 preschoolers, aged 3-5, were observed, 9 of whom were SLI. A total of 60 minutes of observational time per child was collected. In Hadley/Rice (1991), 18 preschoolers, aged 3-5, served as subjects, 8 of whom were SLI, with a total sample time of 24 minutes per child. To the best of our knowledge, these samples are unique in the literature in three respects: (a) naturalistic peer interaction settings, (b) relatively large samples of behavior, and (c) separate samples of SLI children.

The key findings include the following conclusions. Normal children were the preferred partner for all children's social interactions, suggesting that the children were sensitive to their relative communicative competence at an early age. Conversely, children with limited communication skills were ignored more often by their peers (28% of their initiations, compared to 15% for normal children's initiations) and were in turn less responsive to initiations directed to them (they ignored 30% of the initiations to them, as compared to only 7% for the comparison group). Children with speech articulation problems and limited intelligibility shortened their responses (40 to 60% one-word or nonverbal responses for the communicatively limited children compared to 34% for the controls).

On the other hand, the children with communication limitations were more likely to initiate interactions with adults (62% compared to 49% for the normal children) and less likely to initiate interactions with their normally developing peers (38% compared to 51%).

The general impression is that as young as 3 years of age children are sensitive to relative differences in verbal facility, and begin to make adjustments in their social interactions. Children with less skill have difficulty negotiating the interpersonal communicative space. Thus, they develop compensatory strategies, such as reliance on adults for mediation of social interactions and to meet their needs.

These generalizations seem to apply to second-language-learning preschoolers as well as SLI children (cf. Rice et al. 1991; Tabors 1987). The similarities between ESL and SLI children are interesting, in that they bear on a possible counter-interpretation which would propose that the SLI children have subtle social deficits to begin with, and that such deficits contribute to the socioverbal adjustments. As far as we can determine, the ESl children in these studies (who come from all over the world) do not demonstrate in their interactions with native speakers the social adjustment evident in their second language settings. In general, the socioverbal adjustments of ESL children are attributed to limited ommunication skill, not subtle problems in social development. The Social Consequences Account suggests that a similar perspective may be helpful for understanding SLI children.

Adult judgements. How do children arrive at such intuitions about social competencies? Is this a developmental phase, or part of a broader cultural bias that children are capable of incorporating into their perspectives about each other?

The possibility of a general social bias was raised by new evidence about the school promotion policies of kindergarten teachers in the U.S. Catts (1990) is conducting a longitudinal study in which preschool and kindergarten SLI children are being followed into the elementary grades. He reports that 33% of kindergarten children suspected of speech and language problems (i.e., those children referred for evaluation) repeated kindergarten or were placed in developmental first-grade programs. (In the U.S., developmental first grades are an "in-between" transitional year, to provide further preparation for entry to the regular first-grade curriculum; cf. Walsh 1989.) Of the 35 children with *significant* language impairments, 17 or 49% did not advance to regular first-grade classrooms. Discussions with the teachers indicate that many of these placement decisions were based on perceived social immaturity.

We hypothesized that these placements were influenced by social judgements based on the child's use of verbal interactive skills in the classroom (Rice/Alexander/Hadley 1991). The reasoning is like this. Teachers associate high verbal success with bright, popular children, in much the same way that people make assumptions about dialect speakers; those who speak a standard dialect are perceived as being brighter, more socially responsible, and so on, than are speakers of nonstandard dialects (Grosjean 1982; Lambert/Hodgson/Gardner/Fillenbaum 1960).

To test this hypothesis, 1½-min audiotape samples of preschool children's speech were played for adult judges, who were asked to judge the children's intelligence, social maturity, likelihood of success in kindergarten, leadership status, and popularity, as well as the parents' educational levels and social status. The children were drawn from three groups, with one boy and one girl from each group. One group was children with speech problems only, a second was children with language problems as well as speech unintelligibility, and the third was children with age-appropriate speech and language skills. The judges were not informed of the child's communicative status, and the samples were presented in a mixed order. Four groups of adult judges rated the children: 27 kindergarten teachers, 25 women with college educations of the same age as the teachers, 175 undergraduate college students, and 56 practicing speech/language pathologists, for a total of 283 subjects.

The findings reveal strong support for the hypothesis. SLI children were perceived to be less intelligent and less likely to succeed in kindergarten than their normally developing peers. Furthermore, this tendency to lower a child's perceived aptitude was directly related to the extent of apparent communication limitation: the lowest ranked children were those with speech and language problems (see Figure 1). The negative bias was also evident in judgements of the children's parents. The raters judged the parents of SLI children to have less education and lower socioeconomic status than the normally developing children. The same relative orderings applied for these judgements as for the child attributes: Speech and language impairments < speech impairments < normal competency (see Figure 2).

These biases were evident across the four different groups of raters. It is not the case that kindergarten teachers constitute an especially judgmental group. Instead, the association of verbal competence with intelligence, probable success in school, parental education and socioeconomic success is more pervasive. Thus, this association is accessed by teachers, college students, educated housewives, and even speech/language clinicians in their immediate impressions of young children.

It is as if adults, in making these judgements of children's speech, call upon assumptions about the nature of specific language impairment, in which discernible speech/language problems are attributable to more general child deficits (e.g., limited intelligence, delayed social maturity) and/or a lack of adequate resources in the home (e.g., limited parental education or socioeconomic resources). There are several problems with such assumptions. One is that they seriously underestimate the complexity of factors contributing to SLI, including the possibility of impaired language-specific acquisition mechanisms (which would operate somewhat independently of other areas of children's intellectual development, or parental socioeducational status). A second problem is that this model could contribute to serious misinterpretations of a particular child's academic aptitude, a possibility discussed below.

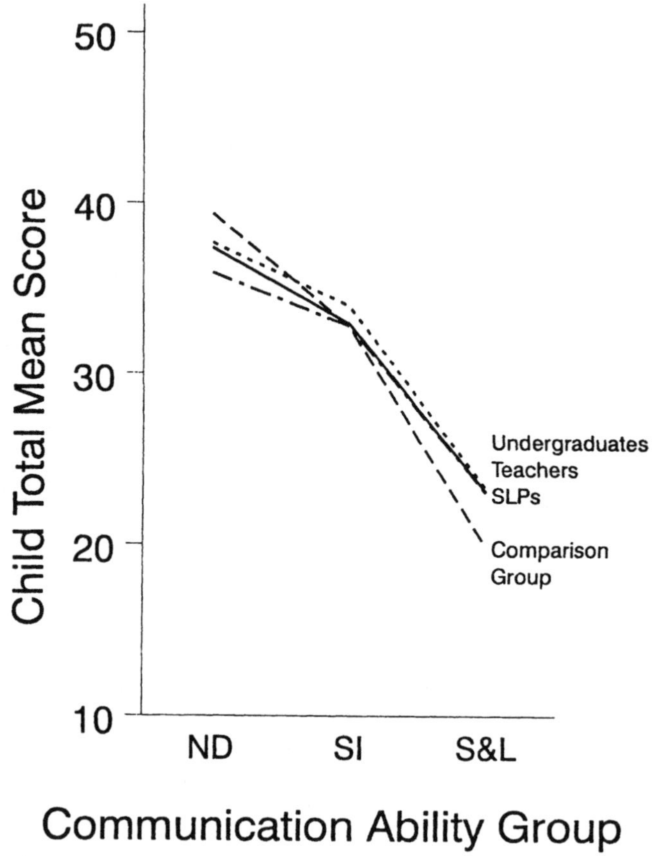

Fig. 1: Child total score by rater groups

As with other biases, its pervasiveness may lie in a strong but incomplete correlation. There is a high correlation of verbal ability and intelligence in the general population (Wechsler 1949). And this association would in turn predict school achievement. The problem, of course, is that this relationship, abstracted across the general population, cannot be presumed of individuals who have specific problems with speech and language. Just as such biases are unrealistic in the case of individuals with nonstandard dialects, they are not realistic for preschoolers with limited communication skill.

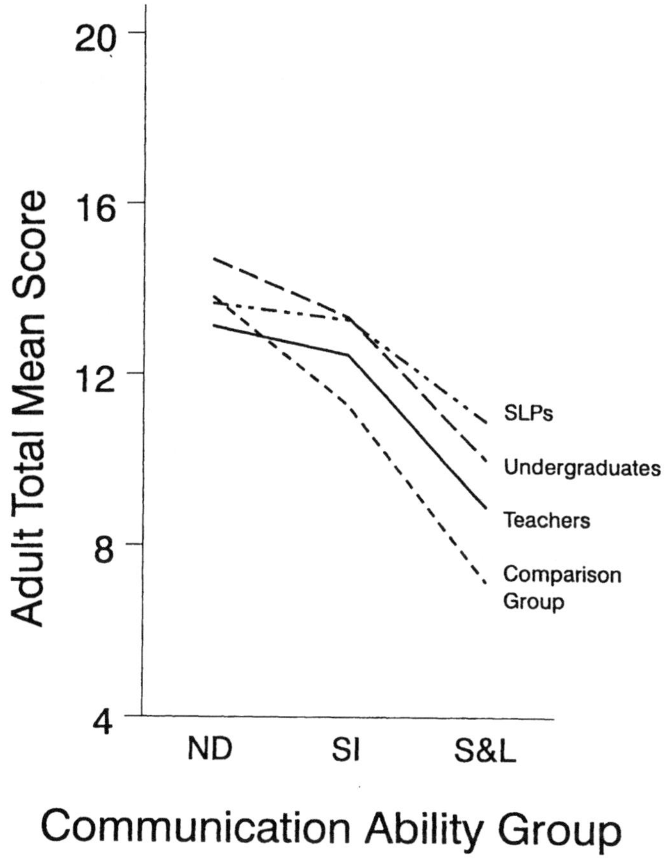

Fig. 2: Adult total score by rater groups

The Social Consequences Account of limited language skill: Reprise, predictions, and caveats

Reprise. Socialization experiences can activate young children's language acquisition. At the same time, early on, language becomes a tool of socialization, and a means of enculturation. Children with limited language seem to be vulnerable from both perspectives. To begin with, they, by definition, are less able to parlay their early social experiences into linguistic skills, or at least they are much slower at doing so. As a consequence of less-than-expected language skills, they are in turn at-risk for participation in the social interactions that serve to drive further language development and social status. They become the victims of an assumed association of verbal skills and social sensitivity, cognitive ability, and social status. Even preschool children are evidently able to make some social assumptions based on verbal skill, and, apparently, adults, including teachers and speech/language pathologists, do so as well.

Predictions. This Social Consequences Account predicts that part of the risk for school achievement of SLI children could be attributable to a combination of low teacher expectations, and a form of learned socio-verbal helplessness on the part of the child. It is well established that language-impaired children (but less so the speech-impaired children) are at-risk for academic achievement and social acceptance (cf. Weiner 1985). In particular, a finding replicated across a number of studies is that SLI children encounter problems with reading (Catts 1989, 1990). And, as described earlier, children with speech and language impairments are more likely to be retained in kindergarten or placed in developmental first grades, a practice that has dubious educational outcomes and a negative effect on children's self-esteem (Peterson/DeGracie/Ayabe 1987).

If an SLI child is initially perceived as socially immature, or less cognitively capable, than his or her peers, those judgements could play out in ways that limit educational opportunities, as well as impair the development of a healthy self-esteem. Based on a sample of U.S. teachers, Walsh (1989) reports that the decision not to promote a child to regular first grade can depend upon the child's perceived social maturity. The most common explanation of teachers for why children were not promoted was as follows: Children who are academically advanced, but socially immature, are promoted to transitional first grade, whereas children who are academically slow are retained in kindergarten. Suspected difficulties with cognitive abilities can be quickly ruled out by appropriate evaluation with nonverbal intelligence measures. The determination of social maturity, however, seems to rest heavily with the judgement of the classroom teacher.

Thus, to the extent that "social immaturity" is inferred from children's conversational interactions, the SLI child could be grievously misrepresented. There are two ways in which their behavior could be misinterpreted. One is if their interactive skills are limited, such that they are less initiative in the classroom, or less successful in their interactions with other children or teachers. Another is if they develop inappropriate compensatory behaviors for coping with their interactive limitations, such as calling out or hitting other children. In either case, a teacher may misinterpret the secondary limitations associated with a communication problem, and its accompanying history of limited success in social interactions, as indicative of a child's social acumen. The irony is that such a pattern of social adjustment would be expected if a child was fully aware of his or her conversational limitations (i.e., if a child was socially astute) as is the case with ESL children. So the SLI child who withdraws or lingers on the edge of peer interactions because of an awareness of limited verbal interactive skills would be at-risk for designation as socially immature and hence in need of accommodations in the academic curriculum, even though many of these children test in the normal range on nonverbal achievement tests. It may turn out that from the very outset the academic achievement of SLI children is jeopardized by a social corollary of their language limitations.

Caveats. Much more information about the details of a Social Consequences Account is needed before its full value can be ascertained. Of primary importance is identification of the ways that the children's particular sociolinguistic deficits impair their ability to initiate turns and maintain conversations. How do these children's limitations play out in the interpersonal exchanges? Where are the deviations from the expected competencies of young children? Of equal and related significance is the need to identify the features that account for the judgements of social and cognitive maturity. Is it something particular to verbal competence, or something in the nonverbal domain, such as latency of response, eye gaze, or some breakdown in the intricate coordination of these two dimensions? Finally, more information is needed to determine the nature of the disparity between these children's verbal competencies and those expected in classrooms. What rules for talking apply in educational settings? Are the interactive expectations in institutional settings significantly different from those of the children's homes? Answers to these questions will inform accounts of children's emerging communicative competencies, their social development, cultural biases toward individuals with communicative differences, educational policy, and intervention for children with communication problems.

Implications for diagnosis and intervention

Among the implications for diagnosis are the following:

1. If adjustments in social interactions are a possible consequence of lan-

guage impairment, children with limited language skills are vulnerable to misdiagnosis as socially immature children, or as children with some form of aberration in social development. Thus, it is essential that these two domains of development be differentiated as much as possible at the time of diagnosis.

2. A comprehensive evaluation, then, should give careful attention to language capabilities, with documentation of a child's linguistic competencies in the areas of syntax, lexical development, phonology, and, as well, pragmatic abilities. Furthermore, observation of children's peer interactions should be included, in order to determine how well the children apply their linguistic skills to ongoing discourse demands. In particular, the pattern of initiations and responses to peers is a promising area of examination, insofar as, in classroom settings, it has demonstrated a differentiation between young children with good communication skills and children with limited competencies.

3. Children regarded as socially immature should receive a careful evaluation for possible speech and language limitations, insofar as the impressions of social deficits could mask an underlying difficulty with communicative competencies.

4. Counselling with caretakers and teachers may be necessary, to clarify the ways in which limited communication ability could influence a youngster's verbo-social interactions. If the adults who care for and teach a youngster can come to appreciate the close relationship between verbal skills and social interactions, they can bring greater compassion and understanding to the child's problems, and be in a better position to encourage peer interactions, and enhance the probable success of a youngster.

As for intervention, the following implications come to mind:

1. It may be necessary to target the development of social interactive skills, such as the ability to initiate conversations with one's peers, as an explicit goal of intervention.

2. The technology for enhancing children's spontaneous interactions, their use of socially appropriate linguistic forms in order to meet their social needs, is relatively undeveloped. Nevertheless, some general observations can be attempted. One is that the setting in which intervention occurs must be as naturalistic as possible. It is very difficult, if not impossible, to contrive interactions between an adult and a child that simulate the kinds of spontaneous interactions that occur between children. Yet the adult (teacher) must somehow set the occasions for interactions that are likely to be successful, and guide a child toward participation. Several levels of child participation are involved. First is the willingness to participate in spon-

taneous interactions with peers. This may have to be cultivated, in the context of the individual setting. Second, is a willingness to initiate conversations, to try to use language in a way that enhances social standing. Without such attempts, children cannot get the necessary experience with social interactions, nor the encouragement provided by occasions of success. Third is the development of some level of metalinguistic skill (although this need not be literally at a fully conscious level), to allow for the development of a child's ability to monitor his or her effectiveness in an interaction, and to make appropriate verbal corrections.

The particulars of the technology for accomplishing these goals are going to depend upon the social and cultural conventions that apply to the group settings, and the roles of the interventionist, the classroom teacher or other adult caretakers, and the children. In our own classroom setting, we are exploring a technique that offers some promise. I offer it here as an example of how social interactions can be "engineered" by adults. Our technique is put into operation when a child initiates a comment or request toward a teacher, a fairly common occurrence in the LAP classroom, as well as in other preschool settings. When the child tells the teacher to "See this!", for example, the teacher redirects that initiation toward another child, as in "Oh, why don't you show your picture to Johnny?," or, more explicitly, "Tell Johnny you drew a nice bird." This simple technique blends easily into the give-and-take of classroom interactions, so does not call attention to some form of explicit "therapy" for a particular child. Yet our findings reveal that teacher redirects of child initiations can lead to a higher proportion of child initiations toward peers, the desired outcome (Schuele/Rice in preparation).

In conclusion, the Social Consequences Account of Specific Language Impairment focuses our attention on the dynamics of children's verbal interactions, and the potential social impact of limited verbal skills. In particular, this model predicts that a child's verbal abilities will influence the probability of success (or failure) in peer interactions. Identification and description of the social consequences of limited language are essential for the formulation of comprehensive and valid models of language acquisition and impairment. Furthermore, knowledge of social consequences will have a direct bearing on our assessment of and intervention with children with limited language competencies.

Note

Portions of this paper appeared in Rice, M.L. (in press). "Don't talk to him: He's weird": The role of language in early social interactions. To appear in A. Kaiser & D. Gray (Eds.), The social use of language: Research foundations for early language intervention. Baltimore: Brookes Publishing Co.

Preparation of this paper supported by USDE award No. H024U80001 to the Kansas Early Childhood Research Institute and NIDCD award No. 5 R29 DC00485 to the author.

References

Anderson, E. (1977). Learning to speak with style. Unpublished doctoral dissertation. Stanford University, Stanford, CA.

Black, B. & Hazen, N.L. (1990). Social status and patterns of communication in acquainted and unacquainted preschool children. Developmental Psychology, 26, 379-387.

Brown, R. (1973). A first language Cambridge, MA: Harvard University Press.

Bunce, B.H., Rice, M.L., & Wilcox, K.A. (1990). LAP update: The effectiveness of language intervention within a classroom setting. Paper presented at the American speech-Language-Hearing Association Annual Convention, Seattle, WA.

Catts, H. (1989). Defining dyslexia as a developmental language disorder. Annals of Dyslexia, 39, 50-64.

Catts, H. (1990). Promoting successful transition to the primary grades: Prediction of reading problems in speech and language handicapped children. In Kansas Early Childhood Research Institute Annual Report. Lawrence, KS: University of Kansas, Life span Institute.

Cooper, C.R., Marquis, A., & Ayers-Lopez, L. (1982). Peer learning in the classroom: Tracing developmental patterns and consequences of children's spontaneous interactions. In L.C. Wilkinson (Ed.), Communication in the classroom. 69-84. New York: Academic Press.

Ervin-Tripp, S. & Gordon, D. (1986). The development of requests. In R.L. Schiefelbusch (Ed.), Language competence: Assessment and intervention. 61-96. San Diego, CA: College-Hill.

Fey, M.E. (1986). Language intervention with young children. San Diego: College-Hill.

Garnica, O.K. (1981). Social dominance and conversational interaction: The omega child in the classroom. In J.L. Green & C. Wallat (Eds.), Ethnography and language in educational settings. 229-250. Norwood, NJ: Ablex.

Grosjean, F. (1982). Life with two languages: An introduction to bilingualism. Cambridge, MA: Harvard University Press.

Hadley, P.A. & Rice, M.L. (1991). Conversational responsiveness in speech and language impaired preschoolers. Journal of Speech and Hearing Research, 34, 1308-1317.

Hazen, N.L. & Black, B. (1989). Preschool peer communication skills: The role of social status and interaction context. Child Development, 60, 867-876.

Heath, S.B. (1989). The learner as cultural member. In M.L. Rice & R.L. Schiefelbusch (Eds.), The teachability of language. 333-350. Baltimore: Brookes Publishing.

Hohmann, M., Bonet, B., & Weikart, D.P. (1978). Young children in action. Ypsilanti, MI: High Scope Press.

Hymes, D. (1972). On communicative competence. In J.B. Pride & J. Holmes (Eds.), Sociolinguistics. Harmondsworth, England: Penguin.

Lahey, M. (1988). Language disorders and language development. New York: MacMillan Publishing.

Lambert, W., Hodgson, R., Gardner, R., & Fillenbaum, R. (1960). Evaluational reactions to spoken languages. Journal of Abnormal and Social Psychology, 60, 44-51.

Peterson, S.E., DeGracie, J.S., & Ayabe, C.R. (1987). A longitudinal study of the effects of retention/promotion on academic achievement. American Educational Research Journal, 24, 107-118.

Rice, M.L., Hadley, P.A., & Alexander, A.L. (1991). Social biases toward children with speech and language impairments: A Naive causal model of language limitations. Manuscript submitted for publication.

Rice, M.L., Sell, M.A., & Hadley, P.A. (1990). The social interactive coding system (SICS): An on-line, clinically relevant descriptive tool. Language, Speech, and Hearing Services in Schools, 21, 2-14.

Rice, M.L., Sell, M.A., & Hadley, P.A. (1991). Social interactions of speech and language impaired children. Journal of Speech and Hearing Research, 34, 1299-1307.

Saville-Troike, M. (1982). The ethnography of communication. Baltimore, MD: University Park Press.

Schieffelin, B.B., & Ochs, E. (Eds.) (1986). Language and socialization across cultures. Cambridge: Cambridge University Press.

Schuele, C.M. & Rice, M.L. (in preparation). The effectiveness of redirected initiations in increasing SLI children's peer interactions. Manuscript in preparation, University of Kansas, Child Language Program.

Tabors, P.O. (1987). The development of communicative competence by second language learners in a nursery school classroom: An ethnolinguistic study. Unpublished doctoral dissertation. Harvard Universty, Cambridge, MA.

Vygotsky, L.S. (1978). Mind in society: The development of higher psychological processes. In M. Cole, V. John-Steiner, V. Scribner, & E. Souberman (Trans. and Eds.) Cambridge: Harvard University Press.

Walsh, D.J. (1989). Changes in kindergarten: Why here? Why now? Early Childhood Research Quarterly, 4, 377-391.

Wechsler, D. (1949). Manual, Wechsler intelligence scale for children. New York: Psychological Corporation.

Weiner, P. (1985). The value of follow-up studies. Topics in Language Disorders, 5, 78-92.

Commentary on Rice: What do we know about the sequelae of socioemotional and cognitive consequences of specific language impairment?

Sabine Weinert

Nearly everybody confronted with the phenomenon of specific language impairment for the first time is struck by its specificity and the mystery of the underlying causes. This is because specifically language impaired (SLI) children are characterized by having profound problems in acquiring the morpho-syntactic aspects of language without displaying any obvious cognitive, emotional, neurological, or sensory disorders that could account directly for their severe language deficits. Thus, SLI children seem to start off with a rather narrowly circumscribed language deficit. But if we look at the later development of these children, there is accumulating evidence that they are at a substantially increased risk for a sequelae of cumulating educational, emotional, and psychosocial problems and thus may end up with a fairly general developmental deficit (e.g. Aram/Nation 1980; Aram/Ekelman/Nation 1984; Baker/Cantwell 1987; Howlin/Rutter 1987).

M. Rice's "Social Consequences Account" bears on this issue. Specifically, she proposes a mechanism that goes beyond correlational evidence by suggesting a negative social spiral that might bridge the gap between language deficits on the one hand and the risk of educational and/or psychosocial problems on the other. Table 1 summarizes the main steps that are assumed to constrain developmental progress in SLI children.

The "Social Consequences Account" addresses a set of points that are especially valuable for a comprehensive view of the topic: In general, it highlights the social-communicative consequences that may result from deficits in verbal skills. This is particularly important since the data patterns obtained in relevant studies on the pragmatic abilities of SLI children have mainly been interpreted as evidence that these children do not suffer from a primary communicative deficit; rather their pragmatic strengths are limited by poor mastery of language structure (e.g. Johnston 1982). But this is not the whole story, as M. Rice shows, and her point is well taken. In particular, the "Social Consequences Account" shifts our view from causes to conse-

Tab. 1: The "Social Consequences Account"

SLI children lack flexibility with language and, thus, often lack the "socially adjusted uses of language". →

They are therefore more likely to be rejected and isolated from peer interactions. →

SLI children recognize this problem and develop compensatory strategies. →

Because of the resultant behavior, the children are regarded as socially immature and cognitively limited. →

These biases, in turn, can constrain the academic options and psychosocial development of the children.

quences of deficits in language use, thereby stressing the importance of the peer group, which is often neglected in developmental research. Specifically, it is suggested that a child of normal intelligence, normal overall developmental progress, and normal communicative sensitivity, who nonetheless lacks verbal flexibility and/or intelligibility, might be at risk for communication problems and social rejection within his or her peer group. This, in turn, starts a negative social spiral based on actions and reactions of both the child and the environment. Thus, as Table 1 shows, the "Social Consequences Account" emphasizes (1) the important function of deficient language behavior with respect to the social and communicative aspects of interpersonal activities, and (2) the mediating function of the social and communicative consequences of specific language impairment for the development of educational and socioemotional problems.

What is the significance and demonstrative power of the available empirical basis for the supposed mechanism? There are at least two general questions: First, are the proposed (social) consequences valid in themselves? This means:

- Are SLI children disposed to be rejected in peer interactions?
- Do they really develop compensatory strategies?
- And, most important, are they perceived as socially immature and cognitively limited?

Second, if these assumptions are empirically valid, what about their interrelations? Do the proposed consequences actually specify the mechanism that determines the shift from language-specific to more general developmental deficits?

To turn to the first general question, M. Rice presents a set of data that is in accordance with the individual consequences proposed by the "Social Consequences Account" (see also Rice/Sell/Hadley 1991; Hadley/Rice 1991). In particular, her empirical results give rise to an intriguing set of theoretically relevant follow-up questions; and I would like to consider just a few of them.

First of all, M. Rice reports on differences in peer interactions between normal-language (NL) and language-impaired children: Compared to NL children, the SLI children were less initiative and less responsive in dialogue and they were more often ignored by their peers. This data pattern is particularly interesting, because it indicates not only quantitative but also qualitative differences. Thus, it should stimulate further research into the quality of peer interactions between NL and SLI children, their specific prerequisites, the typical interactive sequences of (verbal) actions and reactions, and their developmental consequences. Besides focusing on interindividual differences - as M. Rice has done -, the intraindividual variability of interaction patterns will be of theoretical and practical significance as well - especially in homogeneous compared to heterogeneous dyads of children of different language abilities and at different ages. Thus we may ask, for example, whether SLI children are more responsive and initiative when interacting with other language-disordered children than with normal-language children.

As a second main result, M. Rice states that the percentage of initiations directed toward peers and adults varies with language and/or speech ability. The SLI children's greater reliance on adults is interpreted as a compensatory strategy. To draw further conclusions, it is important to know more about the absolute number compared to the relative proportion of initiations: Do SLI children - at least in the long run - withdraw not only from their peers but also from adults? What kinds of nonverbal compensatory strategies do they develop? And what about interrelations between various compensatory strategies and their possible social consequences? Obviously, the range as well as the gains and costs of various compensatory strategies are still quite obscure.

This brings me to the final question to be discussed briefly: namely, the assumption that SLI children might be perceived as socially immature and cognitively limited. As M. Rice shows, there is a tendency to take verbal behavior as an indicator of general cognitive functioning. Of course, this result is interesting in itself. Nevertheless, the reasonable conclusion that SLI children are at risk for unjustified negative expectations is not necessarily true. In fact, the adult subjects in M. Rice's study were only presented with audiotape recordings, that is, their judgments were restricted to just one cue, namely, to differences in verbal behavior. Thus, it is still an open question whether adults in general stick to this cue or whether they are likely to notice the markedly inconsistent cues that may be characteristic of SLI children in real-life situations. In other words: When interacting with SLI children, are their judgments predominantly biased by the language deficits of the child, or do adults take into account the discrepancies between both the deficits and the competencies of these children? In fact, the indicative function of language behavior as well as its communicative social function will only turn into a theoretically conceived mechanism of developmental change if - or as far as - they exert regulatory power upon interactive exchange.

This leads up to the second general question: What do we know about the interconnections between the proposed (social) consequences? To come to the most important point first: In my opinion, the empirical evidence given in M. Rice's paper is especially relevant to singular social consequences, which are obviously important in themselves; but it does not answer the "why" questions and the supposed interrelations between consequences. Actually, I would like to argue that these interrelationships are theoretically more complicated than the "Social Consequences Account" suggests. In addition, I would like to propose a supplementary mediator for educational and socioemotional problems in SLI children that might be of great importance to the negative social spiral as well as to a negative cognitive spiral; namely, a cumulating knowledge deficit.

To begin with, we are still lacking empirical data to specify the interrelations underlying the empirical correlation between speech/language deficits, communication skills, and the quality or quantity of peer interactions in SLI children. From a theoretical point of view, deficient pragmatic communication skills in SLI children may not only be caused by their poor mastery of language structure. Pragmatic and communicative deficits may also result from reduced opportunities for social interactions, especially with peers. Thus, the developmental path is by no means clear cut: Do SLI children ties to acquire flexible pragmatic skills within the peer group, that is, do they lack these skills because they are rejected from peer interactions? Or are they rejected from peer interactions because they lack pragmatic skills? Obviously these alternatives are not mutually exclusive. In fact, it is still an open empirical question whether and how different types of peer experience affect the development of special communication skills in SLI children or whether and how the availability and use of these skills affects peer experiences. To complicate the interrelations further, language deficits are likely to exert a direct influence on peer interactions. This is because productive and/or receptive problems in language processing should make verbal exchange quite laborious. Reduced verbal exchange in turn may impede subsequent language progress. To address these interconnections empirically, a comparative analysis of the developmental changes in SLI children's dyadic interactions in familiar and unfamiliar peer groups seems a promising approach. In addition, M. Rice's quasi-experimental approach ought to be especially relevant to this issue, since it allows for a comparative analysis of dyadic interactions within a 2 x 2-factorial design with children varying (a) in current language skills (NL/ML vs. SLI/ESL, see below) and (b) in their history of communication development (NL/ESL vs. SLI/ML; see also Hadley/Rice 1991). The pattern of differences between SLI children, normal-language children (NL), children learning English as a second language (ESL), and children with a previous history of language impairment, who are now functioning within normal range (ML) could help to separate the functional roles of current language skills compared to the impact of previous communication development.

But which socioemotional consequences are likely to result from the interrelated deficits in speech/language abilities, verbal communication skills, and peer experiences? The empirical evidence on the role of verbal interaction patterns in peer dyads is suggestive, but it is not sufficient to draw the conclusion that these deficits lead to a generalized low social status in the peer group, that is, to conclude that SLI children per se are less popular and regarded as less likable than normal-language children. Thus, future studies will have to show whether observed differences in (verbal) peer interactions are augmented by more enduring negative attitudes toward the SLI child. This question is of special interest since we do not know yet how verbal abilities and communication skills affect socioemotional peer experiences and how these peer experiences in turn affect the development of communication skills and the socioemotional well-being of the child (Black/Hazen 1990). A comparative analysis of the relation between the likability of SLI children and their verbal and nonverbal (pragmatic) skills might provide some insight into the functional relations underlying the empirical connection between language/communication skills and social status in the peer group.

Besides negative attitudes of the social environment, there is another candidate for mediating the impact of deficient peer interactions on socioemotional development: Specifically, we may ask whether peer reputations and problems in communication become internalized into the SLI child's self-concept. In fact, if this were the case, deficits in language and communication skills may be augmented by negative self-expectations that are likely to be generalized to new interaction situations. Although we do not have empirically validated answers to these questions, it is reasonable to assume that SLI children whose language deficits are offset by better cognitive and social abilities are likely to become aware of their language and their (socio-emotional) communication problems and put them together in their intuitive self-theory.

So far I have discussed several factors that possibly constrain psychosocial development. But the consequences of deficits in language processing and of reduced peer interactions may not only be socioemotional in nature; in addition, we can expect negative cognitive consequences mediated by a cumulating knowledge deficit that might be inextricably intertwined with the negative social-communicative outcomes of specific language impairment. In fact, oral communication is one of the important factors in knowledge acquisition. The knowledge acquired so far, however, is an essential precondition for acquiring additional new knowledge. In view of the significant role of the increasing knowledge base in modern theories of cognitive development, restrictions in the acquisition of knowledge may cause more general deficits in cognitive development.

There are at least two reasons why SLI children are especially prone to a cumulating knowledge deficit. First, the acquisition of knowledge is limited by their deficits in language processing. These deficits may not only be restricted to the processing of complexly structured sentences but rather to the processing of texts consisting of quite simple sentences. This is because SLI children seem to have severe deficits in basic information processing as indicated by a much slower speed of item identification for well-known and unknown words (e.g. Weinert 1991, 1992). Bearing in mind R. Case's theory of cognitive development, that is, the assumption that there is a trade off between the efficiency of basic cognitive operations and the availability of functional storage and processing space (e.g. Case/Kurland/Goldberg

1982), a low speed of item identification should prevent SLI children from performing more complex cognitive operations. This could be connected with the fact that SLI children have difficulties in using hierarchical text structures in oral information processing and thus may have problems in acquiring knowledge from oral texts (Weinert/Grimm/Delille/Scholten-Zitzewitz 1989).

Second and moreover, these deficits may well be augmented by reduced environmental support. Specifically, if SLI children are deprived from peer interaction, this may imply reduced opportunities for the acquisition of world knowledge, especially socially relevant knowledge. In view of the proposed compensatory communication strategies of SLI children, we may expect, at first glance, that the SLI children's greater reliance on adults might compensate for the reduced learning opportunities in peer interactions. But this need not to be the case. In fact, there is empirical evidence suggesting that adult-child dialogues with SLI compared to NL children are cognitively less demanding and may be less stimulating. Specifically, Grimm (1991) has suggested that the mothers of SLI children take the most obvious cue, that is, the productive language disability of their child as a basis for adjusting their verbal behavior in general. Although the children were of normal nonverbal intelligence, the mothers did not just adjust the formal aspects of their speech. In addition, they also reduced the cognitive complexity of speech. Obviously, they did not take into account the cognitive competencies of their child. Future research has to show whether this maladaptation is mediated by a negative bias toward the cognitive abilities of SLI children.

But irrespective of the empirical validity of this plausible assumption, we may conclude that the opportunities for acquiring an elaborated knowledge base are restricted not only by peer interactions but also because of poor adult-child interactions. Indeed, there does not seem to be an enriched input that might compensate for the language processing deficits of SLI children.

In summary, even if SLI children start off with a narrowly circumscribed language deficit and with cognitive abilities within the normal range of the age population, they might end up with a rather general cognitive and social deficit. In fact, problems in communication and language processing could produce a negative cognitive spiral that seems to be intrinsically intertwined with the negative social spiral. Deficits in verbal abilities, in flexible language use and last but not least accumulating knowledge deficits are likely to restrict the SLI child's (verbal) activity in dialogue. Additionally mediated by the possible socioemotional consequences (e.g. low social status, negative self-concept) and by reduced social support, these consequences could impede both socioemotional development and the permanent acquisition of new knowledge that is needed to enhance the efficiency of language processing and cognitive functioning. In fact, the socioemotional and the cognitive consequences are likely to aggravate one another.

References

Aram, D.M. & Nation, J.E. (1980). Preschool language disorders and subsequent language and academic difficulties. Journal of Communication Disorders, 13, 159-170.

Aram, D.M., Ekelman, B.L., & Nation, J.E. (1984). Preschoolers with language disorders: Ten years later. Journal of Speech and Hearing Research, 27, 232-244.

Baker, L. & Cantwell, D.P. (1987). Factors associated with the development of psychiatric illness in children with early speech/language problems. Journal of Autism and Developmental Disorders, 17, 499-510.

Black, B. & Hazen, N.L. (1990). Social status and patterns of communication in acquainted and unacquainted preschool children. Developmental Psychology, 26, 379-387.

Case, R., Kurland, D.M., & Goldberg, J. (1982). Operational efficiency and the growth of short-term memory span. Journal of Experimental Child Psychology, 33, 386-404.

Grimm, H. (1991). Entwicklungskritische Dialogmerkmale in Mutter-Kind Dyaden mit dysphasisch sprachgestörten und sprachunauffälligen Kindern. Paper given at the "10. Tagung für Entwicklungspsychologie" in Köln. (To appear in Zeitschrift für Entwicklungspsychologie und Pädagogische Psychologie.)

Hadley, P.A. & Rice, M.L. (1991). Conversational responsiveness of speech- and language-impaired preschoolers. Journal of Speech and Hearing Research, 34, 1308-1317.

Howlin, P. & Rutter, M. (1987). The consequences of language delay for other aspects of development. In W. Yule & M. Rutter (Eds.), Language development and disorders. 271-294. London: MacKeith Press.

Johnston, J.R. (1982). The language disordered child. In N.J. Lass, L.V. McReynolds, J.L. Northern, & D.E. Yoder (Eds.), Speech, language, and hearing: Pathologies of speech and language (Vol.2). 780-801. Philadelphia: W.B. Saunders Company.

Rice, M.L., Sell, M.A., & Hadley, P.A. (1991). Social interactions of speech- and language-impaired children. Journal of Speech and Hearing Research, 34, 1299-1307.

Weinert, S. (1991). Spracherwerb und implizites Lernen. Bern: Huber.

Weinert, S. (1992). Deficits in acquiring language structure: The importance of using prosodic cues. Applied Cognitive Psychology, 6, 545-571.

Weinert, S., Grimm, H., Delille, G. & Scholten-Zitzewitz, R. (1989). Was macht sprachgestörten Kindern das Textverstehen so schwer? Heilpädagogische Forschung, 15, 25-37.

Specific language impairment as a problem of accessing language knowledge

Phil J. Connell
Steven L. Franks
C. Addison Stone

The general purpose of the research to be discussed in this paper is to obtain detailed experimental data on the nature of the language knowledge of specific language-impaired (SLI) children and on how SLI children acquire this knowledge from input received during language teaching sessions. These data serve the broad goals of SLI research: to understand better the discrepancies between the linguistic behaviors of SLI and normal children, to determine whether these discrepancies are due to competence or performance deficits, and to develop teaching methods that can overcome or circumvent them.

The preponderance of evidence that has been gathered to date on SLI children indicates that they have difficulty acquiring language with the ease of normal children in spite of normal intelligence, hearing and social-emotional development (Fey 1986). It appears that the initial and intermediate languages that they construct on their way to acquiring the adult language are the same as those of normal children (see Leonard 1987, for a thorough review of the evidence). Thus, SLI children appear to learn the same language in the same way as normal children except that the onset of acquisition is later, the rate of acquisition is slower, and the final level of achievement is lower. Their problem is apparently one of speed of movement through the same intermediate languages that normal children pass through on their way to acquiring the adult language.

Two distinct but converging lines of research have produced the findings that contradict this view. One line of research has concerned the acquisition of morphological rules by SLI children, an area of deficit that is widely known to characterize the disorder (e.g., Fey 1986; Leonard 1982). The research has focused on the apparent facilitative effects of imitation teaching on SLI children's morphological rule induction. The two major facets of the research have been: (i) an examination of how SLI children induce morphological rules under controlled teaching conditions in which they are either encouraged or prohibited from imitating the input and (ii) a determination of whether the difficulty experienced by the SLI children is actually a problem of rule induction (competence) or a problem of rule access or production (performance). To address these issues, SLI children have been exposed to an invented morpheme under two alternative teaching conditions: modeling and imitation, and under two language modalities: auditory or visual, and their mastery of the morpheme was assessed via both comprehension and production test trials. Their performance has been compared to that of two groups of normally developing children matched to the SLI children on chronological age or on language maturity. In general, the findings indicate that the difference between SLI and normal performance can be primarily attributed to constraints impinging on the linguistic performance of SLI children and only secondarily on their ability to acquire knowledge of a grammar.

The second line of research has concentrated on the distribution and interpretation of reflexive pronouns, a central and well-studied aspect of grammar. The development of the reflexive system provides a window through which the grammar of SLI and normal children can be studied and compared. By taking a limited focus, it has been possible to analyze the linguistic knowledge of these children at sufficient depth to uncover subtleties in their developing language system. The two major facets of the research are: (i) an examination of how SLI children interpret reflexives and (ii) a comparison of their grammars with those of normal children, both in terms of the developmental stages traversed and the properties of these stages, as seen through the perspective of reflexive acquisition. The work that has been accomplished thus far is cross- sectional in design and the stages that have been proposed are tentatively awaiting confirmation from longitudinal research. Nonetheless, important observations can be now made about the grammatical competence of SLI children and comparisons are possible to the grammars of normal children. In general, the findings converge with the those of the other research direction; they show that SLI childrens' knowledge of reflexives is at least on par with normal children of the same age, thus implicating performance constraints as a major reason for the discrepancy in their linguistic behavior.

In the following sections, the two lines of research will be described and the results will be presented. An effort will be made to draw the two lines of research together. Even though the approaches taken and issues raised in the two research directions are quite different, the conclusions suggested by the findings are quite similar.

SLI children's learning of morphemes

A series of studies have now been performed that investigate the apparent facilitative effects of imitation teaching on SLI children's morphological rule induction. The general approach of these studies has been to expose SLI children to language rules under controlled instructional conditions to determine if a difference can be found in the rate and extent of learning. In the more recent work, a comparison between modeling and imitation teaching approaches has been the main focus with rule learning assessed through both comprehension and production test trials. Rule learning performance has been compared to two groups of normally developing children matched to the SLI children on chronological age or on language maturity.

Two assumptions about normal and abnormal language acquisition formed the foundation of the teaching methods compared in these studies. First, it is assumed that at least some part of children's language knowledge, and in particular morphological knowledge, evolves through a process of induction learning (Gleitman/Wanner 1982). Induction learning is a process by which relevant linguistic facts or data are stored in memory and subsequently analyzed to uncover distributional patterns that can be used to classify surface forms into relevant linguistic categories.

Secondly, it was assumed from the results of a previous study that SLI children can induce rules as a result of being exposed to linguistic facts in a structured teaching situation (Connell 1986; Fey 1986). In this study, rule induction occurred only when SLI children were required to imitate and produce the language forms given during teaching sessions as input for the rule. In instances in which they were merely required to interpret the meaning of input sentences (as in picture-pointing comprehension teaching trials), the children gave no evidence of learning the rule. As it is generally assumed that the main avenue through which normal children induce language rules is by listening to input sentences, interpreting their meaning, and relating the meaning to language form (Gleitman/Wanner 1982), the fact that SLI children could learn only in experimental contexts that require overt imitation of the target forms implied that they needed more than the normal type of input to learn language rules.

In a follow-up study to substantiate this finding by directly comparing SLI with normal language learners (Connell 1987b), the induction-learning patterns of 40 SLI children between the ages of 3:10 and 5:11 (years:months) were compared to those of 40 age-matched normals under two experimental-teaching conditions: one in which imitation of the input was encouraged (imitation format) and one in which it was not (modeling format). The rule the children were to induce governed an invented suffixal morpheme meaning "part of" (e.g., cow-a was shown to mean "part of a cow"). Both formats were designed to emulate the basic features of induction learning: the information presented to the learner contained both the meaning and the form of the invented morpheme, and exemplars of suffix attached to several words (nouns) were provided. Given this type of input, the learner could examine the relation between the invented form (/a/) and meaning (part of) of the morpheme across a substantial data set, recognize a pattern, and induce a morphological rule. The imitation teaching format differed from the modeling format only that in the former the children were required to imitate the experimenter's utterances containing the morpheme and in the latter they were not.

The results indicated that SLI children produced the new rule more reliably when they were provided with imitation trials as opposed to modeling trials. Normal children, on the other hand, displayed no such preference. Thus, the superiority of imitation teaching for SLI children suggested by the former study was confirmed, again suggesting that they learn from the language input provided in teaching trials in a manner that is different from normal children.

The unusual difficulty encountered by SLI children in learning a rule through the modeling format was used by Roseberry/Connell (1991) as a marker to identify SLI bilingual (Spanish/English) children. An invented morpheme was taught to 26 children whose first language was Spanish and who had limited proficiency in English. Half of the children had been previously identified as normal language learners who needed more exposure to English and the other half had been identified through rigorous formal and informal testing as SLI. The SLI group learned the morpheme at a significantly slower rate than the normal children after receiving modeling teaching, thus allowing the two groups to be differentiated solely on the grounds of their performance on the invented morpheme learning task. Using the morpheme learning task as a screening procedure for SLI would circumvent many of the obstacles that impede identifying language impairment in the limited English proficiency population; obstacles such as the shortage of bilingual Speech-Language Pathologist and the lack of valid standardized tests for bilingual children. In terms of the goals of the research program, the findings demonstrate that the unusual learning style of SLI children is robust enough to be used as a marker for the condition.

The goal of the subsequent steps in the research program has been to attempt to discover the source of the effect, to determine why SLI children were less able to induce a rule from modeling input. One of the first questions addressed was whether the failure to learn a rule through modeling induction teaching was a matter of competence or performance. In the earlier studies, acquisition of the new rule was assessed only by means of production trials. That is, children were required to produce the new morpheme in appropriate circumstances but no attempt was made to assess their understanding of the new morpheme in comprehension trials. Thus, it could have been that the SLI children in the modeling condition actually induced the new rule (i.e., had competence) but, for some reason (e.g., difficulty with morphological access), failed to produce it on the test trials (i.e., did not exhibit performance). Thus, both comprehension and production test trials were included in the study to examine more fully the morphological knowledge of the children.

A second question addressed was whether the unique nature of SLI children's rule learning was in fact unique to SLI children or rather was a stage of development encountered by normal as well as SLI children. The previous experiments left open the possibility that SLI children's morpheme learning was facilitated by imitation-teaching trials (and was inhibited by modeling-teaching trials) because they happened to be at a language-development level that inherently requires more imitation practice.

To address these issues, Connell/Stone (in press) compared the morpheme learning performance of SLI children to that of two groups of normally developing children matched to the SLI children on chronological age or on language maturity. The comparison was made with data obtained from comprehension and production test trials.

Three groups of children were created on the basis of disorder, age, and level of language development: 32 SLI (C.A. 5:0 to 6:11), 24 age-matched (C.A. 5;0 to 6;11), and 20 language matched (C.A. 3;0 to 4;11) children. These subjects were taught a set of invented morphemes by a computerized language-teaching program designed specifically for this study. All components of the teaching experience including pretesting, presentation of teaching trials and post-testing, were performed by the program. The use of a computer program to perform the teaching guaranteed that subjects received identical learning experiences, within the bounds of the design, so that any differences in performance found could be attributed to group differences and the experimental variables under investigation. The subjects were given four computerized language-teaching sessions over a two-week period. They were taught two morphemes during the sessions, one in two successive modeling teaching sessions which was followed or preceded by two imitation teaching sessions in a counterbalanced plan. Thus, the critical comparison between the effect of modeling- and imitation-teaching trials was performed within the same subject.

Analysis of the comprehension and production data revealed a significant difference between the effect of modeling and imitation for the SLI subjects, but the two normal groups responded similarly to the two methods. This addresses the first issue - whether the unique pattern of SLI children's rule learning was in fact unique to SLI children or rather was a stage of development encountered by normal as well as SLI children. This pattern appeared to be a specific characteristic of SLI children in that neither group of normal children demonstrated it. The results for the comprehension trials, however, did not parallel those for the production trials, and these results address the first question - whether the failure to learn a rule through modeling induction teaching was a matter of competence or performance. There were no differential effects of modeling and imitation for any of the groups meaning that the SLI children responded to instructional method similarly to the children in the other two groups. Thus, the group-specific effect was reliably evident for production trials only, indicating that it was a performance rather than a competence effect.

In summary, the results indicate that the modeling-imitation effect is related to performance or use of the morphological rule not competence or knowledge of it. It also appears that the effect is inherent to the language impairment syndrome itself and not a matter of developmental lag. This, then, allows us to clarify the question posed earlier. Rather than asking "what factors underlie the modeling-imitation difference in SLI children's language learning", the more precise question can be asked "what performance factors underlie the modeling- imitation difference in SLI children's language learning". This does not imply that the learning problems of SLI children result exclusively in problems with production performance. On the contrary, the SLI children's overall morpheme learning performance, that is, in imitation and modeling on comprehension and production probe measures, was less than that of the age-matched group. Rather, it means that the difference between the effect of imitation and modeling teaching procedures is exclusively in the domain of performance, and in particular, production performance.

One rather prominent possible explanation is that the performance effect is linked to an underlying deficiency in access to phonological representation. This interpretation is consistent with other recent findings in implicating phonological access and/or the quality of phonological representations as a key factor in specific language impairment (Kamhi/Catts/Mauer et al. 1988). The act of imitating a target morpheme could serve two functions simultaneously: to refine the phonological representation stored for the morpheme and to provide practice in accessing it from storage. In order to evaluate the plausibility of this explanation, Stone/Connell (in press) performed a study in which the same invented morphemes were taught to SLI and normal children in a visual as opposed to auditory mode. The visual mode was chosen as the logical contrast to isolate the effects that the auditory processing system contributes to the morpheme learning problem. It was reasoned that if SLI subjects showed no pattern of imitation superiority when learning the same rule in a visual language, then the pattern found in the auditory-language data might be attributed to problems in constructing appropriate phonological representations from auditory input or from retrieving these representations once they had been established. If, on the other hand, the same pattern was found in the visual morpheme task that was evident in the auditory morpheme task data, a broader difficulty with storing or accessing symbolic codes would be implicated, a difficulty that was independent of input modality.

Three identical groups of children were created to test this issue. As before, they were grouped on the basis of disorder, age, and level of language development: 21 SLI (C.A. 5:0 to 6:11), 25 age-matched (C.A. 5;0 to 6;11), and 21 language-matched (C.A. 3;0 to 4;11) children. As was the case in the auditory morpheme study, the subjects were taught a set of invented morphemes by a computerized language-teaching program, this time entirely in a visual mode. The fact that both tasks were presented by computer further strengthened the grounds on which the results of the two studies were to be compared. The same invented morphemes were taught, but rather than demonstrating that the morpheme meaning was marked by attaching a suffix to a noun, they were taught to graphically represent the morpheme meaning by placing a geometric shape onto an iconic picture of an object. Thus, the geometric shape was conceived as the analogue of the suffix taught in the auditory morpheme task. As before, the subjects were taught two morphemes during the sessions, one in two successive modeling teaching sessions which was followed or preceded by two imitation teaching sessions in a counterbalanced plan, thus allowing the critical comparison to be performed within subject.

An analysis of the comprehension and production data revealed a pattern that was considerably different from that found in auditory morpheme study. Interestingly, the difference lie not with the SLI children's results, but with the age-matched and language-matched groups results. The imitation advantage found only in the SLI production data in the auditory morpheme study was found in the production responses of both normal groups in the visual morpheme results. The effect was much more prominent with the age-matched subjects. This intriguing finding calls for a reconsideration of the conclusions reached for the auditory morpheme study. It was concluded that imitation practice afforded SLI children a unique advantage in using a newly acquired morpheme form. The source of this advantage was assumed to be the beneficial effect that imitation practice had on an inefficient morpheme retrieval process that was a symptom of SLI. In contrast, the results of the present study indicate that, like SLI children, age-matched normal children also tend to produce a visual morpheme more reliably under the imitation condition as well. Thus, there is no evidence of a unique learning style. The answer to this quandary may lie in the extreme difficulty that the normal children had in learning the visual morpheme. After the same number of teaching trials as provided in the auditory morpheme study, the normal children in the visual study demonstrated knowledge of the morphemes on the comprehension and production probes approximately half as often. It could be that when normal language learners are placed in conditions that act to make learning relatively inefficient, such as in the visual-morpheme task conditions, the efficiency with which they learn/retrieve new forms is enhanced to some degree if they are allowed to imitate them.

Perhaps, though, the learning style is unique to SLI children. Normal children display the style when they encounter language input in a modality that is unfamiliar to them. In contrast, SLI children demonstrate the style when engaged in a learning task that emulates the experiences they have encountered throughout their language learning history. Thus, SLI children performed as if they were unfamiliar with language data presented in the auditory modality.

In sum, the findings from this research program suggest the following tentative conclusion: SLI children may have a modality-specific difficulty with the access to, or storing of, auditory input needed to induce morpheme rules (the group-specific instructional effect for the production data, but not the comprehension data, on the auditory task). Thus, taken as a whole, the results of this line of research provide some important information regarding the underlying cause of the unique instructional needs of the SLI children in the auditory morpheme-learning task initially identified by Connell (1987b). First, from the results of the auditory-morpheme study (Connell/Stone in press), it appears that the instructional effect is not due to general differences in linguistic rule induction, as was presumed in earlier work (Connell 1987b). Instead, the effect relates specifically to production of the newly learned morpheme. Thus, a difficulty of access to phonological representation appears to be implicated. Second, the results of the visual morpheme study suggest that the effect is not found in an analogous learning task in the visual modality, suggesting again that what is at issue is a modality-specific problem of representational adequacy or access. Third, from the results of the former auditory morpheme study, the effect is not found in younger, normally developing children matched to the SLI group on general language maturity. Nor is it evident in the language-matched children in the visual study. Thus, the differential response to instruction is not merely a function of general language maturity. Fourth, from the results of the visual-and auditory-morpheme studies, the effect is independent of a more general difficulty in rule-learning that is manifested as depressed performance on both auditory and visual symbol-learning tasks and that may represent a generally less active approach to the learning of new symbolic relationships. These conclusions should serve to refine future work which hopefully can identify more precisely the exact nature of both the group-specific language-learning difficulty and the broader rule-learning inefficiencies in SLI children documented in the present data.

SLI childrens' knowledge of reflexives

The overall purpose of the second line of research was to investigate the growth of linguistic knowledge in SLI children within the confines of a linguistic model of language acquisition. Most current linguistic theories posit a core component of "universal" principles of human language structure, and the intent of this research was to study how this component is manifested in the language of SLI children (for a general treatment of the theoretical issues see Chomsky 1981; Haegeman 1991; or Radford 1988). In the following section, the kinds of linguistic knowledge that we are examining will be generally described and this will be followed a brief description of the methods and the results of the experiments.

Within this framework, language acquisition is viewed as an interaction between innate principles of language incorporated in a Universal Grammar (UG) and the input a child receives from the environment. These two sources conspire to determine the nature of the adult language that a child eventually acquires. One of the modules that the UG provides is Binding Theory - a system for assigning coreference relationships among NPs. The term "binding" derives from the coreference relationship that "binds" an antecedent NP to pronouns (e.g., him, her, it, etc.) and reflexives (e.g., *himself, herself, itself,* etc.). An antecedent NP is one which the pronoun or reflexive makes reference to. According to Binding Theory, there are three different types of NPs: names, reflexives, and pronouns. As illustrated in (1), names are NPs that have inherent reference such as *Mary* in (1a-d). Pronouns (such as *her* in (1a & c) and reflexives such as *herself* in (1b & d) are NPs that take their reference by binding to other NPs, thus they make no independent reference to objects or events in the real world. In these sentences, the names in parentheses following a pronoun or reflexive indicate the reference intended. Pronouns and reflexives can be seen to be in a reciprocal relation with one another in terms of which NPs can bind them, as is demonstrated by the acceptableness of (1a & b) and the unacceptableness (denoted by the asterisk) of (1c & d). In English, pronouns must be bound to NPs outside of their clause and reflexives must be bound inside their clause. Thus, the *her* in (1c) cannot refer to *Mary* while the *herself* in (1d) cannot refer to someone else.

(1) a. Mary defended her (someone else).
b. Mary defended herself (Mary).
c. *Mary defended her (Mary).
d. *Mary defended herself (someone else).

The part of Binding Theory that is the focus of our research on SLI children concerns the stages of reflexive acquisition. Reflexive acquisition has received considerable attention recently because the issues involved in adult grammars are fairly well understood and because children appear to pass through developmental stages in the acquisition process (Chien/Wexler 1990; Franks/Connell 1991; Grimshaw/Rosen 1990; Lust 1987; Progovac/ Connell 1991, 1992a, 1992b). The characteristics of English reflexives are demonstrated in (2a-c). As can be seen, *herself* can refer only to *April* and not to *Joan* or *Mary*. This fact is captured by the principle that the reflexive must be bound to an NP within its own clause. Thus, *Joan* and *Mary* are prohibited from binding with *herself* because they are outside the clause containing *herself* (the boundaries of the clause containing the reflexive are demarked by square brackets).

(2) a. Joan told Mary [that April poured juice for herself (April)].
b. *Joan told Mary [that April poured juice for herself (Joan)].
c. *Joan told Mary [that April poured juice for herself (Mary)].

This principle of Binding Theory is claimed to be universal meaning that all natural languages and all child versions thereof obey it. There is, however, a certain degree of variation among adult languages how this principle is applied. The sentences in (3) provide an example of this variation. Although the sentences are presented in English, they should be regarded as Chinese sentences translated into English for purposes of this example. As is evident, the allowable range of potential binders in these translated Chinese sentences is different from what would be expected of the comparable English sentences. In particular, in the Chinese sentence (3b), *Joan* is outside of the clause containing the reflexive but can bind with the reflexive, a possibility not available in English. This variation across languages is explained by postulating that English allows the reflexive to corefer only with NPs within its own clause while Chinese allows for coreference both inside and outside of this clause. This variation is of central importance for Binding Theory in regard to acquisition because changes from one domain in which a reflexive can bind to an antecedent NP to another are postulated to be the stages of reflexive acquisition. Thus, studying reflexive acquisition involves, in large part, finding out how children come to know the appropriate binding domain for their language.

(3) a. Joan told Mary [that April poured juice for herself April)].
b. Joan told Mary [that April poured juice for herself (Joan)].
c. *Joan told Mary [that April poured juice for herself (Mary)].

Thus, our investigation addressed two issues: to identify the stages of normal reflexive acquisition and to determine whether SLI children traverse the same stages. To this end, the reflexive binding domains of 20 normal adults, 13 normal children between the ages of 3:7 and 8:6, and 10 SLI children between the ages of 3:9 and 7:8 were studied. The SLI subjects varied in terms of their scores on standardized tests of reception and production but all met the criterion of a score of at least one standard deviation from the mean on either a test of comprehension, production or both. They were all diagnosed as SLI by their attending SLP and were receiving language therapy.

The subjects were presented 14 30-second video-taped vignettes in which three actors interact at a "juice party". While viewing the tape, the subjects were asked questions like "Did Bugs ask Ernie if Mickey poured the juice for himself?" to determine which of the NPs in the question were allowed as antecedents for the reflexive. These questions followed vignettes in which the main characters (Mickey, Ernie, and Bugs) enacted scenes that forced the question to be interpreted in specific ways. For example, one vignette depicted Mickey pouring juice for Bugs, an event which Bugs cannot see, and thus Bugs asks Ernie who Mickey poured the juice for. In response to the question above, the English-speaking adults responded "no" because *himself* in this question could only refer to *Mickey* and the juice was not, in fact, poured for Mickey. On the other hand, if the question were translated to Chinese and asked of a Chinese-speaking adult, the answer would be "yes" because Chinese allows *himself* to refer to *Bugs*. Thus, the subjects' responses to this question and other similar questions was used to discover the kind of reflexive system contained in their grammars.

Again, the size of the binding domain of the SLI and normal children's reflexives was the primary focus of the research because a change in domain size appears to constitute the stages of development. The results indicated that most of the normal children had one or the other type of binding domain. Of the 10 normal subjects who were capable of answering the questions reliably, 5 demonstrated the long distance (Chinese-like) domain (n = 5), 3 the narrow (English-like) domain, and 2 a strategy to bind to the nearest NP. It is assumed that these 2 children were forced to use the strategy because the demands of processing the complex sentences used in the task were too costly, so that for these children the actual domain cannot be determined from the results. The other 3 normal children gave responses that were inconsistent and were judged to be too unreliable to be interpreted. Of the 8 SLI children who were capable of answering the questions reliably, 2 demonstrated the narrow or adult-like domain, and 6 the strategy mentioned above. Like the normal children, 2 gave responses that were judged uninterpretable.

We would assume that the narrow domain is the most linguistically mature given that it is the one displayed by all the adult subjects. Thus it would appear that while some normal children are in the earlier developmental stage in which reflexives are allowed to bind outside of their own clause, and some are in a later one, in which binding is limited to within-clause, the SLI children who could be tested were in the later stage. Since the children in the two groups were approximately the same age, this finding suggests that some of the SLI children were on par or more advanced than some normal children. This finding would imply that the delay in language development usually associated with SLI cannot be found in reflexive acquisition, when acquisition is tested using methods designed to tap language knowledge rather than language performance. Of course, this study examined only one narrow area of language knowledge and it is possible that knowledge in this area does not predict or coincide with knowledge in others. However the data are nonetheless suggestive that when the language knowledge of SLI children is studied using methods that require their interpretation rather than production of sentences, the gap between the language development of normal and SLI children is greatly narrowed.

Conclusions

The question that the results of the these two research directions raise is the cause of the language delay displayed by SLI children - whether it represents an abnormal slowness in acquiring language knowledge as it has usually been characterized or whether it actually represents a deficiency in learning how to access this knowledge. These are two possible ways of characterizing the nature of the delay in their linguistic behavior: the problem is either one of delayed knowledge or of delayed obedience (cf. Grimshaw/Rosen 1990, for a discussion of knowledge vs. obedience of grammatical principles).

The standard approach (Fey 1986; Leonard 1982) has been the delayed knowledge one, which would claim that acquisition, whatever the particular stages involved, proceeds at a slower pace with SLI than with normal children. This delay has been associated with various cognitive deficiencies: in sophistication of play (Lombardino/Stein/Kricos 1986; Roth/Clark 1987), conversational competence (Brinton/Fujiki/Winkler/Loeb 1986), reading and pre-reading skills (Gillam/Johnston 1985; Kamhi/Catts 1986), hypothesis formation and testing (Kamhi/Catts/Koenig/Lewis 1984; Kamhi/Nelson/Lee/Gholson 1985; Stone/Forman 1988), narrative discourse ability (Liles 1985, 1987), inferencing from known facts (Weismer 1985), and metalinguistic abilities (Kamhi/Koenig 1985; Kamhi/Lee/Nelson 1985). Also, SLI children have been shown to have perceptual processing deficiencies when compared to normal children, especially for rapidly presented auditory stimuli (Elliot/Hammer/Scholl 1989; Tallal/Stark/Mellits 1985a, b) and mental imagery ability (Johnston/Weismer 1983; Savich 1984; Whitmire/Stone 1991).

The approach supported by the evidence compiled in these studies on normal and SLI children is that SLI children are delayed in the frequency with which they obey their relatively normal knowledge of language. Thus, while these deficiencies may exist, they do not appear to impinge on SLI children's progress in acquiring language knowledge that is appropriate for their chronological age. This suggests that the process of constructing language knowledge by SLI children is governed to a large extent by factors that are relatively unaffected by the cognitive or perceptual abnormalities that might afflict them (cf. Rosenberg 1984) for similar arguments). The only logical alternative is that it is governed by universal principles of language structure that is innately available to them.

The possibility that SLI children may have language performance problems that tend to mask their actual competence is not a new idea in the field (cf. Curtiss/Tallal 1991). What is different about our conclusions is that SLI children are being portrayed as having competence that may be equivalent in some aspects of language to normal age-peers whereas all former proposals assume a significant delay in competence with an overriding deficiency in performance.

While the possibility that SLI children have relatively intact language competence must be evaluated very carefully before being applied to clinical practice, it provides a testable null hypothesis for clinical practice and future research. Even if further study proves the proposal to be largely true, there will undoubtedly be exceptions and special cases that will have to be systematically sorted out. The contrary assumption, that such children lack appropriate language competence, though, has already had a significant impact on current clinical practice in the field. Take for example the tendency of clinicians to disbelieve parent's reports of their children's ability to interpret many of the sentences spoken to them. Clinicians commonly assume that parents read too much into the occasional appropriate response of their children to commands and questions, placing the blame on the parent's overriding need to have their children be normal. However, it is possible that clinician's have just as strong a bias in the opposite direction, based on their exaggerated focus on language performance, in particular, on language production. Because children fail to say sentences and perform poorly on some standardized tests does not necessarily mean that their language knowledge is less than normal. As demonstrated in the last two sections, they simply may have difficulty accessing their relatively normal language knowledge on such tasks.

This kind of bias may also have affected the research in the field. In the Connell (1986) study previously mentioned, SLI children who were described as being in the one-word stage were asked to point to pictures depicting an action in response to semantically reversible sentences such as "Show me the frog kissing the bunny" and "Show me the bunny kissing the frog" to determine the extent of their knowledge of semantic roles. Their failure to point to the correct picture was used as evidence that they did not know how to interpret these sentences and that they did not know the syntax of semantic roles. This now appears to have been the wrong conclusion, at least with some of the children. In a presently ongoing study, we have been finding that most such children can correctly answer questions such as "Did the frog kiss the bunny", and "Who did the bunny kiss?" asked about appropriate pictures. To answer such questions correctly, a child would have to know how syntax codes semantic roles because one would have to understand what semantic role is assigned to each NP in order to interpret the question correctly. Thus, SLI children who appear to be in the one-word stage based on language sample data and formal test data may actually be in a syntactic stage of language knowledge.

Thus, it may be appropriate to adopt the opposite assumption, to assume that SLI children may have language knowledge that is not much different from that of normal children and proceed accordingly. Such an approach to language evaluation could lead to better ways to test language knowledge, and, because good language teaching is based on a thorough understanding of the language knowledge that the learner already has, this assumption may eventually lead to more effective language teaching methods.

Acknowledgments

The research reported in this paper was supported in part by a grant from NIDCD and a Multidisciplinary Ventures Fund administered by Indiana University. We would like to thank ChiMing Yang for his assistance in the development of the computer programs used to implement the instruction, and Lucy Felbinger, Kalyani Krishnan, Peg Bemen,

Laura Riddle, Barry Wagner, Susan Giger, Lisa Ubben, Marsha Finke, and Robin Barker for their assistance in data collection and analysis.

References

Brinton, B., Fujiki, M., Winkler, E., & Loeb, D. (1986). Response to requests for clarification in linguistically normal and language-impaired children. Journal of Speech and Hearing Disorders, 51, 370-378.

Chien, Y-C. & Wexler, K. (1990). Children's knowledge of locality conditions in binding as evidence for the modularity of syntax and pragmatics. Language Acquisition, 1, 225-295.

Chomsky, N. (1981). Lectures on government and binding. Dordrecht: Foris.

Connell, P. (1986). Acquisition of semantic role by language-disordered children: Differences between production and comprehension. Journal of Speech and Hearing Research, 29, 366-374.

Connell, P. (1987a). Teaching language functions, meanings and utterances to language disordered children. In S. Rosenberg (Ed.), Advances in applied psycholinguistics, (Vol. 1): Disorders of first language acquisition. 40-75. Cambridge, England: Cambridge University Press.

Connell, P. (1987b). An effect of modeling and imitation teaching procedures on children with and without specific language impairment. Journal of Speech and Hearing Research, 30, 105-113.

Connell, P. & Stone, C.A. (in press). Morpheme learning of children with specific language impairment under controlled instructional conditions. Journal of Speech and Hearing Research.

Curtiss, S. & Tallal, P. (1991). On the nature of the impairment in language-imapired children. In J. Miller (Ed.), Research on child language disorders. 189-210. Austin, TX: Pro-Ed.

Elliot, L., Hammer, M., & Scholl, M. (1989). Fine-grained auditory discrimination in normal children and children with language learning patterns. Journal of Speech and Hearing Research, 32, 112-119.

Fey, M. (1986). Language intervention with young children. San Diego: College-Hill Press.

Franks, S. & Connell, P. (1991). Binding, movement and the acquisition of anaphora. Penn Review of Linguistics, 15, 49-62.

Gillam, R. & Johnston, J. (1985). Development of print awareness in language-disordered preschoolers. Journal of Speech and Hearing Research, 28, 521-526.

Gleitman, L. & Wanner, E. (1982). Language acquisition: The state of the state of the art. In E. Wanner & L. Gleitman (Eds), Language acquisition: The state of the art. 3-48. Cambridge: Cambridge University Press.

Grimshaw, J. & Rosen, S. (1990). Knowledge and obedience: The developmental status of Binding Theory. Linguistic Inquiry, 21, 187-222.

Haegeman, L. (1991). Introduction to government & binding theory. Cambridge, MA: Basil Blackwell.

Johnston, J. & Weismer, S. (1983). Mental rotation abilities in language-disordered children. Journal of Speech and Hearing Research, 26, 397-403.

Kamhi, A. & Catts, H. (1986). Toward an understanding of developmental language and reading disorders. Journal of Speech and Hearing Disorders, 51, 337-347.

Kamhi, A., Catts, H., Koenig, L., & Lewis, B. (1984). Hypothesis-testing and nonlinguistic symbolic abilities in language-impaired children. Journal of Speech and Hearing Disorders, 49, 169-176.

Kamhi, A., Catts, H.W., Mauer, D., Apel, K., & Gentry, B.F. (1988). Phonological and spatial processing abilities in language- and reading-impaired children. Journal of Speech and Hearing Disorders, 53, 316-327.

Kamhi, A. & Koenig, L. (1985). Metalinguistic awareness in normal and language-disordered children. Language, Speech and Hearing Services in Schools, 16 199-210.

Kamhi, A., Lee, R., & Nelson, L. (1985). Word, syllable, and sound awareness in language-disordered children. Journal of Speech and Hearing Disorders, 50, 207-212.

Kamhi, A., Nelson, L., Lee, R., & Gholson, B. (1985). The ability of language-disordered children to use and modify hypotheses in discrimination learning. Applied Psycholinguistics, 6, 435-451.

Leonard, L. (1982). The nature of specific language impairment in children. In S. Rosenberg (Ed.), Handbook of applied psycholinguistics: Major thrusts of research and theory. 285-237. Hillsdale, NJ: Erlbaum.

Leonard, L. (1987). Is specific language impairment a useful construct? In S. Rosenberg (Ed.), Advances in applied psycholinguistics, volume 1: Disorders of first-language development. 1-39. Cambridge: Cambridge University Press.

Liles, B. (1985). Production and comprehension of narrative discourse in normal and language-disordered children. Journal of Communication Disorders, 18, 409-427.

Liles, B. (1987). Episode organization and cohesive conjunctives in narratives of children with and without language disorder. Journal of Speech and Hearing Research, 30, 185-196.

Lombardino, L., Stein, J, & Kricos, P. (1986). Play diversity and structural relationships in the play and language of language-impaired and language-normal preschoolers: Preliminary data. Journal of Communication Disorders, 19, 475-489.

Lust, B. (Ed.). (1987). Studies in the acquisition of anaphora. Vols I and II. Dordrecht, Holland: D. Reidel.

Miller, J. & Chapman, R. (1981). The relation between age and the mean length of utterance in morphemes. Journal of Speech and Hearing Research, 24, 154-161.

Progovac, L. & Connell, P. (1991). Long-distance reflexives, Agr SUBJECTS, and acquisition. Proceedings of the Formal Linguistics Society of MidAmerica, Ann Arbor, MI.

Progovac, L. & Connell, P. (1992a). L2 acquisition of reflexives: Evidence for adult access to UG. Proceedings of the UWM Linguistics Symposium, Ann Arbor, MI.

Progovac, L. & Connell, P. (1992b). L2 acquisition of reflexives: Evidence for adult access to UG. Proceedings of the UWM Linguistics Symposium, Ann Arbor, MI.

Radford, A. (1988). Transformational grammar. Cambridge, UK: Cambridge University Press.

Roseberry, C. & Connell, P. (1991). Use of an invented language rule in the differentiation of normal and specific language-impaired Spanish-speaking children. Journal of Speech and Hearing Research, 34, 596-603.

Rosenberg, S. (1984). Disorders of first language development:Trends in research and theory. In E. Gollin (Ed.), Malformations of development: Biological and psychological sources and consequences. 195-237. New York: Academic Press.

Roth, F. & Clark, D. (1987). Symbolic play and social participation abilities of language-impaired and normally developing children. Journal of Speech and Hearing Disorders, 52, 17-29.

Savich, P. (1984). Anticipatory imagery in normal and language-disabled children. Journal of Speech and Hearing Research, 27, 494-502.

Stone, C.A. & Connell, P. (in press). Induction of a visul symbolic rule in children with specific language impairment. Journal of Speech and Hearing Research.

Stone, C.A. & Forman, E.A. (1988). Cognitive development in language-learning-disabled adolescents: A study of problem-solving performance in an isolation-of--variables task. Learning Disabilities Research, 3, 107-114.

Tallal, P., Stark, R., & Mellits, D. (1985a). The relationship between auditory temporal analysis and receptive language development: Evidence form studies of developmental language disorder. Neuropsychologia, 23, 527-534.

Tallal, P., Stark, R., & Mellits, D. (1985b). Identification of language-impaired children on the basis of rapid perception and production skills. Brain and Language, 25, 314-322.

Weismer, S. (1985). Constructive comprehension abilities exhibited by language-disordered children. Journal of Speech and Hearing Research, 28, 175-184.

Whitmire, B.M. & Stone, C.A. (1991). Visual imagery skills and language abilities of normal and language-learning-disabled children. Learning Disability Quarterly, 14, 49-59.

Commentary on Connell, Franks and Stone: A context and some implications

Rita C. Naremore

In discussing the contribution to this volume by Connell, Franks and Stone I have two goals in mind: 1. To place their remarks into the larger context of current theories of language acquisition, and 2. to discuss some of the implications of their remarks for clinical research, assessment of, and intervention with language disorders.

Any discussion of the current state of theory about language acquisition in this context will necessarily be both brief and superficial. However, if we are to understand the nature of the shift in focus represented by Connell et al., some acquaintance with the basic logic of Chomsky's Universal Grammar and his thinking about language acquisition is needed, because it is from this logic that Connell's work derives. Specifically, Chomsky (1986, 1988) has addressed himself to four questions about language knowledge:
1. What constitutes language knowledge?
2. How is language knowledge acquired?
3. How is language knowledge put to use?
4. What are the physical mechanisms for this system of knowledge?

In answering these questions, Chomsky has laid a new set of foundations for the study of language acquisition. These foundations may be summarized as follows: Children are born with innate knowledge of language, that is, with innate structures of mind, which may by described in terms of a Universal Grammar (UG). The UG essentially establishes "a system of conditions deriving from the human biological endowment that identifies the languages that are humanly accessible under normal conditions (Chomsky 1986, 23). In other words, UG provides the parameters within which specific languages of the world must operate. So, children are born with a biological capacity to learn certain things about language. The task of acquisition for the child then becomes one of determining which components of the UG exist in the language of the child's environment. About this process of acquisition, Chomsky says, "The transition ... takes place in a determinate fashion, with no conscious attention or choice. The transition is essentially uniform for individuals in a given speech community despite diverse experience." (Chomsky 1986, 51).

In other words, children have a "language faculty", part of the mind/brain, which acts quite automatically on the environmental input to derive the adult language of the child's speech community. There is much which remains to be elaborated about the operation of the language faculty. As Chomsky (1986, 54) admits, "there is good reason to believe that the language faculty undergoes maturation - in fact, the order and timing of this maturation appear to be rather uniform despite considerable variation in experience and other cognitive faculties." Chomsky and others have noted the possibility that the language faculty may, in fact be dependent on certain mental processes, such as memory, which have their own schedules of maturation and thus have an impact on what the language faculty is able to do for the child at any given point in time. As Chomsky (1986, 53) expresses it, "it might be that because of memory restrictions or whatever, only 'simpler' parts of the evidence that leads to attainment of the (adult language) are available to the child at early stages of acquisition ." Relatively few attempts to study language acquisition within this framework have yet appeared (see, in particular, Hyams 1986; Wexler/Manzini 1987; White 1986). There is no question, however, that the nature of acquisition studies will change if the assumptions of UG are adopted. The focus of such work is likely to shift away from longitudinal studies of children's productions toward smaller, more clearly delineated investigations of specific structures hypothesized to be part of UG, or toward carefully delineated studies of the setting of specific parameters (see, for example, the work of Chien/Wexler 1990; Grimshaw/Rosen 1990; Lust 1987; and much of Connell's previous work as seen in Franks/Connell 1991; Progovac/Connell 1991, 1992).

Connell has adroitly stated the importance of this shift in linguistic theory for studies of language impairment. The goal of our research must first be to determine whether the language impaired child has an impaired language faculty, making him unable to move smoothly from the initial state of innate UG knowledge to the final state of knowledge of a specific language. (A related, but less-discussed hypothesis is that the language impaired child comes into the world with some sort of inadequate innate knowledge.) This first goal represents a direct test of an assumption which has been taken for granted in previous research into language impairment: that the language impaired child is somehow deficient in language knowledge. As Connell's work demonstrates, if we are to continue to work on the basis of this assumption, we need to look for evidence that the language knowledge of these children is somehow incomplete or otherwise different from that of other members of their language communities. This is a clear-cut goal, but the ways of accomplishing it are by no means obvious. One cannot get directly to language knowledge by observing the child's language performance. Chomsky (1988, 47) discusses what might be considered evidence concerning the character of a child's language knowledge and the initial UG. He says it "could come from many different sources apart from judgments concerning the form and meaning of expressions: perceptual experiments, the study of acquisition and deficit or of partially invented languages such as creoles, or of literary usage or language change, neurology, biochemistry, and so on."

Connell has alluded to the difficulty for researchers of getting at language knowledge more than once in his paper. He has stated quite clearly elsewhere (Connell 1992) that standardized tests are not good measures of language knowledge. The task for those interested in understanding children's language disorders is, then, to develop measures of children's language knowledge which are minimally influenced by performance factors, to enable us to determine the nature of these children's language knowledge at any point in their development. Only by using such measures will we be able to determine whether intervention programs should be focused on helping the child activate the parameter settings appropriate to the language of the environment or on helping him develop strategies to use existing language knowledge in the service of communication. In other words, clinical practice is likely to be strongly affected by the results of acquisition research in the next few years. Intervention to teach language knowledge is a very different undertaking from intervention to teach language use. We need to determine which one we should be about, and it is in this effort that the work by Connell et al. is most likely to be useful.

Chomsky (1986, 25) addresses the issue of performance, or of how language is put to use, in the following terms: this question "breaks down into two parts: a 'perception problem' and a 'production problem.' The perception problem would be dealt with by construction of a parser that incorporates the rules of (language knowledge) along with other elements: a certain organization of memory and access, certain heuristics, and so forth." The production problem, he holds to be "considerably more obscure", involving as it does the infinite creativity of the language user and the influence of a set of psychological processes which are much more related to language ability than they are to language knowledge. Two points related to language intervention are worth making here: language disorders may, in fact, have nothing at all to do with language knowledge. The inadequate or delayed language performance we get from the child may be due to some impairment of psychological processes necessary for language use but unrelated to language knowledge. If this is so, then another set of questions must be asked: are these psychological processes impaired in ways that affect only language use, or are they impaired across the board? If the apparent impairment of, say, memory, is related only to auditory linguistic material, then what might we conclude about the nature of the "language faculty"? Perhaps these psychological processes are, in fact, part of that faculty, and affect its operation not only on the output, but also on the input. If this were the case, then we might expect to find some problems with language knowledge, since it is derived in part by the language faculty from the input. If the child has difficulty storing a sentence in short-term memory long enough for the language faculty to use it as data for parameter setting, then language knowledge might, at best, take longer to develop and at worst, be an inadequate representation of the language of the child's environment. On the other hand, if the language faculty itself is not impaired, but the impairment exists only in terms of the child's ability to retrieve or access normal language knowledge, then perhaps we are at fault for terming the child's problem a "specific language impairment". Perhaps it is a memory problem, or something else much more specific.

If we take this second possibility as a guide for our research, then our research goal becomes less clear, and the nature of what we must take as evidence in this research changes. We must first face the inescapable fact of individual variation in language use, and the arbitrary nature of the line we draw between "normal" variation and "disorders". We must then prepare to use the child's language performance as a physician might use a rash - as a fairly gross symptom of something happening in the organism which may not, in itself, be directly observable, but about which we may hypothesize with greater or lesser degrees of confidence. Continuing this analogy, as clinicians we must look for other signs which, taken in conjunction with the rash, might tell us about the nature of what is wrong. For surely the child's abnormally delayed or inappropriate language use is a symptom resulting from as wide a variety of conditions as a rash would be. As Connell points out, this realization changes the nature of clinical language assessment.

If we take Chomsky's model of acquisition as a working framework, and if we come down on the side of performance factors rather than language knowledge being at the root of children's language impairments, as Connell et al. do, then we must examine the purposes for which we assess children's language. First, it no longer seems relevant to conduct an assessment in order to locate a child on some developmental scale. If one assumes (or ascertains) that the child's knowledge of language is the same as that of a normal peer, then the developmental level of the child's language performance, being not connected with knowledge, ceases to be a focus of attention. Instead, what must be asked is which aspects of the child's knowledge are not being manifested in use, whether this problem with language use exists in all contexts or only in some contexts, and what sorts of processes might give rise to it. Assessment, then would focus on determining which processes the child was having difficulty with. In short, the only possible reason for asking questions about the developmental level of a child's language use lies in the assumption that language use reflects in some identifiable way language knowledge. In this model, finding out that a child's language use is at Brown's (1973) Stage II provides a basis for teaching the child the rules needed to proceed to Stage III. If this assumption is false, if a child's problem with language use is a result not of language knowledge but rather of a knowledge retrieval problem, then Stage II and Stage III are completely unrelated to what we must teach, and framing assessment in terms of developmental milestones is essentially a waste of time.

Furthermore, standardized tests become useless instruments, for some of the same reasons. They are not adequate measures of language knowledge, affected as they are by pragmatic, metalinguistic, and other abilities related to language use. Connell (1992) summarizes a body of emerging work demonstrating this fact. At this point, regardless of how we think about models of language acquisition, it is evident that we should abandon any ideas we might have harbored that standardized tests tell us anything about what children know about language. Since these tests have served as the anchors of the assessment enterprise for many clinicians, abandoning them may result in a period of aimless drifting. This makes it all the more necessary that we begin to relate clinical practice to acquisition theory, for it is only from theory that we are likely to be able to plot a course for the future. If we cannot use standardized tests to tell us about a child's language knowledge, then we must develop tasks that are sensitive enough, derived from theoretical descriptions of what such knowledge consists of. And if we decide that language knowledge is not at the root of a child's problem, then we must arrive at an understanding of what factors contribute to the problem, and how to assess these.

It is clear that in our clinical assessment and intervention, as well as in our clinical research, the future is not going to look like the past. The work by Connell, Franks and Stone provides us with some idea of what it might look like, and with some examples of what we must be prepared to search for. For the first time in our history, we may be able to ground our clinical practice securely in a theory of acquisition. That, in itself, will be revolutionary.

References

Brown, R. (1973). A first language: The early stages. London: Allen & Unwin.

Chien, Y-C. & Wexler, K. (1990). Children's knowledge of locality conditions in binding as evidence for the modularity of syntax and pragmatics. Language Acquisition, 1, 225-295.

Chomsky, N. (1986). Knowledge of language: Its nature, origin, and use. New York: Praeger.

Chomsky, N. (1988). Language and problems of knowledge: The Managua lectures. Cambridge: MIT Press.

Connell, P. (1992). Theoretical work in language acquisition and implications for language disorders. Paper presented to the annual meeting of the American Speech-Language-Hearing Association, San Antonio, TX.

Franks, W. & Connell, P. (1991). Binding, movement and the acquisition of anaphora. Penn Review of Linguistics, 15, 49-62.

Grimshaw, J. & Rosen, S. (1990). Knowledge and obedience: The developmental status of Binding Theory. Linguistic Inquiry, 21, 187-222.

Hyams, N. (1986). Language acquisition and the theory of parameters. Dordrecht: Reidel.

Lust, B. (Ed.) (1987). Studies in the acquisition of anaphora. Vols I and II. Dordrecht: Reidel.

Progovac, L. & Connell, P. (1991). Long-distance reflexives, Agr SUBJECTS, and acquisition. Proceedings of the Formal Linguistics Society of MidAmerica, Ann Arbor, MI.

Progovac, L. & Connell, P. (1992). L2 acquisition of reflexives: Evidence for adult access to UG. Proceedings of the UWM Linguistics Symposium, Ann Arbor, MC.

Wexler, K. & Manzini, M.R. (1987). Parameters and learnability. In T. Roeper & E. Williams (Eds.), Parameter setting. 41-76. Dordrecht: Reidel.

White, L. (1986). Implications of parametric variation for adult second language acquisition: An investigation of the pro-drop parameter. In V.J. Cook (Ed.), Experimental approaches to second language acquisition. 141-161. Oxford: Pergamon Press.

The relationship between speech-language impairments and reading disabilities

Hugh W. Catts

During the last 25 years, much interest has been directed toward children with specific reading disabilities (Malatesha/Aaron 1982; Rutter 1978; Thomson 1984). Researchers involved in this work have sought to understand why children with normal cognitive and sensory abilities have significant difficulties in learning to read and write (e.g., Aaron 1978; Miles 1984; Vellutino 1979). Initially, these difficulties were explained on the basis of visual-perceptual deficits (Herman 1959). Most current research suggests, however, that language deficits underlie most cases of reading disabilities (Kamhi/Catts 1989; Liberman/Shankweiler 1985; Stanovich 1988). In fact, some researchers have argued that in many cases reading disabilities are better characterized as a developmental language disorder (Catts 1989a; Chasty 1985; Scarborough 1990).

Also during the last 25 years, attention has been focused on children with speech-language impairments (Johnston 1982; Leonard 1987; Menyuk 1964). These children have normal cognitive and sensory abilities but exhibit significant developmental difficulties in various aspects of speech and language, including articulation, semantics, morphology, and syntax. Numerous theories have been proposed to explain these speech-language impairments (Leonard 1987). These include cognitive, perceptual, and social-interactional accounts (Johnston/Ramstad 1983; Tallal/Piercy 1973; Wyatt 1969). However, to date, no consensus has been reached concerning the underlying cause(s) of speech-language impairments.

Recently, researchers have begun to consider the relationship between speech-language impairments and reading disabilities (see Aram/Hall 1989; Catts 1991 for review). Given the proposed language basis of reading disabilities, an overlap between these developmental disabilities seems likely. Also, speech-language pathologists and other professionals have been aware for years from their clinical practice that young children with speech-language impairments often develop reading disabilities in the primary grades.

Early investigations in this area combined the retrospective analysis of clinical records and the survey of academic functioning to show a strong link between speech-language impairments and reading disabilities (Aram/Nation 1980; Hall/Tomblin 1978). More recently, a number of longitudinal studies have examined the relationship between speech-language impairments and reading problems (Bishop/Adams 1990; Magnusson/Naucler 1990; Menyuk et al. 1991; Tallal et al. 1989). In these studies, children with speech-language impairments have been identified in pre-school or kindergarten and subsequently tested for reading and academic achievement in the primary grades. The results of this work have consistently shown that speech-language impaired children are at risk for reading disabilities.

Although speech-language impaired children, as a group, may be at an increased risk for reading problems, considerable variability in reading outcome appears to exist. Some children with speech-language impairments develop reading disabilities, but others do not. At present, it is unclear what factors are the best predictors of reading outcome in speech-language impaired children. Some researchers have proposed that the severity of language disability, measured in terms of subjects' performance on standardized tests of receptive and expressive language, is closely associated with reading achievement (Bishop/Adams 1990; Tallal et al. 1989; Wilson/Risucci 1988). Others have argued, however, that nontraditional measures of language (e.g., phonological awareness) are better predictors of reading outcome in speech-language impaired children (Magnusson/Naucler 1990; Menyuk et al. 1991).

A longitudinal investigation

In order to further examine the relationship between reading disabilities and speech-language impairments, my colleagues and I recently undertook a longitudinal investigation. In this study, we identified 60 speech-language impaired children (S-LI) and 30 normally developing children in kindergarten and have followed them through the second grade. In kindergarten, subjects were given a battery of standardized speech-language tests and a measure of nonverbal abilities (Table 1). The results of this testing indicated that 43 of the S-LI subjects demonstrated significant impairments on the receptive and/or expressive language tests (referred to as the LI subgroup) and 15 subjects had primarily speech articulation impairments (SI subgroup). All subjects showed normal nonverbal abilities and hearing acuity.

Tab. 1: Standardized tests administered in kindergarten

Receptive Language
Peabody Picture Vocabulary Test
Token Test for Children
Test of Language Development - 2: Grammatical Understanding
Expressive Language
Expressive One Word Picture Vocabulary Test
Structured Photographic Expressive Language Test
TOLD: Sentence Imitation and Grammatical Closure
Articulation
Goldman-Fristoe Test of Articulation
Nonverbal Abilities
Wechsler Preschool and Primary Scale of Intelligence: Block Design and Picture Completion

In addition to the standardized testing, subjects were administered a battery of experimental language measures. These involved measures of what has been referred to as phonological processing (Catts 1989b; Wagner/Torgesen 1987) and included measures of phonological awareness and retrieval of phonological codes from memory. Measures like these have been shown for some time to be related to reading in wide cross sections of children (e.g., Bradley/Bryant 1985; Mann/Liberman 1984; Wolf 1986), but have only recently been employed in studies of S-LI children (Magnusson/Naucler 1990; Tallal et al. 1989). Phonological awareness was assessed by the DELETION and BLENDING tasks. In the DELETION task, subjects were required to delete the first syllable or phoneme from a word and say the remaining sound sequence. In the BLENDING task, subjects blended together and pronounced a series of syllables or phonemes. Retrieval of phonological codes was measured by three rapid automatized naming tasks (Wolf 1986). These assessed subjects' ability to rapidly name or retrieve the phonological name codes of a series of common objects (RANOBJ), colors (RANCOL), or colored animals (RANAN) that were repeatedly displayed on stimulus cards. The time taken to complete the task was the index of performance.

In first and second grade, the Word Identification and Word Attack subtests of the *Woodcock Reading Mastery Tests-R* were administered to the subjects. These subtests measured subjects' ability to read a list of words or pseudowords presented in isolation. In second grade, subjects also received the *Gray Oral Reading Test-Revised (GORT-R)*. On the latter test, subjects received an overall score as well as separate scores for reading comprehension and speed/accuracy of word recognition in context.

Two S-LI subjects moved out of district prior to the first grade and one S-LI and one control subject moved prior to second grade. A large proportion of the S-LI subjects (43%) repeated their kindergarten year or were placed in developmental first grade classes (D-1 classes) prior to going to first grade. D-1 classes have recently been instituted in many school districts in the United States to allow young or slowly developing children (often vaguely defined) an extra year of maturation before first grade. Children in D-1 programs repeat kindergarten classes during half of the school day and attend nonacademic portions of first grade (e.g., music) during the remainder. For the above subjects, the results of the standardized language tests and measures of phonological processing from their second year of kindergarten (or D-1 classes) were used for data analyses. Also, the latter subjects had not completed second grade at the time of this report. Thus, second grade reading data were available only for the regularly matriculating subjects.

The group means and standard deviations for reading achievement in first and second grades are displayed in Table 2. As can be observed, the S-LI subjects demonstrated poorer reading achievement than the normal control subjects in both first and second grades. However, further inspection reveals that these differences are primarily the result of the poor performance of the subgroup of subjects with language impairments (i.e., LI subgroup). Many of the LI subjects were demonstrating reading difficulties in first and second grades, and as a group, performed significantly less well than the control subjects ($\underline{p}<.01$). The children with speech articulation problems alone (i.e., SI subgroup), on the other hand, generally had reading scores within the normal range and did not differ significantly from the control subjects ($\underline{p}>.05$).

Table 3 displays the correlational coefficients between reading achievement in first grade and measures of speech-language and phonological processing in kindergarten. In this analysis, subjects' performances on standardized tests were partitioned into measures of receptive language (RECL), expressive language (EXPL), articulation abilities (ARTIC) and nonverbal abilities

Tab. 2: Mean standard scores (and standard deviations) on tests of reading achievements for the normal control and S-LI groups, as well as for the LI and SI subgroups within the S-LI group.

	Normal	S-LI	LI	SI
First Grade	N = 30	N = 58	N = 43	N = 15
Word Id	110.4 (15.4)	95.8 (17.3)	91.4 (16.3)	108.3 (14.0)
Word Attack	99.1 (14.2)	86.4 (14.3)	83.3 (13.8)	95.5 (14.0)
Second Grade	N = 29	N = 32	N = 20	N = 12
Word Id	107.6 (14.5)	96.7 (18.1)	90.1 (18.4)	107.8 (11.1)
Word Attack	97.0 (14.9)	86.1 (15.7)	80.0 (16.3)	96.3 (7.5)
Gray Oral Reading	97.7 (13.8)	89.9 (18.1)	79.6 (13.4)	107.0 (9.9)

Tab. 3: Correlation coefficients between kindergarten measures and first grade reading achievement (N=58)

	Word ID	Word Attack
Deletion	.59	.60
Blending	.45	.52
Rapid Naming of Animals	.52	.41
Rapid Naming of Objects	.52	.44
Rapid Naming of Colors	.48	.36
Listening Comprehension	.37	.25
Nonverbal IQ	NS	NS

Correlation coefficients for rapid naming tasks expressed in terms of absolute values.

(NONVERBAL). As indicated, no significant relationship was observed between reading achievement and articulation or between reading and non-verbal abilities. Low-moderate correlations were found between reading achievement and receptive and expressive language measures. Higher correlations, however, were generally obtained for the phonological processing measures, with the DELETION task showing the highest correlation with the Word Id and Word Attack subtests.

In order to examine the relative contributions of the kindergarten measures in explaining the variance in reading achievement, multiple regression analyses were performed. In these analyses, omnibus measures of phonological awareness and rapid automatized naming were employed. The omnibus measure of phonological awareness (PA) was created by first converting subjects' performance on the DELETION and BLENDING tasks to z-scores and then combining and averaging these scores. A similar procedure was used to convert the three measures of rapid automatized naming into an omnibus measure (RAN). Also included in these analyses were the omnibus measures of expressive (EXPL) and receptive language (RECL). In order to simplify the presentation and discussion of the results, measures of articulation and nonverbal abilities were not considered. As noted above, these measures were not found to be significantly correlated with reading achievement.

The results of the regression analyses indicated that when entered first, the measures of phonological processing accounted for 46% of the variance in Word Id and 42% of the variance in Word Attack (see Table 4). Once the measures of phonological processing were entered into the regression analyses, neither RECL nor EXPL accounted for a significant amount of variance in the reading measures. When measures of language ability (i.e., RECL & EXPL) were entered first, they did account for a significant amount of the variance. A large amount of variance, however, remained and was explained in part by the phonological processing measures (see Table 4). These results thus indicate that measures of phonological processing better accounted for variance in first grade reading achievement than measures of language ability/disability.

Table 5 displays the correlations between reading achievement in second grade and speech-language and phonological processing measures in kindergarten. As can be observed, the measures of phonological processing continue to be good predictors of reading achievement. Measures of phonological awareness and rapid automatized naming showed moderate to moderately high correlations with all measures of reading achievement in second grade. As was generally the case in first grade, measures of receptive and expressive language were less correlated with measures of word recog-

Tab. 4: R^2 change in fixed order multiple regression analyses for first grade reading achievement

	Reading Achievement	
Steps in regression	Word Id	Word Attack
1. PA	.32	.37
2. RAN	.14	.05*
3. RECL	NS	NS
4. EXPL	NS	NS
3. EXPL	NS	NS
4. RECL	NS	NS
1. EXPL	.14	.24
2. RECL	NS	NS
3. PA	.18	.15
4. RAN	.13	.05*
3. RAN	.19	.09
4. PA	.11	.11

* $p < .05$, all remaining significant R^2 $p < .01$.

Tab. 5: Pearson product-moment correlation coefficients between standardized tests of language and measures of phonological processing administered in kindergarten and reading achievement measured in 2nd grade

	Word ID	Word Attack	GORT-R (SA)[a]	GORT-R (C)
RECL	.39	.43	.62	.74
EXPL	.45	.46	.67	.71
ART	NS	NS	NS	NS
NONVERBAL	NS	NS	NS	NS
DELETION	.57	.64	.64	.64
BLENDING	.32*	.57	.48	.56
RANAN[b]	.78	.68	.61	.54
RANOBJ	.76	.74	.74	.58
RANCOL	.69	.65	.66	.54

[a] S/A = Speed/Accuracy C = Comprehension
[b] Pearson r for rapid naming tasks are expressed in absolute values
* $P < .05$, all other significant correlations $p < .01$

nition in isolation (i.e., Word Id and Word Attack) than were the phonological processing tasks. Receptive and expressive language measures, however, were found to have comparable, and in some cases, higher correlations with the GORT-R reading scores than that found for the phonological processing measures. These various relationships were further borne out in regression analyses.

The results of the fixed order multiple regression analyses for second grade reading achievement are displayed in Table 6. A similar pattern of results to that in first grade was obtained for the measures of word recognition, that is, Word Id, Word Attack, and additionally in second grade, GORT-R Speed/Accuracy. In regression analyses involving these measures, phonological processing tasks proved to be better predictors than measures of language ability/disability. Phonological processing tasks accounted for a large proportion of the variance in word recognition measures, and once the effects of these tasks had been parcelled out, EXPL and RECL accounted for none or very little of the remaining variance. If, on the other hand, lan-

Tab. 6: R^2 changes in fixed order multiple regression analyses for second grade reading achievement

Steps in regression	Reading achievement			
	Word Id	Word Attack	GORT-R (S/A)[a]	GORT-R (C)
1. PA	.24	.44	.38	.44
2. RAN	.43	.26	.26	.12
3. RECL	NS	NS	NS	.11
4. EXPL	NS	.05*	NS	NS
3. EXPL	NS	.07	NS	NS
4. RECL	NS	NS	NS	.07*
1. EXPL	.20	.21	.44	.50
2. RECL	NS	NS	NS	.11
3. PA	NS	.22	NS	NS
4. RAN	.43	.31	.17	NS
3. RAN	.44	.33	NS	NS
4. PA	NS	.20	.17	NS

[a] S/A = Speed/Accuracy C = Comprehension

* $p < .05$, all other significant R^2 changes $p < .01$.

guage measures were entered first, measures of phonological processing continued to account for a significant portion of the variance in word recognition measures.

A different pattern of results was obtained for the measure of reading comprehension on the GORT-R. In this case, the language measures proved to be better predictors. The standardized language measures combined to accounted for 61% of the variance in reading comprehension. As shown in Table 6, when EXPL was entered first, it explained 50% of the variance and RECL accounted for an additional 11%. If the language variables were entered in the reverse order, only RECL accounted for a significant amount of variance in reading comprehension (56%). Regardless of the order of entry, once the effects of these language measures had been partialed out, R^2 changes for the phonological processing measures were nonsignificant. When the phonological processing measures were entered first, they accounted for a large proportion of the variance, but 11% was still attributable to RECL. These results indicate, therefore, that variability in reading comprehension was best accounted for by individual differences in language abilities/disabilities, especially receptive language abilities.

Speech-language impairments and reading disabilities

The results from the present study further document the relationship between speech-language impairments and reading disabilities. Our findings indicate that children with speech-language impairments are at risk for reading disabilities. Many of our S-LI subjects had begun by the early school grades to fall behind their normal peers in reading achievement. These deficits were observed both in measures of word recognition and reading comprehension. Whereas many of our S-LI subjects were experiencing reading problems, others were not. Our results indicated that approximately 50% of the S-LI subjects were reading within normal limits in the first and second grades. Other studies have reported similar percentages of unimpaired readers among their speech-language impaired subjects (Aram/Ekelman/Nation 1984; Garvey/Gorden 1973; Padget 1988; Tallal et al. 1989; Wilson/Risucci 1988).

What factors account for the variability in reading outcome among S-LI children? Our findings indicate that certain speech-language abilities are related to reading achievement, while others are not. Our results indicate that articulation ability may bear little relationship to reading achievement. Correlations between articulation ability and reading achievement were found to be low and nonsignificant both in the first and second grades. In addition, children with articulation impairments alone (i.e., SI subgroup) consistently performed at or above the level of the normal control group in reading achievement. These findings are consistent with numerous other studies that have failed to observe a relationship between articulation impairments (at least as traditionally defined; but see Catts 1989b) and reading disabilities (Bishop/Adams 1990; Hall/Tomblin 1978; Levi et al. 1982).

Whereas articulation abilities were found to be unrelated to reading achievement, measures of expressive/receptive language and phonological processing were observed to be associated with reading outcome. The specific relationships of these measures to reading achievement, however, depended on how reading was measured. When reading was assessed in terms of word recognition, both in isolation and in context, measures of phonological processing proved to be the best predictors of reading outcome. Once phonological awareness and rapid naming were considered in regression analyses, measures of expressive/receptive language accounted for very little variance in tests of word recognition.

A large body of research involving children with no history of speech-language impairments has also documented a relationship between phonological processing abilities and word recognition (Catts 1989b; Wagner/Torgesen 1987). This work has shown that deficits in phonological awareness and retrieval of phonological codes often precede and are closely associated with problems in learning to recognize printed words (e.g., Bradley/Bryant 1985; Wolf 1986). On the basis of this research, it has been proposed that phonological processing deficits lie at the core of reading disabilities in young children (Catts 1989b; Stanovich 1988). Our results as well as those of others (Magnusson/Naucler 1990; Menyuk et al. 1991) indicate that these same deficits may also account for word recognition difficulties in S-LI children.

In the present study, phonological processing abilities were also found to be related to a measure of reading comprehension given in second grade. This relationship, however, was not independent of other language abilities. It was observed that standardized measures of language abilities, especially receptive language ability, accounted for individual differences in reading comprehension over and above that accounted for by phonological processing measures. Such a finding would certainly be predicted on the basis of most theories of reading comprehension (e.g., Perfetti 1985). Comprehension of printed text requires an adequate ability to process the semantic-syntactic aspects of language. Thus it is not surprising that the degree of language ability or severity of language disability, especially receptive language ability/disability, was found to be related to reading comprehension. There was uncertainty, however, whether or not this relationship would be observed as early as the second grade. Reading comprehension in the early grades is heavily dependent on word recognition skills and somewhat less so on higher language abilities (Stanovich/Cunningham/Feeman 1984). Nevertheless, our results suggest that as early as the second grade, the language deficits of S-LI children may adversely affect their reading comprehension. We plan to follow our subjects into the later elementary school grades. As we do, we expect that the relationship between language abilities and reading comprehension will become even more apparent.

In conclusion, our results indicate a strong relationship between speech-language impairments and reading disabilities. This relationship, however, does not appear to be a static one, but rather one that changes over time. In the early school grades, when instruction and assessment focus on word recognition, many S-LI children will experience difficulties in reading. Whereas children's performance on standardized language tests may be related to word recognition problems, phonological processing deficits appear to be better predictors of these problems. S-LI children with good phonological awareness and retrieval abilities will tend to be good word decoders, whereas those with problems in phonological processing will tend to have difficulties in word recognition. As S-LI children progress in school and more focus in instruction and assessment is placed on reading comprehension, a different relationship will emerge. At this time, reading success/failure will become more closely related to degree of language ability/disability and less related to phonological processing abilities. Children with the most severe language problems will likely have the greatest difficulties in reading, whereas those with less severe language problems will show more success in reading. Also, when more emphasis is placed on reading comprehension, some S-LI children may show reading difficulties for the first time. These children will be those who demonstrate good phonological processing and word recognition skills, but who continue to have language problems. As demands in reading are placed on higher level language abilities, these children will fall behind their normal peers. Evidence from the present study suggests this process may begin as early as the second grade.

References

Aaron, P.G. (1978). Dyslexia, an imbalance in cerebral information processing strategies. Perceptual and Motor Skills, 47, 699-706.

Aaron, P.G., Olsen, J., & Baker, C. (1985). The dyslexic college student: Is he also dysphasic? Cognitive Neuropsychology, 2, 115-147.

Aram, D.M., Ekelman, B.L., & Nation, J.E. (1984). Preschoolers with language disorders: 10 years later. Journal of Speech and Hearing Research, 27, 232-244.

Aram, D.M. & Hall, N. (1989). Longitudinal follow-up of children with preschool communication disorders: Treatment implications. School Psychology Review, 18, 487-501.

Aram, D.M. & Nation, J. (1980). Preschool language disorders and subsequent language and academic difficulties. Journal of Communication Disorders, 13, 159-179.

Bishop, D. & Adams, C. (1990). A prospective study of the relationship between specific language impairment, phonological disorders and reading retardation. Journal of Child Psychology and Psychiatry, 31, 1027-1050.

Bradley, L. & Bryant, P. (1985). Rhyme and reason in reading and spelling. International Academy for Research in Learning Disabilities Monograph Series, No. 1. Ann Arbor, MI: University of Michigan Press.

Catts, H. (1989a). Defining dyslexia as a developmental language disorder. Annals of Dyslexia, 39, 50-64.

Catts, H. (1989b). Phonological processing deficits and reading disabilities. In A. Kamhi & H. Catts (Eds.), Reading disabilities: A developmental language perspective. 101-132. Austin, TX: Pro-Ed.

Catts, H. (1991). Early identification of reading disabilities. Topics in Language Disorder, 12, 1-16.

Chasty, H. (1985). What is dyslexia? A developmental language perspective. In M. Snowling (Ed.), Children's written language difficulties: Assessment and management. 11-28. Windsor: NFER-Nelson Publishing Co.

Doehring, D., Trites, R., Patel, P., & Fiedorowicz, C. (1981). Reading disabilities: The interaction of reading, language, and neuropsychological deficits. New York: Academic Press.

Garvey, M. & Gorden, N. (1973). A follow-up study of children with disorders of speech development. British Journal of Communication Disorders, 8, 17-28.

Hall, P. & Tomblin, J. (1978). A follow-up study of children with articulation and language disorders. Journal of Speech and Hearing Disorders, 43, 227-241.

Herman, K. (1959). Reading disability. Copenhagen: Munksgaard.

Ingram, T.T.S., Mason, M., & Blackburn, I. (1970). A retrospective study of 82 children with reading disabilities. Developmental Medical Child Neurology, 12, 271-281.

Johnston, J. (1982). Interpreting the Leiter IQ: Performance profiles of young normal and language-disordered children. Journal of Speech and Hearing Research, 25, 291-296.

Johnston, J. & Ramstad, V. (1983). Cognitive development in preadolescent language impaired children. British Journal of Disorders of Communication, 18, 49-55.

Kamhi, A. & Catts, H. (1986). Toward an understanding of developmental language and reading disorders. Journal of Speech and Hearing Disorders, 51, 337-347.

Kamhi, A. & Catts, H. (1989). Reading disabilities: A developmental language perspective. Austin, TX: Pro-Ed.

Leonard, L.B. (1987). Is specific language impairment a useful construct? In S. Rosenberg (Ed.), Advances in applied psycholinguistics. Vol 1: Disorders of first-language development. 1-39. New York: Cambridge.

Levi, G., Capozzi, F., Fabrizi, A., & Sechi, E. (1982). Language disorders and prognosis for reading disabilities in developmental age. Perceptual and Motor Skills, 54, 1119-1122.

Liberman, I. & Shankweiler, D. (1985). Phonology and the problems of learning to read and write. Remedial and Special Education, 6, 8-17.

Magnusson, E. & Naucler, K. (1990). Reading and spelling in language-disordered children — linguistic and metalinguistic prerequisites: report on a longitudinal study. Clinical Linguistics and Phonetics, 4, 49-61.

Malatesha, R.N. & Aaron, P.G. (1982). Reading disorders: Varieties and treatments. New York: Academic Press.

Mann, V. & Liberman, I. (1984). Phonological awareness and verbal short-term memory. Journal of Learning Disabilities, 17, 592-599.

Menyuk, P. (1964). Comparison of grammar of children with functionally deviant and normal speech. Journal of Speech and Hearing Research, 7, 109-121.

Menyuk, P., Chesnick, M., Liebergott, J.W., Korngold, B., D'Agostino, R., & Belanger, A. (1991). Predicting reading problems in at-risk children. Journal of Speech and Hearing Research, 34, 893-903.

Miles, T.R. (1984). Dyslexia: The pattern of difficulties. Springfield, IL: Thomas Books.

Padget, S.Y. (1988). Speech- and language-impaired three and four year olds: A five year follow-up study. In R.L. Masland & M.W. Masland (Eds.), Prevention of reading failure. 52-77. Parkton, MD: York Press.

Perfetti, C. (1985). Reading ability. New York: Oxford.

Rutter, M. (1978). Prevalence and types of dyslexia. In A. Benton & D. Pearl (Eds.), Dyslexia: An appraisal of current knowledge. 145-167. New York and London: Oxford University Press.

Rutter, M. & Yule, W. (1973). The concept of specific reading retardation. Journal of Child Psychology and Psychiatry, 16, 181-197.

Scarborough, H. (1990). Very early language deficits in dyslexic children. Child Development, 61, 1728-1743.

Stanovich, K. (1988). The right and the wrong places to look for the cognitive locus of reading disability. Annals of Dyslexia, 38, 154-180.

Stanovich, K., Cunningham, A., & Feeman, D. (1984). Intelligence, cognitive skills, and early reading progress. Reading Research Quarterly, 19, 278-300.

Tallal, P. & Piercy, M. (1973). Developmental aphasia: Impaired rate of non-verbal processing as a function of sensory modality. Neuropsychologia, 11, 389-398.

Tallal, P., Curtiss, S., & Kaplan, R. (1989). The San Diego longitudinal study: Evaluating the outcomes of preschool impairment in language development. Final Report, NINCDS.

Thomson, M. (1984). Developmental dyslexia: Its nature, assessment, and remediation. London: Edward Arnold.

Vellutino, F. (1979). Dyslexia: Theory and research. Cambridge, MA: MIT Press.

Wagner, R. & Torgesen, J. (1987). The nature of phonological processing and its causal role in the acquisition of reading skills. Psychological Bulletin, 101, 192-212.

Wilson, B. & Risucci, D. (1988). The early identification of developmental language disorders and the prediction of the acquisition of reading skills. In R. Masland & M. Masland (Eds.), Preschool prevention of reading failure. 187-203. Parkton, MD: York Press.

Wolf, M. (1986). Rapid alternating stimulus naming in the developmental dyslexias. Brain and Language, 27, 360-379.

Wyatt, G. (1969). Language learning and communication disorders in children. New York: Free Press.

Commentary on Catts: How to characterize continuity between preschool language disorders and reading disorders at school age

Dorothy M. Aram

Prediction of reading disorders among preschoolers with language disorders

That many, probably the majority of preschoolers with language disorders subsequently experience reading problems at school-age is now well-established. Depending on the population studied and the definitions of language and reading disorders used, numerous studies have reported that between 40% and 70% of children with preschool language disorders have subsequent reading disorders (see Aram/Hall 1989 for a review of over 20 of these studies). What has not been well understood is what aspects of preschool language disorders are related to subsequent reading disorders or how to predict specifically which language disordered children are at risk for later reading disorders and why.

Until recently, the primary predictors of later reading difficulty among language disordered children targeted extra-linguistic characteristics, for example nonverbal intelligence, social competence or neurological status (Aram/Hall 1989). Only recently have studies begun to examine the linguistic or cognitive factors common to both. An initial, but largely unsupported hypothesis was that because a common phonological system underlies both reading and speaking, early disorders of speech would be associated with later reading problems. Catts' findings reported here provide further evidence to a growing number of studies demonstrating that early speech disorders alone do not predict reading problems (Bishop/Adams 1990; Hall/Tomblin 1978; Levi et al. 1982; Magnusson/Naucler 1990). A relationship between more pervasive language comprehension and production deficits and later reading problems has been evidenced in several studies (e.g. Levi et al. 1982; Menyuk et al. 1991; Scarborough 1990), yet the actual nature of this relationship between more generalized language disorders and later reading problems has been largely unspecified.

It is precisely in addressing this issue - characterizing the actual relationship between preschool language disorders and later reading disorders - that the data reported by Catts is of importance. As one of the few prospective longitudinal studies to examine this issue, Catts' findings aid our theoretical understanding of the connection between earlier appearing language disorders and later emerging reading disorders, and help us clinically to identify and intervene with young language disordered children at risk for reading disorders. Catts has told us that similar to children without language disorders, it is the young language disordered child's ability on phonological processing tasks, not tasks of lexical or syntactic comprehension or production, that best predicts decoding. It is not until reading comprehension measures are used to define reading disorders, that earlier lexical or syntactic deficits are helpful in predicting later reading problems. Catts has also been in the forefront of characterizing reading disorders as a "developmental language disorder that involves a deficit(s) in phonological processing" (Catts 1989, p. 50). In contrast to others who classify reading disorders as developmental language disorders, Catts has been careful throughout his series of publications to specify the aspect of language involved (phonological processing), rather than globally lumping reading disorders with other forms of developmental language disorders. The importance of taking Catts' lead and more narrowly defining reading disorders as phonological processing disorders, as opposed to undifferentiated developmental language disorders, is a topic expanded upon in the following section.

Problems in characterizing reading disabilities as developmental language disorders

At least two major problems are apparent in trying to characterize reading disabilities as developmental language disorders, without specifying that aspect of language involved, namely phonological processing. The first is that the overlap between language disordered and reading disabled populations is not isomorphic. The second is that characterization as a language disorder is too broad to be helpful, but characterization as a phonological processing disorder more adequately defines the involved domain. Turning to each of these issues below.

If one's view of reading disabilities is as a developmental language disorder, then one corollary would be that all reading disabled children have or had language disorders and that all language disordered children will have reading disabilities. Clearly this is not the case. Although the specific proportion varies among studies, all follow-up studies of children with early language disorders report a group of children who do not have later reading problems (Aram/Hall 1989). Similarly, a substantial portion of reading disabled children have not been identified as having earlier or concomitant language disorders. How then does one differentiate between those children having both a language and a reading problem and those having one but not the other, and more importantly how are those children with one but not both different from those children with both? Are they all language disordered? Viewing reading disorders as disorders in phonological processing specifies that it is only when a subset of language processes are involved that a language disordered child will be reading deficient. Such a specification makes it clear why all children with language disorders do not have reading problems.

Catts' data have suggested that it is a language disordered child's phonological processing ability that best determines whether or not reading will be disabled, not the child's more traditionally defined language comprehension or production abilities. Similarly, numerous studies with children not identified as having language disorders also have shown that these children's ability on various phonological processing tasks best predicts reading ability. Viewing these children as having disorders of phonological processing would appear to clarify rather than cloud the relationship. One might ask then, how does going to a higher level of generalization and classifying phonological processing deficits as all having developmental language disorders clarify the relationship?

One retort to this question is that phonological processing is one specific aspect of language or language learning, and therefore a deficit in phonological processing by definition is also a language disorder. The level of generality thus appealed to through this argument is so broad, that it is often empty of much meaning - except perhaps to distinguish language from visual perceptual processes. A parallel argument would be that it is better to characterize developmental language disorders as learning disorders. Clearly language disorders are one form of learning disorder, and for some purposes such a broad classification may be useful - for example for including language therapy within learning disabled services. But does defining language disorders at this level of generality further our understanding of either language or other forms of learning disabilities? Only if one is predominantly interested in broad, general relationships. That a child has a developmental language disorder does not go far in explaining differences in outcome related to reading ability; that a child has difficulty with phonological processing does - with or without an accompanying more traditionally defined "language disorder". Thus characterizing incipient reading disabled children as having phonological processing deficits as Catts has done, would appear to hold much more predictive and explanatory power than stating that they have developmental language disorders.

Nonetheless, the fact that the risk for reading disorders is substantially higher in populations with developmental language disorders than among children developing language normally, suggests that there are factors beyond phonological processing that place language disordered children at higher risk for reading disabilities. Yet Catts' data, demonstrating lexical and syntactic comprehension and production skills as measured by the tasks described, are not predictive of decoding. The question is how might we proceed in attempting to understand why language disordered children (i.e. children with lexical and syntactic comprehension and production disorders) are at higher risk for reading deficits than are children without language disorder, even though the lexical and syntactic deficits have not yet been found to predict reading decoding skills.

Additional approaches for identifying relations between language disorders and reading deficits

Three additional approaches are suggested as possibilities for further advancing understanding of why children with lexical and syntactic comprehension and production deficits were not found to be at risk for decoding deficits. The first approach is to confine analysis of predictive relationships only to young language disordered children who do encounter decoding deficits. Although we know that a range of decoding abilities are presented by language disordered children, examination of only those children who do have decoding problems may reveal relationships not yet appreciated.

A second approach would aim to address the hypothesized heterogeneous nature of children with developmental language disorders (Aram/Nation 1975; Rapin/Allen 1983) and suggests that the same set of relationships between early status and outcome may not hold for all language disordered children. From this perspective, it may be that different relationships exist for different subtypes of language disordered children. It may be that, for example, phonological awareness measures are more highly predictive of reading decoding among language disordered children with predominantly language comprehension disorders; or that rapid automatized naming tasks may be more predictive of reading decoding among language disordered children whose disorders are predominantly output disorders involving lexical retrieval and possibly syntactic production. Further, a subtype approach to establishing relationships between early predictors and later outcome may identify specific aspects of language comprehension and production that are predictive of reading decoding, relationships potentially obscured by averaging across all language disordered children as if they present comparable language and reading deficits. Catts' data presented here provide evidence that looking for relationships between subgroups of language disordered children and differing phonological processing tasks may be a productive research avenue. He has shown us in Table 4 (p. 173) that when phonological awareness is entered first into a regression analysis that the perfomance of the language disordered children on the Rapid Automatized Naming Test explained an additional 14% of the variance. The importance of this is that these two measures, the phonological awareness and rapid naming tasks, were sensitive to different phonological processing abilities in different children. How these children's phonological processing is related to their specific pattern of language deficit is an important question to address.

A third approach for further addressing the relationship between early language disorders and later reading disorders arises from the premise that it may be that the reason phonological awareness tasks predict later decoding is that the phonological awareness tasks used require metalinguistic ability beyond what was assessed for the receptive and expressive language tasks. As is being explored by Chesnick, Menyuk and collaborators (1992; and Menyuk this volume), it is possible that had more metalinguistic lexical or syntactic comprehension tasks been employed, stronger relationships between early syntactic and lexical abilities and later decoding may have been revealed.

Although each of these avenues requires a different study, Catts' data advances our understanding of how to predict reading disorders among language disordered children in at least two crucial respects. First and for the present, it appears that tests of phonological awareness are the best predictors of decoding among language disordered children; and second, lexical and syntactic comprehension and production deficits may relate to later difficulty with reading comprehension. Catts has helped us go this far. Can he help us go a little farther with his uncommon, longitudinal data base?

Future requests

Given the rarity and potential richness of prospective longitudinal studies addressing these issues, the existing studies need to be reported in as much detail as possible, to permit better interpretation and clinical application of these data and to prepare the base for further studies. In future reports, Catts is encouraged to share with us more information in three areas.

The first is more detailed description of the speech disordered children's speech. That children with speech disorders do not typically have decoding disorders continues to seem counter-intuitive, despite the growing evidence against such a relationship. What is missing from all studies, including Catts', is a sufficiently enough detailed description of the speech disorders presented to allow interpretation by the reader as to whether the disorder is predominantly articulatory or motor speech based, or if it is a disorder of phonological representation. Although Magnusson/Naucler (1990) suggested that more articulatory-based phonological errors may not be associated with later reading problems while more rule-based errors may, this writer is aware of no studies which have actually detailed such a relationship, much less detailed the nature of "speech" disorders among the children studied. It may be that speech disorders are not related to later decoding, yet until the lack of such a relationship has been demonstrated among a group of significantly phonologically impaired children (as opposed to articulatorily impaired), the issue is not settled.

A second area in which we might ask for more, is to examine specific aspects of language as each relates to reading, rather than to collapse across all receptive and all expressive language measures. Here, for example, the relationship between expressive vocabulary, as measured by the *Expressive One Word Picture Vocabulary Test*, and the rapid automatized naming tasks may be of more interest than the relationship between a composite receptive or expressive language function, which only blunts any differences that may be present between different aspects of language and reading.

A final hope for future reports of Catts' data is to be explicit about the natural reading history of individual children. High on the wish list is to know what the overlap is between children who had decoding deficits at first grade and also second grade; and what the overlap is in children having both decoding and reading comprehension disorders at second grade. Reporting data by individual subjects, when the sample size permits as for the second grade group, allows us to see relationships not captured by statistical treatment and opens the search to all readers. While the present volume probably is not the best forum for raw data, other contexts may better permit this level of detail to be shared.

Important unanswered questions remain to be unraveled bearing on the relationship between speech-language impairments and reading disabilities. Catts' work has given us predictors which have present-day application and has steered us in productive directions for continued research into this important relationship.

References

Aram, D.M. & Hall, N.E. (1989). Longitudinal follow-up of children with preschool communication disorders: Treatment implications. School Psychology Review, 18, 487-501.

Aram, D.M. & Nation, J.E. (1975). Patterns of language behavior in children with developmental language disorders. Journal of Speech and Hearing Research, 18, 229-241.

Bishop, D.V.M. & Adams, C. (1990). A prospective study of the relationship between specific language impairment, phonological disorders and reading retardation. Journal of Child Psychology and Psychiatry, 31, 1027-1050.

Catts, H.W. (1989). Defining dyslexia as a developmental language disorder. Annals of Dyslexia, 39, 50-64.

Chesnick, M.A., Menyuk, P., D'Agostino, R., & Belanger, A. (1992). Development of metalinguistic skills in children of varying language ability. Paper presented at the American Speech-Language Hearing Association Meetings, San Antonio, Texas.

Hall, P.K. & Tomblin, J.B. (1978). A follow-up study of children with articulation and language disorders. Journal of Speech and Hearing Disorders, 43, 227-241.

Levi, G., Capozzi, F., Fabrizi, A., & Sechi, E. (1982). Language disorders and prognosis for reading disabilities in developmental age. Perceptual and Motor Skills, 54, 1119-1122.

Magnusson, E. & Naucler, K. (1990). Can preschool data predict language-disordered children's reading and spelling at school? Folia Phoniatria, 42, 277-282.

Menyuk, P., Chesnick, M., Liebergott, J.W., Korngold, B., D'Agostino, R., & Belanger, A. (1991). Predicting reading problems in at-risk children. Journal of Speech and Hearing Research, 34, 893-903.

Scarborough, H.S. (1990). Very early language deficits in dyslexic children. Child Development, 61, 1728-1743.

Rapin, I. & Allen, D.A. (1983). Developmental language disorders: Nosologic considerations. In V. Kirk (Ed.), Neuropsychology of language, reading, and spelling. 155-184. New York: Academic Press.

Part 2:

Disorders of written language (developmental dyslexia)

Implications of the Pittsburgh Study for issues of risk

Charles A. Perfetti
Mara C. Georgi
Isabel Beck

"Who is at risk in learning to read?" This question invites an encompassing answer, because the risk factors extend beyond cognitive and instructional problems to factors of opportunity and literacy environments. In fact, it is likely that the cognitive risk factors and the noncognitive risk factors interact in some pernicious ways. Children at great risk due to lowered opportunities for literacy support are those for whom the cognitive and instructional factors will turn out to be most important.

We will focus in this chapter on what we see as the most critical cognitive component for learning to read - the acquisition of the alphabetic principle. The children from whom the alphabetic principle remains hidden are those children most likely to fail at learning to read.

This should not be news. The alphabetic principle, the principle of writing system design that associates meaningless graphic units with meaningless speech units, is the key to reading in an orthographic writing system, a fact widely recognized, thanks to the arguments of Liberman/Shankweiler (1979), Gough/Hillinger (1980), and others. Both the logic of writing systems and a wealth of data underpin this claim (see Bradley/Bryant 1991; Byrne 1991; Ehri 1991 and other work in collections edited by Brady/Shankweiler 1991 and Rieben/Perfetti 1991). Furthermore, the data are increasingly clear on the critical event allowing children to discover and use the alphabetic principle - the development of phonemic awareness (Bryant/Bradley 1980; Lundberg/Frost/Petersen 1988; Mann 1991; Treiman/Baron 1983). To use the principle that letters associate with phonemes, the child must acquire some awareness of the phonemes.

Some children will acquire the alphabetic principle on their own. Children who are advantaged by literate homes may be in a good position to discover the alphabetic principle, and others will discover it despite instruction that does not make it especially easy. Still, other children will not discover the alphabetic principle and their ability to read will be severely hampered.

Some years ago, we became interested in a couple of critical questions connected with phonemic awareness and reading instruction. We were intrigued by what we saw as a paradox. We were convinced that phonemic awareness was logically necessary for learning how to read, despite the fact that, at that time, there was no convincing evidence that this was the case. (The evidence was correlational.) At the same time, we wondered, as had Morais/Cary/Alegria/Bertelson (1979), where a child could obtain phonemic awareness outside of literacy. There is little either in the structure of language or in the child's environment to make such awareness inevitable. So we set out to investigate our own hypothesis, which was that a fairly dim and inexplicit form of phonemic awareness was necessary for making initial progress at true reading, whereas reading *itself* was necessary for a fuller blossoming of explicit phonemic awareness. We were also interested in an instructional angle on this question. Since a program that explicitly teaches decoding - in effect teaching the alphabetic principle - appears to use phonemic awareness, an interesting question arises: Will children in such a program show more or less dependence on early phonemic awareness than children not taught directly? On the one hand, such children may fail to grasp the key instructional events without phonemic awareness. On the other hand, perhaps they would be less dependent upon early phonemic awareness if the instructional method itself promoted its acquisition.

Our attempts to answer these questions resulted in a longitudinal study of first grade children, with the results first presented in 1981 and finally published in 1987 (Perfetti/Beck/Bell/Hughes 1987) and referred to here as the Pittsburgh Study. The answer to the first question was yes, there appears to be the reciprocal relationship we expected. Children's progress in learning to read is initially predicted by their prior progress on a simple synthetic phoneme blending task but is not dependent on prior progress in a more analytic phoneme deletion task. Performance on the deletion task itself was predicted by early progress in learning to decode, but then, in turn, predicted still later progress in decoding.

The second question was answered in the following way: Children who were taught decoding directly by a synthetic phonics program (Beck/Mitroff 1972), showed a weaker relationship between early phonemic awareness (measured by the synthesis/blending task) and final reading achievement than did students taught by a basal program that did not include direct code instruction. This result suggests that children whose instruction does not emphasize coding may turn out to be more dependent on early phonemic awareness than children who learn phonemic awareness and decoding together.

This latter result brings us to our first conclusion regarding at-risk children. We suspect that children are at risk when their instruction is not directed at teaching them the code. Other results from the Pittsburgh Study, including some results never reported, will provide the basis for our further attempt to deal with the question of at-risk readers.

After we briefly review some of the important results published in Perfetti et al. (1987), we will focus on a group of subjects whose data were not reported. These are a group of clearly at-risk children: 17 children who had failed to read in the first grade and were "repeating" first grade during their second year of school. Their second attempt at learning to read (but not their first attempt) was through a direct code program (Beck/Mitroff 1972).

Key findings of the Pittsburgh Study

The Pittsburgh Study had three purposes. 1) To try to untangle cause and effect in the relationship between phonemic awareness and learning to read, and specifically to try to obtain evidence for a reciprocal relationship in which the two abilities are mutually supporting. 2) To observe two methods of reading instruction in connection to the relationship between phonemic awareness and learning to read. 3) To show that there are different cognitive components in various phonemic awareness tasks. In reviewing the key findings, we will focus only on the first two questions.

Subjects

There were 99 first grade students involved in the study. Results from 82 of the students were published previously in Perfetti et al. (1987). The remaining 17 students were the Repeaters, the children repeating first grade because they had not learned to read, and whose data are reported in this paper for the first time.

The subjects were classified into three groups based on the type of reading instruction they received. One group was the Direct Code group, n=25. This group of students was instructed by the New Reading System (NRS) (Beck/Mitroff 1972). Students in this system are explicitly taught to "blend" phonemes and they directly learn letter-sound correspondences. 16 of the students were boys and 9 were girls. Their mean age was 6 years, 5 months at the beginning of the school year. 14 of the students were African-American and 11 were white. They were from an urban public school in a community of primarily lower-middle income families.

The largest group was 57 Basal students who were divided in two sub-groups based on their "reading readiness". One of the sub-groups had been placed in a reading readiness curriculum based on school placement, in effect beginning their school year with drills and exercises but without reading stories from the basal readers until somewhat later. This group of 31 students is referred to as the low Basal group. Their classroom instruction had very little direct code instruction but there was some phonics included. After completing the reading readiness program, the students began the basal readers. Most students began the basal readers by early November. The 31 lower level students were comparable to the Direct Code group in socio-economic status and reading readiness. 13 of the students were girls and 18 were boys. At the beginning of the study, the students' mean age was 6 years, 2 months. 15 of the students were African-American and 16 were white.

The second subgroup of the Basal students was 26 students with a higher reading ability at the beginning of the school year. They started with the basal readers instead of a reading readiness program. The initial mean age of the students was 6 years, 3 months. 11 of the students were girls and 15 were boys. Although this group, which we will refer to as the high Basal group, was from the same school (and therefore the same SES) as the low Basal group, only 4 students were African-American, the remaining 22 were white.

The final group was the 17 Repeaters. After their first, unsuccessful year of reading instruction, they were placed in a Direct Code Program for their second year. The Repeaters were a mean age of 7 years, 2 months at the beginning of the school year. There were 10 boys and 7 girls. 11 of the students were African-American and 6 were white. The Repeaters were from the same school as both Basal groups. Because they had a year of reading instruction before entering the study, they do not provide clean data for the question of the relationship between learning to read and phonemic awareness.

Tasks

Measures were taken on both reading achievement and phonemic awareness for each student. Reading achievement was assessed by the Wide Range Achievement Test (WRAT) after 33 weeks of school (end of the year). All students also completed a pseudoword reading task at each testing point (approximately at weeks 8, 19, and 33 of the school year). This task consisted of four simple, orthographically regular pseudowords which the student had to pronounce. The purpose of the pseudoword reading task was to track the development of decoding skills for each child. Finally, at the end of the year, the students' progress in the curriculum was assessed by noting how far into their respective curricula they had gone.

Three phonological tasks were designed to test the students' phonemic awareness. Two of the tasks examined phoneme analysis and the third evaluated phoneme synthesis. Each student completed all three tasks during the pretest (week 1) and the three testing points.

One of the analysis tasks required the student to tap a pencil once for each phoneme in a word. For example, the experimenter would say the word cat and the student was supposed to tap the pencil three times. There were eight words followed by eight pseudowords in this task. The words were either two, three, or four segment words. Half the subjects performed the tapping task first in the testing session.

The other analysis task was a phoneme deletion task. Students were to delete either the initial or final phoneme of a given word and respond with the result. For example, the experimenter would say *cat* and ask the child to produce cat without the /t/. After the student responded, s/he was then asked to produce cat without the /k/. The same eight words from the tapping task were used. In four cases, students were asked to delete the initial phoneme first. For the other four words, students were to delete the final phoneme first. In each testing session, half the students began with the deletion task. There were no pseudowords in the deletion task.

The synthesis task asked the students to verbalize a word or pseudoword after the experimenter said each phonemic segment in isolation. For example, the experimenter said /k/ /ae/ /t/ with a pause of about one second between each phoneme and the student was supposed to respond with the word *cat*. There were eight words followed by four pseudowords in this task.

Results

The phonological awareness tasks are moderately correlated to each other (see Table 1; when calculating correlations, both high and low Basal groups were included to take advantage of the larger sample size. Generally, however, the high Basal group is not referred to because they were demographically different than the other groups in the study). However, both the cognitive demands of the three tasks and their measurement properties were different. Whatever common phonemic abilities that might underlie the tasks are partly masked. Moreover, there is a fundamental difference in being able to *synthesize* or blend segments and being able to *analyze* syllables into constituent segments. It is the latter that comes closer to the intuitive idea of awareness.

Tab. 1: Correlations between synthesis and deletion tasks at each testing point

	T_0	T_1	T_2	T_3
Basal:	.65	.59	.61	.62
Direct:	.57	.45	.28	.37

Note: For Basal group (n=57), correlations above .22 are significant at $p<.05$.
For Direct Code group (n=25), correlations above .33 are significant at $p<.05$.

The correlation between Deletion and Synthesis actually starts out about the same for the two groups. But for the Direct Code group, this correlation decreases over the year because the Direct Code group explicitly learns how to synthesize phonemes but not how to analyze them. Over the year, the Direct Code group shows more improvement on the synthesis task than on the deletion task. On the other hand, the Basal group improves almost equally in both tasks. The students learn both how to synthesize and delete phonemes as they learn to read, but they don't receive direct instruction for either task.

The relationship between the phonological awareness tasks and end of year reading skill changes as the school year progresses (see Table 2). For the Basal group, both Synthesis and Deletion are initially good predictors of end of year reading skill. For both tasks, the correlation between the task and the WRAT is about .60 at the pretest. However, the correlations diverge with instruction. By the end of the school year, Deletion and reading correlate r=.75, while Synthesis and reading correlate r=.47. This reduced correlation reflects mastery of synthesis and reduction of its discriminability.

Tab. 2: Correlations between phonological awareness tasks and year-end reading achievement for Basal group

	T_0	T_3
Synthesis	.62	.47
Deletion	.59	.75

Note: T_0 - pretest T_3 - final testing point

For the Direct Code group, Synthesis is never a good predictor of year end reading skill (see Table 3). At the pretest, prior to instruction, it correlates with year-end reading only r=.21. The correlation stays at this level until the end of the school year, when it is r=.47, the same as for the Basal group.

Deletion also does not predict end of the year reading skill as well for the Direct Code group as it did for the Basal group (r=.43). Although the correlation rises at the intermediate test points to r=.72, it is again modest, r=.53, at year end (see Table 3).

Tab. 3: Correlations between phonological awareness tasks and year-end reading achievement for Direct Code group

	T_0	T_3
Synthesis	.21	.47
Deletion	.43	.53

Note: T_0- pretest T_3 - final testing point

The relationship between phonological awareness and pseudoword reading is particularly interesting because it allows predictions about progress in learning to read. This is so because of multiple test points, rather than a single year end measure. Here, the interesting data are partial time lag correlations - correlations between a phonemic awareness measure at time n with a pseudoword reading measure at time n+1. Partialed out is the same time correlation between the two measures.

For the Basal group, Synthesis predicts pseudoword reading at the next test point. The largest partial correlation is between the Synthesis score at T_1 (October) and the pseudoword reading score at T_2 (January). This is significant, partial r=.33. For students learning to read with Basal instruction, synthesis is a one-way relationship. Improvements in synthesis skills signal an increase in reading skill.

For Deletion, at least with Basal students, there is a reciprocal relationship over time. First, gains in pseudoword reading at T_1 predict gains in phonemic awareness at T_2 (October to January). Then, gains in phonemic awareness at T_2 lead to further gains in reading at T_3 (January to April). So, as Basal group students progress through their curriculum, gains in pseudoword reading and gains in synthesis supplement each other, and the student learns to read.

For the Direct Code group, both Synthesis and Deletion have one-way relationships with pseudoword reading. Synthesis is similar to that for the Basal group but it occurs later. T_2 (January) Synthesis predicts T_4 (April) reading. Deletion also has a one-way relationship but it is slower. Early gains in pseudoword reading at T_1 (October) predict later gains in phonemic awareness at T_4 (April). Here, we have clear evidence for the role of reading itself in promoting phonemic awareness.

The results of the Deletion task also address the question of whether the acquisition of phonemic awareness is an all or none process. If acquisition is all or none, most students should either be totally unsuccessful or completely successful on the Deletion task. This does not seem to be the case, as can be seen in Figures 1 and 2. At the second testing point, most of the students were doing very badly at Deletion. Figure 1 shows 9 of the 31 low Basal students did not get any words correct. However, there are some students showing partial knowledge. Seven students got between 31% and 69% of the words in the Deletion task correct. By the final testing point (see Fig. 2), there were even more students who showed some sort of partial ability on the Deletion task. 12 of the 31 low Basal students scored between 20% and 80% correct in Deletion. These Deletion results suggest that acquiring phonemic awareness is not all or none but incremental. It may be possible to "sort of" have phonemic awareness.

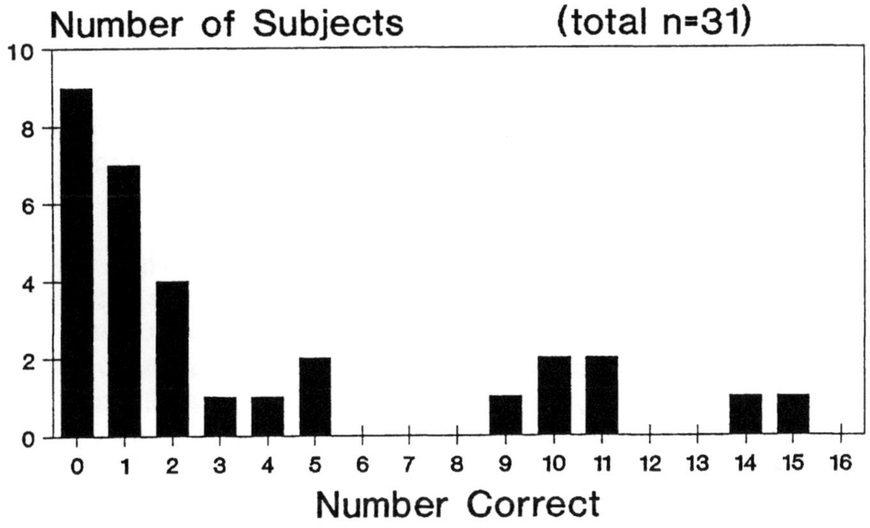

Fig. 1: *Distribution of Deletion scores for the low Basal group at the second testing period*

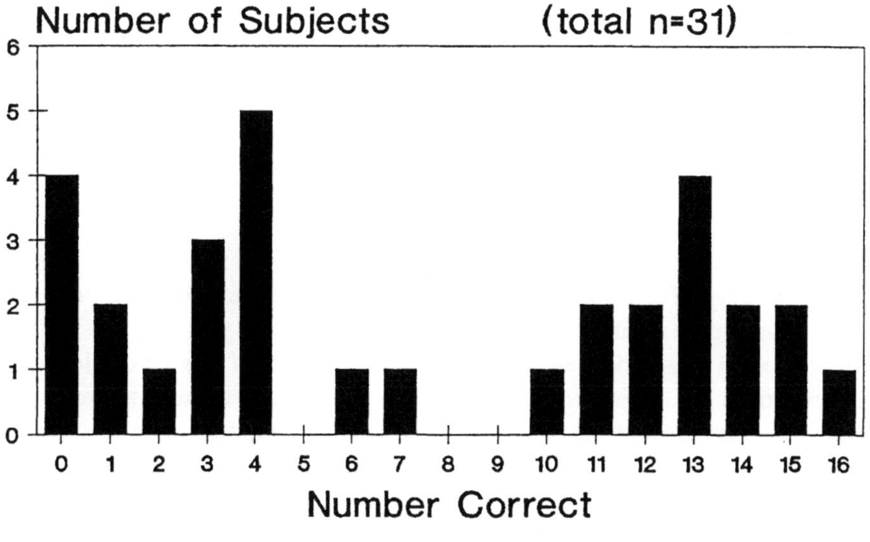

Fig. 2: *Distribution of Deletion scores for the low Basal group at the third testing period*

Issues of risk

These results (Perfetti et al. 1987) along with other work (Mann 1986), indicate that a reciprocal relationship exists between phonemic awareness and learning to read. Reading instruction builds on phonemic awareness and vice versa. To become an expert reader, students must acquire phonemic awareness, use those phonemic skills to begin learning to read and then, as they read, strengthen their phonemic awareness.

Students who risk failure at learning to read are those who enter school without phonemic awareness and then are exposed to reading instruction that does not correct the problem. This is contrary to the belief that phonemic awareness is important only for students who will be instructed by direct decoding methods. Instead, the results of the study suggest that teaching the alphabetic principle is especially important to those students who do not learn direct decoding. Phonemic awareness prior to instruction was more important for students who were to be taught by basal readers than students taught direct code. That is, children who do not learn to decode are more dependent on their early phonemic awareness than children who explicitly learn to decode. This can be seen in Tables 2 and 3. The correlation between phonemic tasks (Deletion and Synthesis) and year-end reading achievement is higher for the Basal group than for the Direct Code group. The correlation difference is especially noticeable in Synthesis. For the Basal group, $r=.62$ but $r=.21$ for the Direct Code group. Since the Direct Code students were taught blending, their initial Synthesis skills were not as important to their reading achievement at the end of the school year.

The Repeaters

The Repeaters were a group of 17 children who had failed to learn to read in their first try. They were in a basal program for their first year of reading instruction and in a direct code program their second year. At the beginning of this second year, they were truly nonreaders. 16 of the 17 could not read all the words of a very simple sentence composed of words from a first grade list. The exception was one child, whom we fear teachers had misclassified.

Although the Repeaters were similar to the incoming first graders in that none of them could read, there were some differences between each group. In the beginning of the school year, the Repeaters had different phonemic abilities than the entering first graders. Comparisons between the Repeaters, both high and low Basal groups, and the Direct Code group for each phonemic task are given below. Comparisons between the low Basal group and the Repeaters are especially useful because these two groups were similar in gender and race makeup as well as SES.

The Repeaters were better at Synthesis than any of the others (the Direct Code group and both Basal groups). In Deletion, the Repeaters were not as good as either the Direct Code or high Basal groups. The Repeaters and the low Basal group had similar Deletion scores but the Repeaters were better at getting words right, but much worse at getting nonwords right. The final phonemic task was Tapping, which is not a good task to use with children who have had any reading instruction because they tend to tap for each letter of the word instead of each phoneme. The Repeaters demonstrated the limits of the tapping task since they were much better than all of the other groups.

As the school year progressed, the Repeaters continued to perform well in Synthesis. They were consistently better than both Basal groups. However, by T_2 (week 19) the Repeaters were equalled by the Direct Code group and surpassed by the Direct Code group at the end of the school year.

For Deletion, however, the story is different. The Repeaters showed less gain over the course of the school year than expected. In fact, the Repeaters showed no improvement in Deletion from T_2 to T_3. Their performance on the deletion task was comparable overall to the low Basal group and much worse than the Direct Code group and the high Basal group. By T_3 (final testing point), even the low Basal group had surpassed the Repeaters in Deletion.

At year end, the Repeaters also were not reading as well as the other groups (see Fig. 3). Reading skill was measured by the WRAT. The Repeaters were reading at a very low second grade level (2.1) whereas the low Basal Group was reading at a 2.4 grade equivalent. The difference between the Repeaters and the Direct Code was even more pronounced.

Unlike real word reading performance, the Repeaters were dramatically better at pseudoword reading than the low Basal group. The Repeaters were comparable to the Direct Code group at all test points and equal to the high Basal group by T_2. (The high Basal group is not included in Figure 4).

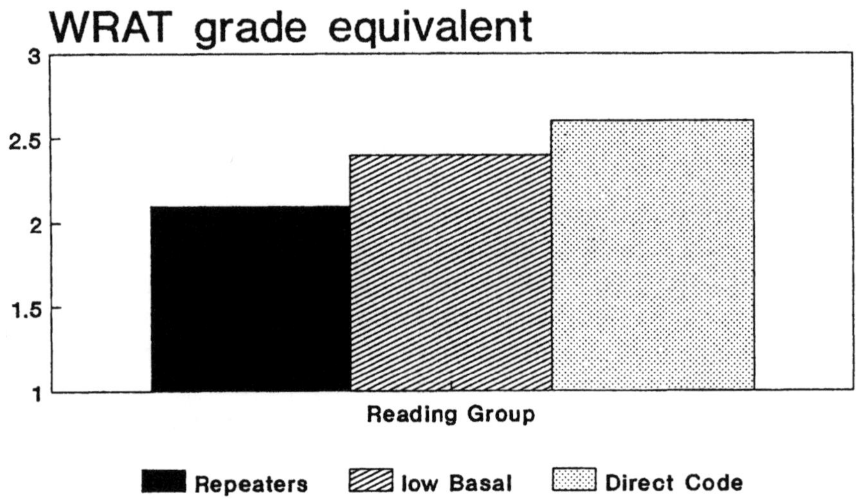

Fig. 3: Year-end reading grade equivalent for each reading group

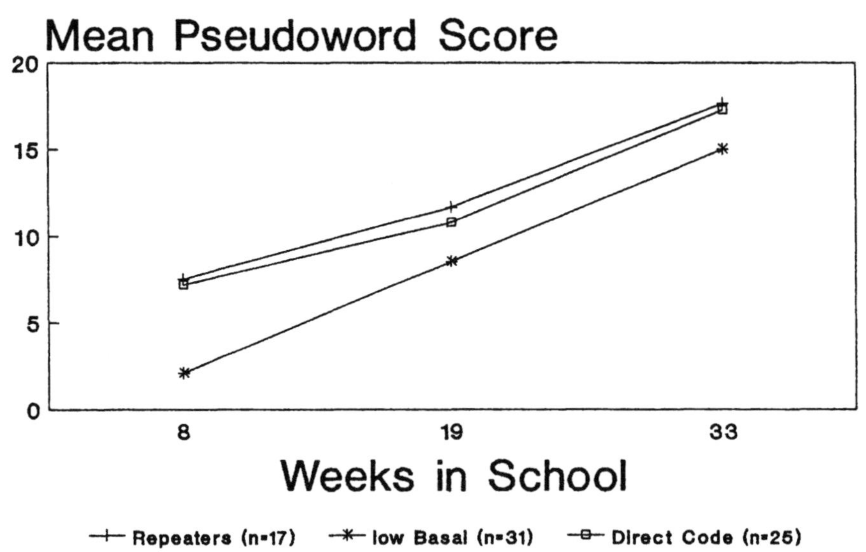

Fig. 4: Mean pseudoword reading score for each reading group at each testing period

Although the Repeaters' results on the phonological tasks are interesting, we cannot make conclusions about the predictive value of these phonological tasks because the sample size is small (n=17). The correlations of Synthesis and Deletion with reading skill were less stable for the Repeaters than for the other groups. Also, the partial time-lag correlations tend to be nonsignificant for this small sample size.

However, there are simple correlations that are informative. The simple relationship between phonological awareness and pseudoword reading can be seen in Table 4. It is the same reciprocal relationship that was found in the Pittsburgh study with the Basal and Direct Code groups. Early ability in Synthesis predicts pseudoword reading at the next point, but Synthesis quickly loses its ability to predict reading. The correlation between Synthesis performance at the first testing point and pseudoword reading performance at the second testing point is r=.74, but there is no relationship between Synthesis at test 2 and pseudoword reading at test 3.

Tab. 4: Correlations between phonological tasks and pseudoword reading from one test point to the next

SYN-1 and R-2, r=.74
SYN-2 and R-3, r= 0
R-1 and SYN-2, r=.48 (partial r=.27)
R-2 and SYN-3, r=.27
R-1 and DEL-2, r=.69
R-2 and DEL-3, r=.41 (partial r= .25)

Note: R is pseudoword reading. The numbers refer to test point 1, 2, or 3.

Table 4 also shows the relationship between pseudoword reading and Deletion. Pseudoword reading at testing points 1 and 2 predicts Deletion performance at testing points 2 and 3. At least two of the partial correlations are greater than zero.

In summary, the Repeaters were able to learn to read with Direct Code instruction. They were especially good at pseudoword reading, quickly matching the Direct Code students and surpassing the low Basal group. The Repeaters did not match either the low Basal group or the Direct Code group in their ability to read the words of the WRAT, but they came respectably close given their obvious handicap. With respect to phonemic awareness, the Repeaters had synthesis abilities prior to the year but not deletion abilities. This verifies that synthesis ability is *not* sufficient for success in reading, although it may be necessary. The Repeaters improved in deletion but not as much as the other groups. The relationship between awareness and progress in learning to read was comparable to the other groups, with reading predicted by Synthesis and reading itself predicting Deletion.

Some conclusions regarding risk

The contribution of the Pittsburgh study is primarily to our understanding of the reciprocal relationship between phonological awareness and learning to read. The results for all the students, regardless of type of instruction, showed that some kind of phonemic awareness was necessary for most students to learn to read. In addition, progress in reading was needed before further advances in phonemic awareness could occur. These results reinforce the critical importance played by phonological awareness in learning to read an alphabetic orthography. In addition, they show the reciprocal relation between phonological awareness and learning to read.

The study also allowed us to assess two different types of reading instruction and to draw conclusions about their effectiveness. The results indicate that children taught to decode are less dependent on their early phonemic awareness than are children in basal programs. This is a sensible conclusion because Direct Code students explicitly learn about phonemes and how to blend sounds. Children who initially lack this knowledge will be taught it in a Direct Code classroom. Their Basal counterparts won't receive training about phonemes. Children in Basal classrooms must rely on their initial knowledge of phonemes to help them learn to read. As their reading skills increase, they will be able to make conclusions about phonemes but many of the children will be at a disadvantage compared to the Direct code students.

The implications of this study for at-risk children are indirect. There was a wide range of reading achievement after one year, and it was predictable in part by earlier abilities in phonemic segmentation. Clearly, children who have not acquired phonological awareness are at risk for not learning to read. In addition, reading ability strengthens phonological awareness, which is needed before reading progress continues. Children without phonemic awareness risk not being able to take the first steps toward learning to read and as a result, their phonemic awareness is further handicapped.

The additional data reported here show that good instruction can bring both reading and phonemic awareness. Good instruction is particularly important for at-risk children because without it, they might not learn to read. Many at-risk children are children who lack phonemic awareness and they may need to be explicitly taught phonemic awareness to learn to read. For such children, some direct instruction in coding may be helpful.

Children who initially failed to learn to read are a special case. Although our results suggest some success with direct code instruction for Repeaters, we should emphasize that any child who fails to learn to read with his/her age-peers is put further at risk. Indeed, some children develop compensatory, nonanalytic skills that become habit. These nonanalytic habits may be hard to overcome and further hamper a child's ability to learn to read.

The best way to guarantee that a child will successfully learn to read is to insure strong reading instruction early in the child's schooling.

References

Beck, I.L., Perfetti, C.A., & Hughes, C. (1981). Phonemic knowledge and learning to read: A longitudinal study of first-graders. Presented at the Society for Research in Child Development, Boston, MA.

Beck, I.L. & Mitroff, D. (1972). The rationale and design of a primary grades reading system for an individualized classroom. Pittsburgh: Publication Series, Learning Research and Development Center, University of Pittsburgh.

Bradley, L. & Bryant, P. (1991). Phonological skills before and after learning to read. In S.A. Brady & D.P. Shankweiler (Eds.). Phonological processes in literacy: A tribute to Isabelle Y. Liberman. 37-53. Hillsdale, NJ: Lawrence Erlbaum Associates.

Brady, S.A. & Shankweiler, D. (Eds.) (1991). Phonological processes in literacy: A tribute to Isabelle Y. Liberman. Hillsdale, NJ: Lawrence Erlbaum Associates.

Bryant, P.E. & Bradley, L. (1980). Why children sometimes write words which they do not read. In U. Frith (Ed.), Cognitive processes in spelling. 355-370. London: Academic Press.

Byrne, B. (1991). Experimental analysis of the child's discovery of the alphabetic principle. In L. Rieben & C.A. Perfetti (Eds.), Learning to read: Basic research and its implications. 75-84. Hillsdale, NJ: Lawrence Erlbaum Associates.

Ehri, L.C. (1991). Learning to read and spell words. In L. Rieben & C.A. Perfetti (Eds.), Learning to read: Basic research and its implications. 57-73. Hillsdale, NJ: Lawrence Erlbaum Associates.

Gough, P.B. & Hillinger, M.L. (1980). Learning to read: An unnatural act. Bulletin of the Orton Society, 20, 179-196.

Liberman, I.Y. & Shankweiler, D. (1979). Speech, the alphabet, and teaching to read. In L.B. Resnick & P.A. Weaver (Eds.), Theory and practice of early reading, Vol. 2. 109-132. Hillsdale, NJ: Lawrence Erlbaum Associates.

Lundberg, I., Frost, J., & Petersen, O-P. (1988). Effects of an extensive program for stimulating phonological awareness in preschool children. Reading Research Quarterly, 23, 264-284.

Mann, V.A. (1986). Phonological awareness: The role of reading experience. Cognition, 21, 65-92.

Mann, V.A. (1991). Phonological abilities: Effective predictors of future reading ability. In L. Rieben & C.A. Perfetti (Eds.), Learning to read: Basic research and its implications. 121-133. Hillsdale, NJ: Lawrence Erlbaum Associates.

Morais, J., Cary, L., Alegria, J., & Bertelson, P. (1979). Does awareness of speech as a sequence of phones arise spontaneously? Cognition, 7, 323-331.

Perfetti, C.A., Beck, I.L., Bell, L., & Hughes, C. (1987). Phonemic knowledge and learning to read are reciprocal: A longitudinal study of first grade children. Merrill Palmer Quarterly, 33, 283-319.

Rieben, L. & Perfetti, C.A. (Eds.). (1991). Learning to read: Basic research and its implications. Hillsdale, NJ: Lawrence Erlbaum Associates.

Treiman, R. & Baron, J. (1983). Phonemic-analysis training helps children benefit from spelling-sound rules. Memory and Cognition, 11, 382-389.

Commentary on Perfetti, Georgi and Beck: Children without phonemic awareness before learning to read. Are they at risk?

Heinz Wimmer

The Pittsburgh study (published 1987 by Perfetti/Beck/Bell/Hughes, but first presented 1981) was one of the earliest and most detailed studies on the relationship between phonemic awareness and learning to read. The findings from this study and from numerous other studies are commonly interpreted as evidence for a kind of causal role of phonemic awareness in learning to read. It is not surprising, therefore, that Perfetti/Georgi/Beck (present volume) see lack of phonemic awareness as the main risk factor for reading difficulties: "Children who have not acquired phonological awareness are at risk for not learning to read" (p. 206) and similarly "children without phonemic awareness risk not being able to take the first steps toward learning to read and as a result, their phonemic awareness is further handicapped" (p. 206).

This implication of the Pittsburgh study for the issue of risk follows from the main message, indeed from the title of the original publication: "Phonemic awareness and learning to read are reciprocal..." (Perfetti/Beck/Bell/Hughes 1987). The present formulation of this reciprocal relationship is: "a fairly dim and inexplicit form of phonemic awareness was necessary for making initial progress at true reading, whereas reading itself was necessary for a fuller blossoming of explicit phonemic awareness" (p. 194).

In my comment I will dispute the claim that any form of awareness of the phonemic segments of speech *precedes* acquisition of alphabetic reading, and consequently I will dispute the implication that children without phonemic awareness are at risk. In doing so I will bring in some findings from a recent study showing that phonemic awareness was more a consequence than a precondition of learning to read, but important nevertheless (Wimmer/Landerl/Linortner/Hummer 1991). My proposal is that the ease or the difficulty with which phonemic awareness can be induced by learning to read is in fact the critical factor.

An evaluation of the reciprocal view

The reciprocal view on the relationship between phonemic awareness and learning to read is a kind of compromise position between two earlier and contradictory views on this relationship. When in the seventies psycholinguists became seriously interested in research on learning to read, the underlying assumption was that the child must be able to segment the speech wave into phonemic constituents *before* alphabetic word representations could be related to these segments (Liberman/Shankweiler/Liberman et al. 1977; Rozin/Gleitman 1977). However, it soon turned out that this *prerequisite view* on the relationship between phonemic awareness and reading could not be correct. Morais/Cary/Alegria/Bertelson (1979) found that adult Portuguese illiterates showed no or little phonemic awareness. Converging evidence came from adult Chinese readers who were also found to exhibit lack of phonemic awareness (Read/Zhang/Nie/Ding 1986). These findings were in direct contradiction to the prerequisite view and suggested instead that phonemic awareness is a *consequence* of learning to read an alphabetic writing system.

However, there was also support for the prerequisite view. It came from longitudinal studies which assessed phonemic awareness before children started school and related the phonemic awareness scores to later reading achievement. Typically substantial correlations were found (see review by Wagner/Torgesen 1987). Exemplary for such longitudinal correlations are those of about .60 between phonemic awareness at the beginning of grade one and reading achievement at the end of grade one reported by Perfetti et al. (present volume, p. 199, Tab. 2). Obviously, there is a contradiction between the longitudinal findings and the findings from the illiterates and the logographic readers. The longitudinal correlations would imply that a substantial number of children has acquired phonemic awareness before learning to read, while the studies with illiterates and logographic readers show that there is no phonemic awareness in persons who have not learned to read an alphabetic orthography.

Perfetti et al.'s reciprocal view attempts to reconcile these apparently contradictory findings. Basically it does so by positing two forms of phonemic awareness. The explicit form is seen as the result of learning to read (thus taking into account the lack of phonemic awareness found among illiterates and logographic readers), while the "dim, inexplicit form" is posited as prerequisite for learning to read (thus accounting for the longitudinal correlations).

While I admire the theoretical elegance of the reciprocal view, I am less convinced that the data provided by Perfetti et al. provide strong support. The main problem is that the observed relationship between "inexplicit" and "explicit" phonemic awareness at the beginning of grade one does not conform to the expectation following from the reciprocal view. To explicate this point it is important how the two forms of phonemic awareness were assessed. The inexplicit form of phonemic awareness was measured by a phoneme synthesis task. For example, the child was given the phonemes /k/ - /a/ - /t/ and had to respond with "cat". Explicit phonemic awareness was measured with a phoneme deletion task, where, for example, the child had to say "cat" without the /k/. The implication of the reciprocal view is that before learning to read phoneme synthesis should be easy, since it measures only inexplicit phonemic awareness, while phoneme deletion should be difficult. This, however, was not the case. Unfortunately, there are no direct data on task difficulty, but Figure 1 of the original publication of the Pittsburgh study (Perfetti et al., 1987) shows that at the beginning of grade one not a single child reached the criterion of at least 9 of 12 points correct on the phoneme synthesis task. Furthermore, from Figure 4 in Perfetti et al. (1987), which compares the percentages of children reaching criterion on the two tasks, no difference in difficulty is discernible between inexplicit and explicit phonemic awareness. This high difficulty of inexplicit phonemic awareness is a serious problem, since the reciprocal view rests on the assumption that before learning to read the inexplicit form should be largely present, while the explicit form should be absent.

One plausible interpretation the similar high difficulty of both phoneme synthesis and phoneme deletion observed by Perfetti et al. is that both tasks may reflect the low level of early reading skills among their children at the beginning of grade one. The relationship between early reading skills (such as extended knowledge of letter-sound associations) and performance on the phonemic awareness tasks was not directly examined. It is not implausible, however, that the children with better knowledge of letter-sound associations at the beginning of grade one were the ones with somewhat higher scores on the phonemic awareness tasks. If this was the case, then it may well be that the reported longitudinal correlations between phoneme synthesis and later reading score are spurious ones, reflecting the true correlations between early letter knowledge (resulting in somewhat better phonemic awareness) and later reading.

This is not a far-fetched speculation. A longitudinal study by Lundberg/Olofsson/Wall (1980) also had reported substantial correlations between phonemic awareness scores at the beginning of grade one and later reading scores. However, when in a reanalysis of this study Wagner/Torgesen (1987) controlled for reading abilities at the beginning of grade one, then most of the former significant predictions dropped to zero.

An alternative formulation of the reciprocal view: Early awareness of syllable-onset and syllable-rime

My critical comment on the reciprocal view was particularly directed against the formulation that a "dim, inexplicit form of phonemic awareness" assessed by phoneme synthesis is necessary for learning to read. It should, however, be noted that there is another formulation of the reciprocal view.

Summarizing impressive longitudinal studies done in Oxford in the last decade, Goswami/Bryant (1990; see also Bryant/Alegria 1989) concluded that early awareness of alliteration and rhyme is a precursor for early progress in reading, while phonemic awareness is a consequence of reading acquisition (the second clause was more explicit in Bryant/Alegria 1989). Alliteration and rhyme was later identified with natural divisions of syllables (syllable-onsets and syllable-rimes) which are typically larger than single phonemes. The /tr/ in "trick" and "trap" is an example for a syllable onset, the /-ight/ in "fight" and "right" is an example of a syllable rime.

In the longitudinal studies of the Oxford group, predictive relationships were found between knowledge of nursery rhymes and early sensitivity for onsets and rimes tested among 3- and 4-year-olds and reading achievement scores several years later. These predictions were found even when several possible confounds of the phonological predictors were controlled for, and, of course, it cannot be argued that knowledge of nursery rhymes among 3- and 4-year-olds might be a consequence of already existing reading abilities. My only critical comment against the Oxford formulation of the reciprocal view has to do with the role of syllable-onsets and -rimes in early reading. I suspect that sensitivity for these constituents of syllables is more important for the early phases of learning to read English, with its exceptionally low consistency between graphemes and phonemes, than for learning to read a more regular orthography.

There is some evidence for this suspicion. In a longitudinal study with children learning to read German, we found little relationship between sensitivity for syllable-onsets and -rimes assessed at the beginning of grade one and reading achievement measures at the end of grade one (Landerl/Linortner/Wimmer 1992; Wimmer/Landerl/Schneider 1992). This may have been due to the fact that the young reader of the consistent German writing system rely much more on grapheme-phoneme translation than the young English reader (Wimmer/Frith 1992; Wimmer/Goswami 1992). The mentioned finding of no reliable correlation between phonological sensitivity and later reading implies that lack of or low levels of sensitivity for syllable-onsets and -rimes before school does not prevent children from a successful start into reading - at least when children are introduced to reading via grapheme-phoneme translation, and when the writing system is fairly consistent. However, it is interesting to note that although early sensitivity for syllable segments was not predictive for reading at the end of grade one, it became predictive for reading speed at the end of grade three (Wimmer/Landerl/Schneider 1992).

Phonemic awareness as a consequence of learning to read, but of critical importance nevertheless

Further scepticism against the reciprocal view and its implications for the issue of risk comes from longitudinal studies where we directly examined the relationship between phonemic awareness before reading instruction and progress in learning to read and to write (Wimmer/Landerl/Linortner/Hummer 1991). Again our subjects were learning to read German. For the evaluation of their performance on the phonemic awareness task at the beginning of grade one, it is important to note that the majority of these children were unable to decode the simplest word and knew only few letters at the beginning of grade one. This results from the fact that in Austrian and also in German kindergartens, there are strict rules against reading preparation. Given these circumstances, it is not suprising from the perspective of the consequence view that our children quite often showed lack of or little phonemic awareness at the beginning of grade one, although phonemic awareness was measured with a task that appeared to be quite easy and natural. We used a vowel substitution task which mimicks a natural linguistic process (e.g. sing sang sung) and which was in fact easier than the more widely used phoneme counting task. According to the reciprocal view the mentioned finding would have implied that the majority of our children lacked the prerequisite for success in learning to read and were therefore at risk for reading failure. However, this was not the case. With few exceptions our children showed high reading and spelling achievements at the end of grade one. In particular, many of the children with lack of or little phonemic awareness at the beginning of grade one showed high reading and spelling achievements at the end of grade one. Not suprisingly, the few children with high phonemic awareness at the beginning of grade one (most of them readers) scored uniformly high at the end of grade one. Quite in agreement with the consequence view on the relationship between phonemic awareness and learning to read, it was found that nearly all children with some reading ability before school scored high on the phonemic awareness task, and that at least from the middle of grade one onwards most children scored at ceiling level.

However, there were indications that phonemic awareness is not simply an irrelevant side effect of learning to read. We found that children with less satisfying progress in learning to read and to spell at the end of grade one also tended to score lower on the phonemic awareness task, although they all relied on grapheme-phoneme translation in reading and spelling. A study with older dyslexic German children also found somewhat impaired phonemic awareness despite heavy reliance on indirect reading and spelling strategies (Wimmer 1993). The most straightforward interpretation of this pattern of findings is supplied by the assumption that phonemic awareness is a critical component of learning to read an alphabetic orthography. This view agrees with the consequence view in assuming that without learning to read an alphabetic writing system there is little chance that the phonemic structure of spoken language may ever become explicit for a child. In contrast to a "mere" consequence view, it stresses the critical involvement of phonemic awareness in learning to read. In particular, it assumes serious reading difficulties when the child is confronted with alphabetic word representations and thus is given an optimal opportunity, but still does not gain high levels of phonemic awareness.

After having formulated this critical component view in Wimmer et al. (1991) we found that Perfetti (1991) had arrived at a similar conclusion: "Downgrading phonological awareness from causal status to reciprocal status does not diminish its importance for reading. Indeed it allows it to be seen as a *central* component of reading instead of as a prerequisite" (p. 40). The present position goes further and downgrades phonemic awareness from reciprocal to consequence status, but also sees phonemic awareness as *the* central component. Nevertheless there is a difference between these two similar formulations for the question of risk. The reciprocal view implies that lack of phonemic awareness before learning to read puts children at risk for reading failure, the critical component view does not. From the critical component view it would only follow that the few children, who had acquired phonemic awareness even before learning to read, must have an optimal start into reading. For the large number of children without phonemic awareness one would not expect difficulties. The educational implication would be "wait and see" with the specific addition of "don't wait too long". If introduction to an alphabetic writing system does not induce phonemic awareness in a child, as it does for the large majority of children in very short time, then there definitely is a need for quick intervention.

References

Bryant, P. & Alegria, J. (1989). The transition from spoken to written language. In A. Ribaupierre (Ed.), Transition mechanism in child development: The longitudinal perspective. 126-144. Cambridge: University Press.

Goswami, U. & Bryant, P. (1990). Phonological skills and learning to read. Hove: Erlbaum.

Landerl, K., Linortner, R., & Wimmer, H. (1992). Phonologische Bewußtheit und Schriftspracherwerb im Deutschen. [Phonological awareness and acquisition of literacy in German]. Zeitschrift für Pädagogische Psychologie, 6(1), 17-33.

Liberman, I.Y., Shankweiler, D., Liberman, A.M., Fowler, C., & Fischer, F.W. (1977). Phonetic segmentation and recoding in the beginning reader. In A.S. Reber & D.L. Scarborough (Eds.), Towards a psychology of reading. 297-225. Hillsdale, N.Y.: Erlbaum.

Lundberg, L., Olofsson, A., & Wall, S. (1980). Reading and spelling skills in the first school years predicted from phonemic awareness skills in kindergarden. Scandinavian Journal of Psychology, 21, 159-173.

Morais, J., Cary, L., Alegria, J., & Bertelson, P. (1979). Does awareness of speech as a sequence of phones arise spontaneously? Cognition, 7, 323-331.

Perfetti, C.A. (1991). Representations and awareness in the acquisition of reading competence. In L. Rieben & C.A. Perfetti (Eds.), Learning to read: Basic research and its implications. 33-44. Hillsdale, N. Y.: Erlbaum.

Perfetti, C.A., Beck, I., Bell, L.C., & Hughes, C. (1987). Phonemic knowledge and learning to read are reciprocal: A longitudinal study of first grade children. Merrill-Palmer Quarterly, 33, 283-319.

Read, C., Zhang, Y., Nie, H., & Ding, B. (1986). The ability to manipulate speech sounds depends on knowing alphabetic reading. Cognition, 24, 31-44.

Rozin, P. & Gleitman, L. R. (1977). The structure and acquisition of reading II: The reading process and the alphabetic principle. In A.S. Reber & D.L. Scarborough (Eds.), Toward a psychology of reading. 55-141. Hillsdale, N.Y.: Erlbaum.

Wagner, R.K. & Torgesen, J.K. (1987). The nature of phonological processing and its causal role in the acquisition of reading skills. Psychological Bulletin, 101, 192-212.

Wimmer, H. (1993). Characteristics of developmental dyslexia in a regular writing system. Applied Psycholinguistics. (In press).

Wimmer, H. & Frith, U. (1992). Orthographies and learning to read: An English - German comparison. Unpublished manuscript, University of Salzburg.

Wimmer, H. & Goswami, U. (1992). The influence of orthographic consistency on reading development: Word recognition in English and German children. Manuscript submitted for publication.

Wimmer, H., Landerl, K., Linortner, R., & Hummer, P. (1991). The relationship of phonemic awareness to reading acquisition: More consequence than precondition but still important. Cognition, 40, 219-249.

Wimmer, H., Landerl, K., & Schneider, W. (1992). The role of alliteration and rhyme in learning to read a regular orthography. Manuscript submitted for publication.

Prediction of difficulties in reading and spelling on the basis of the Bielefeld Screening[1]

Harald Marx
Heiner Jansen
Gerd Mannhaupt
Helmut Skowronek

Difficulties in the acquisition of literacy are a worldwide problem. Children in cultures with an alphabetic script face serious and similar problems, even though the specific spelling-sound relations in a given language and the specific features of the national schooling system may have different effects.

Because of the societal importance of this problem there is a long lasting tradition of research on early detection and prevention of reading and spelling difficulties. The course of this research is characterized by a specification of those predictors proposed to be relevant. Starting with medically and going on to functionally oriented models the research nowadays favours predictor models that comprise abilities and skills deduced from an analysis of the early reading and spelling development (cf. Skowronek/Marx 1993). Early prediction - to be followed by preventive and interventive measures - is important since reading/spelling disorders are cumulative and increasingly resistent to remediation with years of schooling (Kretschmann/Lindner-Achenbach/Puffahrt et al. 1990; Stanovich 1986). To identify children at risk for reading/spelling difficulties at preschool age and in line with the current research orientation mentioned above we developed a screening device ("Bielefeld Screening") and applied it in a three year predictive longitudinal study.

Theoretical background and predictor selection

Up to now there are many theoretical attempts to explain developmental aspects of reading and spelling acquisition on the one hand (Chall 1983; Frith 1985, 1986; Gough/Hillinger 1980; Günther 1986; Høien/Lundberg

1988; Marsh/Friedman/Welch/Desberg 1981) and processing aspects on the other hand (Høien/Lundberg 1989; for an overview see Skowronek/Marx 1993). The integration of developmental and processing models has started recently. For example, Scheerer-Neumann (1989a, b) uses developmental stage models (Frith 1985) and processing models (Coltheart 1978; Humphreys/Evett 1985; Scheerer-Neumann 1981) in combination to explain reading development in individual cases. Both theoretical frameworks are used to identify relevant preschool predictors which are as close as possible to reading and spelling processes (Berninger 1986).

Stages must not be seen as emerging "by nature". For instance, Ehri (1991) points out - referring to stages of "cue reading" ("logographic") and "cipher reading" ("alphabetic") as delineated by Gough/Hillinger (1980) - that method of instruction, i.e. phonics vs. sight word approaches, can make important differences. Children instructed by a phonics approach don't rely so much on visual-logographic strategies but soon can use particular letter-sound relations for recognizing simple words. Focussing on letter-sound relations the child begins to develop important components of language awareness: "(1) objectivation or the ability to reflect on language forms while abstracting from the meaning aspect and paying attention to sound properties of language and (2) the ability to identify phonemes and to manipulate phonemic segments" (Valtin 1984, 228). Accordingly, arguments from the analysis of beginning reading an alphabetic script and massive evidence from studies predicting literacy achievement underline phonological awareness to play a central role in early literacy acquisition (Lundberg/Olofsson/Wall 1980; Mann 1991; Perfetti/Beck/Bell/Hughes 1987; Stanovich/Cunningham/Cramer 1984).

On the other hand, process models based on dual-route theory (Høien/Lundberg 1989) differentiate two different reading processes: the orthographic and the prelexical phonological coding route. Despite the criticisms of dual-route theory (Van Orden/Pennington/Stone 1990) one may assume this model to be of heuristic value to identify relevant processing components of early reading acquisition (see also Scheerer-Neumann 1989a, b). Høien/Lundberg (1989) postulate several interrelated components in word recognition. First the reader has to analyse the graphic letter string visually (letter identification, parsing processes). If the orthographic route is used the orthographic word-recognition system activates the semantic information and, finally, leads to word-retrieval.

If the prelexical phonological coding route is used, the visual elements must be transformed, first, into phonological codes; second, the phonological elements must be synthesized to sound-images which can be used to search for appropiate phonological patterns in lexicon, and, third, the related semantic content is retrieved. The ability to segment spoken words into their phonological segments as well as various short-term memory functions are of critical importance during this process. Viewing the dual-route model from a developmental perspective, the beginning reader mainly uses the phonological coding route (phonetic cue reading or alphabetic stage). Consequently, the phonological coding route must be emphasized in analysing early literacy development.

These arguments from early reading processes are supported and differentiated by a critical discussion of empirical research relating to dimensions of phonological processing (Wagner/Torgesen 1987). According to these authors, phonological processing may be distinguished into phonological awareness, phonological recoding in lexical access and phonetic recoding to maintain information in working memory. The Bielefeld Screening refers explicitly to these three aspects (see Skowronek/Marx 1989). To assess phonological awareness we used four tasks (recognition of rhyming word pairs, syllable segmentation, initial phoneme to word matching and phoneme blending). Additionally, measures of phonetic recoding (repeating pseudowords), attention to visual sequences of symbols (word matching), lexical recoding speed (two scores from rapid naming of the colours of objects) and memory for object attributes (knowledge of object colours) were used as predictor variables.

Comments on methodology

Prediction studies vary considerably in design. First, the most critical difference between purely correlational studies and studies using individual prediction must be emphasized. To maximize the reliability of individual predictions Cronbach/Gleser (1965), Lichtenstein/Ireton (1984), Marx (1992b, c), and Silver (1978) recommend as an ideal pattern: screening and preselection, careful testing and precise selection of the "at risk" subjects and, finally, criterion measurement and identification of the problem subjects.

Since left unconsidered in many classification studies, it needs to be explicitly stated that the final decision on children at risk should be based on two combined measurements.

Despite the early and repeated delineation of requirements for classificatory prediction the most common type of prediction study is still the purely correlational approach. However significant and impressive the correlational evidence from these studies might be, conclusions concerning the prediction of individual failures in literacy acquisition cannot be drawn (cf. Leach 1980, 1983; Rubin/Balow/Dorle/Rosen 1978). Quite to the contrary, correlations may even be misleading. Share/Silva (1986) reported correlations of selected predictor and criterion tests in reading as high as r = .71, but the corresponding results of classificatory predictions (of problem children) were disappointing.

To discover efficient combinations of predictors by post-hoc multivariate analysis may be seen as an intermediate step from simple and multiple correlational analysis towards genuine classificatory prediction. When results from studies of this type are not cross-validated artefacts cannot be ruled out, as Feshbach/Adelman/Fuller (1974) have shown in the case of the screening index of Jansky/de Hirsch (1972), and Morrison/Mantzicopoulos/Stone (1988) have shown in the case of the screening of Silver/Hagin (1981). Therefore, when prediction aims at valid identification of at risk subjects in real situations - as is the primary purpose of our longitudinal research - and not in analyzing general relations between predictors and criteria, the identification should be based solely on genuine classificatory research.

Indiscriminate use of the classificatory approach, i.e. failing to consider its methodological pitfalls, may often lead to an overestimation of predictive validity. Key parameters are the base rate and the selection rate. When they are both too high and/or differ too much it is almost impossible to evaluate the quality of prediction. Table 1 gives examples of studies which are charged with methodological problems of this kind.

An appropriate estimate of predictive quality is provided by RIOC, i.e. the relative improvement over chance (Loeber/Dishion 1983; cf. Marx 1992c), which may even correct some difference between selection and base rate.

For instance, the study of Ferinden/Jacobson (1970), with a selection rate of 27 % and a base rate of 61 % points to the problem of economy in classification and intervention. This base rate suggests that more than 60 % of the school children examined face learning problems. Obviously, an empirical base rate as high as this is extremely unrealistic compared to the much more modest base rates of learning disabilities in the population. In cases

Tab. 1: *Results of classification studies to predict academic achievement*

Study	Sel. Rate (SR)%	Base Rate (BR)%	Max. Corr. (MC)%	N	Classifications[1] val pos a	fal pos b	fal neg c	val neg d	Total Corr. (TC)%	Rand. Corr. (RC)%	RIOC
	26.9	61.2	65.7	67	17	1	24	25	62.7	44.8	85.6
Ferinden/	58.2	56.7	98.5	67	35	4	3	25	89.6	51.1	81.2
Jacobson (1970)	44.8	58.2	86.6	67	27	3	12	25	77.6	49.1	76.0
Feshbach/	11.1	30.6	80.5	585	54	11	125	395	78.8	65.1	83.5
Adelman/	12.6	29.7	82.9	572	44	28	126	374	73.1	65.1	44.9
Fuller (1974)	5.8	29.8	76.0	571	28	5	142	396	74.3	55.6	91.7
Feshbach/	10.7	10.7	100.0	549	27	32	32	458	88.3	80.9	38.7
Adelman/	11.9	9.7	97.8	536	20	44	32	440	85.8	80.7	29.8
Fuller	8.6	9.8	98.8	451	19	20	25	387	83.2	80.8	43.2
(1977)	10.9	9.7	98.8	431	12	35	30	354	84.9	81.5	19.7
Lindeman/Good-	85.5	13.1	27.6	214	28	155	0	31	27.6	23.8	100.0
stein/Sachs et al.	59.8	13.1	53.3	214	28	100	0	86	53.3	42.7	100.0
(1984)	36.9	13.1	76.2	214	24	55	4	131	72.4	59.6	77.1
Satz/Friel	24.3	3.8	79.5	473	18	97	0	358	79.5	73.7	100.0
(1974)	24.3	15.4	91.1	473	57	58	16	342	84.4	67.8	71.2

Legend and calculation formulas: a = valid positives; b = false positives; c = false negatives; d = valid negatives
SR = Selection Rate = (a + b) / N; BR = Base Rate = (a + c) / N; MC = Maximum Correct = 1 - (|SR - BR|);
TC = Total Correct = (a + d) / N; RC = Random Correct = ((a + b) * (a + c) / N + (c + d) * (b + b) / N) / N;
IOC = Improvement Over Chance = |TC - RC|; RIOC = Relative Improvement Over Chance = IOC / (MC - RC) x 100

[1] Classifications are limited to 2 x 2 groupings. In case of more partitions subcategories are combined.

like this, conclusions about the usefulness of the predictors must either be drawn very carefully or dropped altogether.

Using base rates three times as high as the realistic selection rate, for example (see Table 1: Feshbach/Adelman/Fuller 1974), boosts the RIOC compared to studies with nearly identical base and selection rates (see Table 1: Feshbach/Adelman/Fuller 1977). In addition, the opposite relation of base and selection rate, i.e. a too high selection rate compared to a realistic base rate (see Table 1: Lindeman/Goodstein/Sachs/Young 1984; Satz/Friel 1974), results in a high number of correct predictions of problem cases, but also in a high number of false positive predictions. Concluding reviews of the relevant research Leach (1983) as well as Lindsay/Wedell (1982) appear disappointed by the low standards in classification studies and recommend abandoning research of this type altogether. In our view, this recommendation is not warranted, although it points to the need to follow methodological requirements more strictly (cf. Marx 1992a, b, c).

Cultural differences in early reading/spelling instruction

In contrast to Germany and other European countries (e.g. Sweden), preschool children in the USA and Canada start - often informally - to learn reading and spelling one year prior to school. In many parts of Australia children also get their first reading lessons during kindergarten, at age five. At least, children are taught specific verbal skills to prepare for the acquisition of reading/spelling, e.g. analyzing and synthesizing syllables and words. Often kindergarten children know quite a lot of letters or are even able to read a few simple words. Consequently, oral segmentation of words into phonemes or blending of sounds to words are chosen as predictors from the phonological awareness domain in Anglo-American studies.

Referring to the well-known discussion (cf. Morais/Alegria/Content 1987a, b) about phonological skills being (causal) antecedents or, to the contrary, consequents of early reading achievement, one may suspect that first measurements from most Anglo-American predictive studies do not relate to prerequisite skills sensu stricto but already are confounded with first results of informal reading instruction. Consequently, in studies of kindergarten children the best predictors of reading and spelling achievement turn out to be basic literacy skills like letter knowledge, reading, and spelling of sight vocabulary words (Tramontana/Hooper/Selzer 1988). More correctly, these skills have to be interpreted as early criterion variables (Bowey/Francis 1991; Marx 1989, 1992c).

From the practical point of view of finding out the best "at risk"-predictors in kindergarten age one has to admit, of course, that some overlap of predictors and criteria will not weigh too heavily since the major point is the reliable identification of children at risk to assign them to adequate prevention programs.

At all events, prediction of reading/spelling difficulties in Germany, Sweden or Austria differs from prediction in Anglo-American countries. Preparation for any school-type learning skill is strictly rejected in German kindergartens. Therefore, the literacy-related skills in German children are much less developed (Jansen 1992; Jansen/Mannhaupt/Marx 1993; Klicpera 1989; Wimmer/Hartl/Moser 1990; Wimmer/Hummer 1990), and are, most probably, comparable to those of four-year-olds in Anglo-American studies.

In conclusion, no straight and simple solution to the problem of intercultural comparison can be offered. The differences between some European and Anglo-American school systems can and should be seen as two realizations of the independent variable "school system" in the global quasi-experimental design leading to different effects in reading/spelling development of children.

The Bielefeld Longitudinal Study

Design

As shown in Table 2, the children were tested six times between November of the preschool year and the end of second grade. As a rule, measurement intervals were about six months.

The children were tested ten and four months before they entered first grade. During the first two years assessment took place about one month before the end of each term. For predictive results presented in this paper the final measurement at the end of the second grade was used. We report a selection of results which is restricted to data from measurements at T1 and T2 (predictors) and T6 (criteria).

Tab. 2: Time-schedule of assessments

Event	Measurement	Month	Year	Assessment
Begin of last preschool year		September	1986	
	T 1	October - December		Screening
	T 2	March - May	1987	Screening retest, intelligence
School entrance		September		
	T 3	November - December		
	T 4	June	1988	
Begin of 2nd grade		August		
	T 5	November - December		
	T 6 (longitudinal assessment)	April - May	1989	Math achievement
	T 6 (survey assessment)	May - June		Spelling, reading, intelligence

Preschool instruments

A screening device has to satisfy some technical requirements (e.g. practicality, economy; see Skowronek/Marx 1989). But most important is specificness, i.e. the screening taps essential prerequisite process components of reading/spelling acquisition; therefore, later reading/spelling achievement is more precisely predicted than achievement in other subjects, and competing predictors, e.g. general or nonverbal intelligence, predict reading/spelling achievement significantly less well.

The Bielefeld Screening. The screening consists of eight subtests in two domains and two control variables (naming of letters and numbers). Table

3 shows the final selection of the predictor variables. The first domain relates to "phonological awareness", but taps only its most elementary components (cf. Lewcowicz 1980; Wagner/Torgesen 1987; Yopp 1988), since pretests had shown that German kindergarten children are less competent in phonemic analysis than Anglo-American children (cf. Mannhaupt/Jansen 1989, Marx 1991a, b). The second domain contains components of attention to visually presented material and assesses various aspects of memory. Details of administration and scoring are given in Skowronek/Marx (1989) and Marx (1992c).

The classification of children at risk vs. non risk was done as follows: First, for each predictor task the cut-off for a risk score was set, irrespective of testing time (see Table 3 for details). Setting of risk scores was either based on random probabilities of guessing/success or on empirical distributions (lowest 15 %) of each task.

At T1, a child who in sum attained four and more risk scores was classified as "at risk". According to a supplementary discriminant analysis, children who ranged at or below the 15th percentile of the total distribution of screening raw scores were classified as borderline cases and added to the "at risk" group. Remaining children were classified as "non risk".

At T2, a child was classified as "at risk", when she/he got four or more risk scores. Children with three risk scores were classified as borderline, and having two or less risk scores was considered to be "non risk". As a final step, both classifications were summed to come up with the final "at risk" vs. "non risk" prediction. All children classified as "at risk" at T2 were finally classified as "at risk", as were children classified as "at risk" at T1 and, subsequently, as borderline at T2. All remaining children were finally classified as "non risk".

Preschool intelligence. To test for differential validity of the Bielefeld Screening, preschool intelligence was assessed by the German adaptation of Culture Fair Test (CFT1; Weiß/Osterland 1980). The test was administered individually at T2. Children scoring equal to or below 91 were classified as "IQ at risk". The cut-off allows for a selection rate comparable to the screening.

School instruments. At the end of second grade (T6) more than 2400 Bielefeld children, including the children from our longitudinal study, from almost all elementary schools in Bielefeld were tested in spelling, reading,

Tab. 3: Domains and subtests of the Bielefeld Screening including the risk score for each variable at T 1 and T 2.

Domain	Screening Task	Number of items	Variable related	Risk score limit and method of determination[1]			
				R/D	T 1	R/D	T 2
Phonological Awareness	Recognition of rhyming words	10	Correct decision	R	< 7	D	< 8
	Syllable Segmentation	10	Correct pronunciation	R	< 7	D	< 8
	Phoneme-word matching	10	Correct decision	R	< 7	D	< 8
	Sound blending with pictures	10	Decision with same vowel	R	< 7	D	< 8
Attention and Memory	Repeating Words	10	Correct repetition	D	< 4	D	< 5
	Knowledge of object colors	8	Correct naming	D	< 7	D	< 8[2]
	Rapid naming of the colors		Naming time in seconds				
	1. uncolored objects	24	Original time 1	D	> 63	D	> 53[2]
	2. color-incongruent objects	24	Time difference 2 - 1	D	> 40	D	> 34[2]
	Visual word matching		Choice of alternatives				
	1. accuracy of decision	12	75-100% identical alternatives	R	< 8	D	< 10
	2. response time per item	12	Median time in seconds	D	< 3.8	D	< 4.5[3]

[1] Risk scores are based either on the probabilities of random solutions (R) or on the 15 % cut-off of the empirical distribution (D).
[2] In the color task only two risk scores were possible to avoid stating a borderline case (three risk scores) by a single subtest.
[3] No risk score was given when there were more than eight 100 % correct responses.

and intelligence. Intervals between the three testing sessions were two weeks, at the most. Three weeks prior to the first survey session children from the longitudinal sample only were tested for math achievement.

Achievement in reading and spelling. The standardized spelling test, administered in the first testing session, required the children to spell 32 words from second grade vocabulary ("Diagnostischer Rechtschreibtest 2"; Müller 1982). In addition, an informal word dictation of eight twosyllable-words was administered. Reading skills were examined by a specially developed group reading test ("Knuspels Leseaufgaben", Marx in preparation). In the provisional form the test consisted of six subtests, of which three were used in the present study: First, in testing word recoding skill the child is asked to recognize sound consistencies in word pairs of differing orthographic similarity (e.g., "Meer - mehr", "alte - alle"). Second, tapping word decoding skills, meaningful words have to be recognized from letter sequences which differ in orthographic acceptability (e.g., "Fluuk", "üppen"). Third, reading comprehension was examined by children's answers to short written instructions.

To calculate composite criterion scores that were independent of the representative sample the raw test scores of all children except those from the representative sample were transformed to T-norms. The two spelling scores went with equal weight into a composite spelling score. The same procedure was applied to the three reading scores. Finally, a literacy score was composed from the T-transformed spelling and reading scores and again transformed to T-norms. After these norms were established, raw scores of the representative sample were also transformed to T-scores.

Math achievement. Three weeks prior to the survey the children from the longitudinal sample were given an informal math test, assessing basic math skills like addition, subtraction, and multiplication of two-digit numbers. Raw scores of children from the representative sample were T-transformed as described above.

School age intelligence. Intelligence was tested by the German adaptation of the Columbia Mental Maturity Scale (CMM 1-3, Schuck/Eggert/Raatz 1975). Raw scores were T-transformed, except for the representative sample. As described above, raw scores of this sample were transformed after T-norms had been independently established.

Children from the representative sample who ranged in the bottom 15 % in any of the criterion or control variable distributions were classified as problem cases.

Samples

The Bielefeld Screening was administered to 1120 children (about 75 % of the Bielefeld kindergarten population at age five in 1986) ten months before they entered school. The average age was 70.1 months (s = 3.69). Irrespective of the results of this first testing children were divided by chance into two subsamples that contained 85% (sample 1) and 15% (sample 2), respectively. The entire sample 2 (n = 169) was allocated to the longitudinal study. A group of 171 children of sample 1, who were classified as "at risk" or borderline cases, on the basis of T1 screening, were also selected for the longitudinal study. Finally, of these 340 children 240 participated in the longitudinal study, dependent on the parents' consent.

As the longitudinal study generally aimed at prediction and intervention, the sample just mentioned was again divided into a representative and an intervention sample. 54 at risk children took part in an intervention study (for details see Mannhaupt 1992). Finally, the representative sample consisted of 186 children (147 "non risk", 39 "at risk").

Results

Correlational results

As the screening subtests were designed to discriminate well at the lower end of the distribution they show clear ceiling effects. Therefore, correlations on subtest level would severely underestimate the true relations of variables. But on the level of composite scores, where individual performance profiles may compensate for skewness, correlations will nevertheless carry some valuable information. Composite scores were set up for all children (of total longitudinal sample) by standardizing and summing up subtest scores with equal weight.

Total screening scores of the Bielefeld Screening from T1 and T2 correlate at $r = .82$ ($p < .001$) (uncorrected Pearson retest correlation coefficient). Thus, stability of the Bielefeld Screening seems to be fairly good. The correlation of screening and intelligence is $r = .61$ ($p < .001$) at T1 and $r = .52$ ($p < .001$) at T2. Total screening score at T1 correlates at $r = .60$ ($p < .001$) with total literacy score at T6; the corresponding coefficient for screening at T2 is $r = .62$ ($p < .001$). The correlations between preschool intelligence, on the one hand, and school age intelligence, total literacy score, and math achievement are r = .43 (p < .001), r = .32 (p < .001), and r = .38 (p < .001), respectively.

Predictive results

Prediction based on the Bielefeld Screening. The prediction of criterion and control performances by the composite score from the Bielefeld Screening is shown in Table 4.

Intelligence at T6 is predicted by the composite score from the Bielefeld Screening at a total correct rate of 76.0 % which is close to the random correct rate of 73.9 %. The RIOC is correspondingly low (9.5 %). Prediction of problem vs. normal children in math achievement is remarkably better: RIOC increases to 34.8 %. Coming to prediction of specific criteria, spelling is predicted at a total correct rate of 86.3 % which yields a RIOC of 52.9 %. The result for reading is even better: total correct rate is 90.2 %, with a correspondingly high RIOC of 71.3 %. Combined literacy achievement is predicted best, at a total correct rate of 92.2 %, high above random rate by a RIOC of 72.2 %.

Summing up, the rate of correct predictions for intelligence is close to chance effects. Math achievement is predicted a little better. However, results for these control predictions are clearly exceeded by the rates of correct prediction for spelling, reading, and the composite literacy score.

Unspecific prediction based on intelligence. Performance in spelling and reading is predicted by preschool intelligence at the total correct rate of 73.0 % and 76.3 %, respectively, as is shown in Table 5.

Literacy (reading and spelling combined) is correctly predicted at 75.0 %. However, these rates practically do not differ from chance rates when children are divided randomly into "IQ at risk" and "IQ non risk" groups. Rates of random corrects for reading and spelling are 75.7 % and 76.2 %, respectively. Surprisingly, intelligence at the end of second grade is not predicted by preschool intelligence to a satisfactory degree. The correlation is as low as r = .43. The best prediction by means of the intelligence classification is that for math achievement, although not significantly differing from chance.

Tab. 4: ***Results of the classificatory prediction of reading, spelling, and control variables at T6 (end of 2nd grade) on the basis of the Bielefeld Screening composite score of T1/T2***

Variables at T6 (end of 2nd grade)	Classifications										
	Sel. Rate (SR) %	Base Rate (BR) %	Max. Corr. (MC) %	N	val pos a	fal pos b	fal neg c	val neg d	Total Corr. (TC) %	Rand. Corr. (RC) %	RIOC
Intelligence											
CMM 1-3	17.1	13.7	96.6	146	5	20	15	106	76.0	73.9	9.5
Control											
Maths	15.6	16.3	99.3	141	10	12	13	106	82.3	73.2	34.8
Criterion											
Spelling	17.0	15.0	98.0	153	14	12	9	118	86.3	73.1	52.9
Reading	17.0	13.7	96.7	153	16	10	5	122	90.2	73.9	71.3
Literacy	17.0	17.0	100.0	153	20	6	6	121	92.2	71.8	72.2

Legend and calculation formulas:
a = valid positives; b = false positives; c = false negatives; d = valid negatives
SR = Selection Rate = (a + b) / N; BR = Base Rate = (a + c) / N; MC = Maximum Correct = 1 - (|SR - BR|);
TC = Total Correct = (a + d) / N; RC = Random Correct = ((a + b) * (a + c) / N + (c + d) * (b + b) / N) / N;
IOC = Improvement Over Chance = |TC - RC|; RIOC = Relative Improvement Over Chance = IOC / (MC - RC) x 100

Tab. 5: ***Results of the classificatory prediction of reading, spelling, and control variables at T6 (end of 2nd grade) on the basis of intelligence (CFT1) at T2***

Variables at T6 (end of 2nd grade)	Classifications										
	Sel. Rate (SR) %	Base Rate (BR) %	Max. Corr. (MC) %	N	val pos a	fal pos b	fal neg c	val neg d	Total Corr. (TC) %	Rand. Corr. (RC) %	R I O C
Intelligence											
CMM 1-3	14.5	13.1	98.6	145	3	18	16	108	76.6	76.2	1.5
Control											
Maths	14.3	15.7	98.6	140	5	15	17	103	77.1	74.5	11.0
Criterion											
Spelling	13.8	14.5	99.3	152	1	20	21	110	73.0	75.7	<0.0
Reading	13.8	13.8	100.0	152	3	18	18	113	76.3	76.2	0.5
Literacy	13.8	16.4	92.2	152	4	17	21	110	75.0	74.3	3.1

Legend and calculation formulas:
a = valid positives; b = false positives; c = false negatives; d = valid negatives
SR = Selection Rate = (a + b) / N; BR = Base Rate = (a + c) / N; MC = Maximum Correct = 1 - (|SR - BR|);
TC = Total Correct = (a + d) / N; RC = Random Correct = ((a + b) * (a + c) / N + (c + d) * (b + b) / N) / N;
IOC = Improvement Over Chance = |TC - RC|; RIOC = Relative Improvement Over Chance = IOC / (MC - RC) x 100

Discussion

Taking into account the correlational results reported here, the Bielefeld Screening proves to be a preschool instrument that specifically predicts the development of literacy acquisition. Even though all correlations of predictors and criteria, specific and unspecific, are highly significant, yet the correlations representing the specific relation, i.e. between screening composite scores and literacy, show the highest values, the differences being highly significant. Furthermore, the stability over half a year is quite satisfactory. The relation between specific literacy predictors and general cognitive achievement is far from zero, with a common variance of 36 %. This supports the idea that in preschool age specific cognitive skills do not develop independently from broader cognitive development.

Our assumption that literacy achievement at end of second grade is specifically predicted has been borne out by the classificatory results. Obviously, preschool intelligence is not a satisfactory predictor for any specific school achievement, neither for spelling, reading, literacy nor for math achievement and not even for later intelligence itself, at the end of second grade. On the other hand, the Bielefeld Screening demonstrates its validity: by RIOCs of 70 % for prediction of literacy vs. about 35 % for math and just some 10 % for intelligence at the end of second grade.

At first glance, these impressive results of classificatory prediction support a dispositional interpretation of reading and spelling difficulties, such that problems will most probably occur when a basic level of adequate skills in phonological awareness and/or in the organization of attention and memory for symbol sequences is not met at school entrance. Will "weak" dispositions in the two precursor domains of phonological awareness and attention/memory organization necessarily lead to reading and spelling difficulties? Is the fate of being a reading/spelling disordered child inevitable and predetermined from the very beginning of school? Definitely not. In our view, it is true that the state of relevant language processing as it is validly assessed by the screening is the result of a child's individual past development towards alphabetic script. An inadequate state of readiness may be based in insufficient stimulation. The other way round, such a state may be influenced to the better by parents, kindergarten teachers and, most important, by teachers, from the very first days of literacy instruction. On the other hand and judging realistically, under present conditions of elementary instruction, for a child identified as "at risk" the points seem to be shifted. Elementary school still needs to invent and practise specific instructional and/or organizational support for slow learners in literacy acquisition.

In conclusion, we judge the merits of our study from a practical as well as from a theoretical point of view. Under theoretical aspects, referring to the controversy about causal direction in the relation of phonological awareness to literacy acquisition the present study is appropriate to push the answer a bit further. On the one hand, it seems possible to use skills of phonological awareness and of attention/memory *combined* as valid, not-confounded predictors of failure in literacy acquisition. On the other hand, one has to admit that the phonological awareness skills measured are located at the very bottom in the hierarchy of relevant skills (Lewkowicz 1980; Skowronek/ Marx 1989). Thus, two answers seem adequate. First, that even children with almost no literacy experience have phonological precursors at their disposal. These are very basic and simple, i.e. rhyming; syllable segmentation; and sound to word matching, when the first sound constitutes the first syllable. Second, higher levels of phonological awareness, i.e. sound blending or phoneme segmentation evolve, at least in German children, as a consequence of literacy instruction in school. From a comparative point of view, in Anglo-American children the developmental pattern, in transition from kindergarten to school, appears to be less discontinuous and clear-cut.

At first glance, the German situation seems to make prediction more difficult. But it turned out less of an obstacle to satisfactory results than was expected. Although the predictors to be chosen are more distant to criterion performance compared with the Anglo-American studies, the classificatory results are very encouraging, notabene with the qualification that we combined two assessments, six months apart, to one prediction. We are currently constructing a more economical one-point prediction. Bearing in mind that as a rule test administration in Germany just prior to elementary school consists of assessments of general school readiness, the reported results on poor predictive quality of intelligence tests raise the question whether specific predictors of reading/spelling and, perhaps, math could replace these general school readiness tests. Administering subject specific preschool screenings could also improve the diagnosis of individual, subject-related weaknesses. Thus, preschool assessment could become more relevant to instruction. It could even be an instrument of support to instruction, complementary to the currently dominant selective orientation.

With regard to the temporal and organizational placement of prevention and/or early remediation, the conclusions from reported results seem obvious. Since the identification of "at risk" children is validly possible prior to school entrance, prevention prior to school seems indicated. However, the route to an adequate state of readiness for alphabetic script in children at risk for reading/spelling difficulties might be more extended than the contrived sample of tasks and stimuli from the screening can convey. The study of Lundberg/Frost/Petersen (1988) speaks for an enormous amount of effort needed to attain significant effects that will persist into second grade. Eventually early remediation in school may be more efficient because types of learning tasks aimed to trigger the missing prerequisites may be more easily developed from tasks closely related to literacy acquisition. However, which types of tasks serve this purpose best is still an open question.

Note

[1]The current study is part of the project "Early identification and intervention in risks of learning disorder in reading and spelling" of the Special Research Unit 227 at the Bielefeld University.

References

Berninger, V.W. (1986). Normal variation in reading acquisition. Perceptual and Motor Skills, 62, 691-721.

Bowey, J.A. & Francis, J. (1991). Phonological analysis as a function of age and exposure to reading instruction. Applied Psycholinguistics, 12, 91-121.

Chall, J.S. (1983). Stages of reading development. New York: McGraw-Hill Book Company.

Coltheart, M. (1978). Lexical access in a simple reading task. In G. Underwood (Ed.), Strategies in information processing. 151-216. New York: Academic Press.

Cronbach, L.J. & Gleser, G.C. (1965). Psychological tests and personnel decisions. Urbana: University of Illinois Press.

Ehri, L.C. (1991). Learning to read and spell words. In L. Rieben & C. Perfetti (Eds.), Learning to read: Basic research and its implications. 57-73. Hillsdale, N.J.: Lawrence Erlbaum Associates.

Ferinden, W.E. & Jacobson, S. (1970). Early identification of learning disabilities. Journal of Learning Disabilities, 11, 48-52.

Feshbach, S., Adelman, H., & Fuller, W. (1974). Early identification of children with high risk for reading failure. Journal of Learning Disabilities, 7, 639-644.

Feshbach, S., Adelman, H., & Fuller, W. (1977). Prediction of reading and related academic problems. Journal of Educational Psychology, 69, 299-308.

Frith, U. (1985). Beneath the surface of developmental dyslexia. Are comparisons between developmental and acquired disorders meaningful? In K.E. Patterson, J.C. Marshall, & M. Coltheart (Eds.), Surface dyslexia. 301-330. London: Erlbaum.

Frith, U. (1986). Psychologische Aspekte des orthographischen Wissens: Entwicklung und Entwicklungsstörung. In G. Augst (Ed.), New trends in graphemics and orthography. 218-233. Berlin: de Gruyter.

Gough, P.B. & Hillinger, M.L. (1980). Learning to read: an unnatural act. Bulletin of the Orton Society, 30, 179-195.

Günther, K.B. (1986). Ein Stufenmodell der Entwicklung kindlicher Lese- und Schreibstrategien. In H. Brügelmann (Ed.), ABC und Schriftsprache: Rätsel für Kinder, Lehrer und Forscher. 32-54. Konstanz: Faude.

Høien, T. & Lundberg, I. (1988). Stages of word recognition in early reading development. Scandinavian Journal of Educational Research, 32, 163-182.

Høien, T. & Lundberg, I. (1989). A strategy for assessing problems in word recognition among dyslexics. Scandinavian Journal of Educational Research, 33, 185-201.

Humphreys, G.W. & Evett, L.J. (1985). Are there independent lexical and nonlexical routes in word processing? An evaluation of the dual route theory of reading. Behavioral and Brain Sciences, 8, 689-705.

Jansen, H. (1992). Untersuchungen zur Entwicklung lautsynthetischer Verarbeitungsprozesse im Vorschul- und frühen Grundschulalter. Egelsbach, Köln, New York: Hänsel-Hohenhausen.

Jansen, H., Mannhaupt, G., & Marx, H. (1993). Probleme bei der Übertragbarkeit angloamerikanischer Entwicklungsmodelle des Lesens und Rechtschreibens auf deutschsprachige Schulkinder. In R. Bromme & H. Bauersfeld (Eds.), Bildung und Aufklärung. Studien zur Rationalität des Lehrens und Lernens. 69-88. Münster: Waxmann.

Jansky, J.J. & de Hirsch, K. (1972). Preventing reading failure. New York: Harper & Row.

Klicpera, C. (1989). The reading development of normal and poor readers in the first grade: How helpful is the concept of developmental stages for the understanding of reading acquisition in German-speaking children? In M. Brambring, F. Lösel, & H. Skowronek (Eds.), Children at risk: assessment, longitudinal research and intervention. 97-118. Berlin, New York: de Gruyter.

Kretschmann, R., Lindner-Achenbach, S., Puffahrt, A., Möhlmann, G., & Achenbach, J. (1990). Analphabetismus bei Jugendlichen. Stuttgart: Kohlhammer.

Leach, D.J. (1980). Considerations in screening for school learning difficulties: An overview of practice. Educational Studies, 6, 181-197.

Leach, D.J. (1983). Early screening procedures. School Psychology International, 4, 47-55.

Lewkowicz, N.K. (1980). Phonemic awareness training: What to teach and how to teach it. Journal of Educational Psychology, 72, 686-700.

Lichtenstein, R. & Ireton, H. (1984). Preschool screening. Identifying young children with developmental and educational problems. Orlando: Grune & Stratton.

Lindeman, D.P., Goodstein, H.A., Sachs, A., & Young, C.C. (1984). An evaluation of the Yellow Brick Road Test through a full prediction-performance comparison matrix. Journal of School Psychology, 22, 111-117.

Lindsay, G.A. & Wedell, K. (1982). The early identification of educationally 'at risk' children revisited. Journal of Learning Disabilities, 15, 212-217.

Loeber, R. & Dishion, T. (1983). Early predictors of male delinquency: A review. Psychological Bulletin, 94, 68-99.

Lundberg, I., Frost, J., & Petersen, O.P. (1988). Effects of an extensive program for stimulating phonological awareness in preschool children. Reading Research Quarterly, 23, 263-284.

Lundberg, I., Olofsson, A., & Wall, S. (1980). Reading and spelling skills in the first school year predicted from phonemic awareness skills in kindergarten. Scandinavian Journal of Psychology, 21, 159-173.

Mann, V.A. (1991). Phonological abilities: Effective predictors of future reading ability. In L. Rieben & C.A. Perfetti (Eds.), Learning to read: Basic research and its implications. 121-133. Hillsdale, New Jersey: Lawrence Erlbaum Associates.

Mannhaupt, G. (1992). Strategisches Lernen: eine empirische Studie zur Ausbildung von Monitoring im frühen Schriftspracherwerb. Heidelberg: Asanger.

Mannhaupt, G. & Jansen, H. (1989). Phonologische Bewußtheit: Aufgabenentwicklung und Leistungen im Vorschulalter. Heilpädagogische Forschung, 15, 50-56.

Marsh, G., Friedman, M., Welch, V., & Desberg, P. (1981). A cognitive developmental theory of reading acquisition. In T. Waller & G. MacKinnon (Eds.), Reading research: Advances in theory and practice. 199-221. New York: Academic Press.

Marx, H. (1989). Zeitliche Ausgangspunkte und ihre Auswirkungen auf Anlage und Aussage von Längsschnittstudien zur frühen Identifikation und Prädiktion von Lese-Rechtschreibschwierigkeiten. Universität Bielefeld: SFB 227, Preprint Nr. 22.

Marx, H. (1991a). Entwicklungsbedingte Verarbeitungsunterschiede bei phonologischen Syntheseaufgaben. Zeitschrift für Entwicklungspsychologie und Pädagogische Psychologie, 23, 330-349.

Marx, H. (1991b). Abhängigkeit der Richtiglösungen im Lauteverbinden von Anzahl und Art der Bildinformation. Zeitschrift für experimentelle und angewandte Psychologie, 38, 620-633.

Marx, H. (1992a). Frühe Identifikation und Prädiktion von Lese-Rechtschreibschwierigkeiten: Bestandsaufnahme bisheriger Bewertungsgesichtspunkte von Längsschnittstudien. Zeitschrift für Pädagogische Psychologie, 6, 35-48.

Marx, H. (1992b). Methodische und inhaltliche Argumente für und wider eine frühe Identifikation und Prädiktion von Lese-Rechtschreibschwierigkeiten. Diagnostica, 38, 249-268.

Marx, H. (1992c). Vorhersage von Lese-Rechtschreibschwierigkeiten in Theorie und Anwendung. Habilitationsschrift. Universität Bielefeld.

Marx, H. (in preparation). Knuspels Leseaufgaben. Manual zu einem Gruppenlesetest für Kinder Ende des ersten bis vierten Schuljahres.

Morais, J., Alegria, J., & Content, A. (1987a). The relationships between segmental analysis and alphabetic literacy: An interactive view. Cahiers de Psychologie Cognitive, 7, 415-438.

Morais, J., Alegria, J., & Content, A. (1987b). Segmental awareness: Respectable, useful, and almost always necessary. Cahiers de Psychologie Cognitive, 7, 530-556.

Morrison, D., Mantzicopoulos, P., & Stone, E. (1988). Screening for reading problems: The utility of SEARCH. Annals of Dyslexia, 38, 181-192.

Müller, R. (1982). Diagnostischer Rechtschreibtest DRT 2. Weinheim: Beltz.

Perfetti, C.A., Beck, I., Bell, L., & Hughes, C. (1987). Phonemic knowledge and learning to read are reciprocal: A longitudinal study of first grade children. Merrill-Palmer Quarterly, 33, 283-319.

Rubin, R.A., Balow, B., Dorle, J., & Rosen, M. (1978). Preschool prediction of low achievement in basic school skills. Journal of Learning Disabilities, 11, 664-667.

Satz, P. & Friel, J. (1974). Some predictive antecedents of specific reading disability: A preliminary two-year follow-up. Journal of Learning Disabilities, 7, 48-55.

Scheerer-Neumann, G. (1981). Prozeßanalyse der Leseschwäche. In R. Valtin, U.O.H. Jung & G. Scheerer-Neumann (Eds.), Legasthenie in Wissenschaft und Unterricht. Darmstadt: Wissenschaftliche Buchgesellschaft, 183-240.

Scheerer-Neumann, G. (1989a). Entwicklungsprozesse beim Lesenlernen: Eine Fallstudie. In M. Beck (Ed.), Schriftspracherwerb - Lese-Rechtschreibschwäche. 15-38. Tübingen: Deutsche Gesellschaft für Verhaltenstherapie.

Scheerer-Neumann, G. (1989b). The representation of developmental stages in a model of word recognition. Paper presented at the 6th European Conference on Reading from July 31st to August 3rd 1989, Berlin.

Schuck, K.D., Eggert, D., & Raatz, U. (1975). Columbia Mental Maturity Scale CMM 1-3. Sprachfreier Gruppenintelligenztest für die Grundschule. Weinheim: Beltz.

Share, D.L. & Silva, P.A. (1986). The stability and classification of specific reading retardation: A longitudinal study from age 7 to 11. British Journal of Educational Psychology, 56, 32-39.

Silver, A.A. (1978). Prevention. In A.L. Benton & D. Pearl (Eds.), Dyslexia: An appraisal of current knowledge. 349-376. New York: Oxford University Press.

Silver, A.A. & Hagin, R.A. (1981). SEARCH Manual. New York: Walker Educational Corporation.

Skowronek, H. & Marx, H. (1989). The Bielefeld longitudinal study on early identification of risks in learning read and write: Theoretical backround and first results. In M. Brambring, F. Lösel, & H. Skowronek (Eds.), Children at risk: assessment, longitudinal research and intervention. 268-294. Berlin, New York: de Gruyter.

Skowronek, H. & Marx, H. (1993). Disorders of written language development: Definitions and overview. In G. Blanken, J. Dittmann, H. Grimm, J.C. Marshall, & C.-W. Wallesch (Eds.), Linguistic disorders and pathologies. An international handbook. 711-724. Berlin, New York: de Gruyter.

Stanovich, K.E. (1986). Matthew effects in reading: Some consequences of individual differences in the acquisition of literacy. Reading Research Quarterly, 21, 360-406.

Stanovich, K.E., Cunningham, A.E., & Cramer, B.B. (1984). Assessing phonological awareness in kindergarten children: Issues of task comparability. Journal of Experimental Child Psychology, 38, 175-190.

Tramontana, M.G., Hooper, S.R., & Selzer, S.C. (1988). Research on the preschool prediction of later academic achievement: A review. Developmental Review, 8, 89-146.

Valtin, R. (1984). Awareness of features and functions of language. In J. Downing & R. Valtin (Eds.), Language awareness and learning to read. 227-260. Berlin: Springer.

Van Orden, G.C., Pennington, B.F., & Stone, G.O. (1990). Word identification in reading and the promise of subsymbolic psycholinguistics. Psychological Review, 97, 488-522.

Wagner, R.K. & Torgesen, J.K. (1987). The nature of phonological processing and its causal role in the acquisition of reading skills. Psychological Bulletin, 101, 192-212.

Weiß, R. & Osterland, J. (1980). Grundintelligenztest CFT1, Skala 1. Braunschweig: Georg Westermann Verlag.

Wimmer, H., Hartl, M., & Moser, E. (1990). Passen "englische" Modelle des Schriftspracherwerbs auf "deutsche" Kinder? Zweifel an der Bedeutsamkeit der logographischen Stufe. Zeitschrift für Entwicklungspsychologie und Pädagogische Psychologie, 22, 136-154.

Wimmer, H. & Hummer, P. (1990). How German-speaking first graders read and spell: Doubts on the importance of the logographic stage. Applied Psycholinguistics, 11, 349-368.

Yopp, H.K. (1988). The validity and reliability of phonemic awareness tests. Reading Research Quarterly, 23, 159-177.

Commentary on Marx, Jansen, Mannhaupt and Skowronek: The Bielefeld Screening Battery to predict reading and spelling difficulties

Linnea C. Ehri

A multitude of perspectives might be adopted to discuss the Bielefeld longitudinal prediction study. It is a study rich in ideas, data, and implications. My perspective arises from my work as a researcher attempting to understand the processes and course of development in learning to read and spell. These processes include metalinguistic capabilities, particularly lexical and phonemic awareness, and how these relate to acquisition, how children develop word reading skill, particularly sight word learning processes, and how spelling develops and contributes to word reading.

My findings combined with research by others have led me to take sides on several issues. One position associated with my work is that the bulk of metalinguistic knowledge evolves during the course of learning to read and spell an alphabetic orthography and hence is a consequence of literacy acquisition (Ehri 1979, 1984; Morais/Cary/Alegria/Bertelson 1979; Read/Zhang/Nie/Ding 1986). This is particularly true at the phonemic level of language where readers' conception of words as sequences of phonemes is heavily influenced by their knowledge of how the spelling system symbolizes phonemes and how specific words are spelled (Ehri/Wilce 1980, 1986). However, my research has also indicated that phonemic awareness plays a central role in the acquisition of word reading and spelling skill. Thus, I view metalinguistic awareness as both a cause and a consequence of literacy acquisition (Ehri 1979, 1991). The two claims are not mutually exclusive.

A second position that I have defended and documented (Ehri 1991, 1992) is that sight word learning is not a strictly visual process in which word forms are linked to meanings via rote memory as dual route theory claims. Also it is not a process in which words are phonologically recoded from print to sound to meaning. Rather sight word learning is a process in which grapheme-phoneme knowledge is applied to secure specific spellings of words to their pronunciations in lexical memory.

A third position I have argued in the literature (Ehri 1989) is that the core deficit which prevents disabled readers from becoming adequate readers and spellers in an alphabetic system is a failure to learn how the alphabetic system symbolizes speech at the phonemic and lexical levels well enough so that this knowledge functions automatically as part of the reading process (Ehri/Wilce 1983). Whether "at risk" students become disabled readers depends more upon the quality of instruction and practice that they receive in learning to read and spell than upon any limitations in their processing capabilities (Ehri 1989).

These views will be apparent in my analyses of the Bielefeld study. My reflections include pointing out some strengths and shortcomings, elaborating on important features of the study and issues that were only briefly mentioned, considering reasons for the battery's success in predicting reading failure, and suggesting directions for future research.

The Bielefeld Study

The Bielefeld longitudinal study to predict reading disability tested children six times over a three-year period from preschool through second grade. The screening battery consisted of measures of phonological processing, attention, and memory and was given twice in preschool. Performance criteria applied to both testings were used to distinguish those students "at risk." Intelligence was also measured in preschool and second grade. Achievement in reading, spelling and math was assessed at the end of second grade. The screening battery proved highly effective for predicting which students became the poorest readers and spellers at the end of second grade. It was much more effective than the preschool intelligence test which yielded predictions of reading disability close to chance. The predictive success of the battery was literacy specific as it displayed only limited accuracy at identifying students who became math-disabled.

The Bielefeld study has several strengths making its results especially valuable. Whereas most of our predictive studies have been conducted with English-speaking subjects, this study examined German-speaking students. Many preschoolers were tested in order to obtain a sizeable sample of students "at risk" for reading failure. The predictive instruments were administered before students had learned much about letters or literacy so their performances were not contaminated by informally acquired knowledge about print. The screening tests were designed to be sensitive to levels of performance characterizing "at risk" students at the lower ends of distributions. Predictions were based on two performances on the battery.

To assess the battery's success at predicting reading disability, cut-off scores were defined, and classification accuracy was assessed relative to that expected by chance. The advantage of this approach over a correlational approach is that success rests only on the battery's accuracy at distinguishing disabled readers. Success is not confounded by accuracy at discriminating among good readers at the upper levels of performance. This is a common weakness of predictive tests (Badian 1988). For example, Jansky/Hoffman/Layton et al. (1989) found that their kindergarten screening battery was better at predicting which students became good readers than which students became poor readers.

The Bielefeld researchers have much more data than are presented in their chapter. We look forward to learning about other findings. Of particular interest is the relative contribution that each of the tasks makes in predicting reading failure. In my perusal of the authors' unpublished data, I noticed that the rapid naming speed task was more highly correlated with criterion measures of literacy in second grade than the phonological awareness tests. Of course, it may be that the phonological correlations were suppressed by ceiling effects, or the naming correlations were inflated by good reader differences, so we need something other than correlations to find out how successful each task was for distinguishing disabled readers. This information would be helpful to others making decisions about which tasks to include in their screening batteries. Also it would be helpful for drawing comparisons among studies to get an idea whether the success of specific predictor tasks might be influenced by other variables, for example, whether the orthography is alphabetic, syllabic or logographic, how much the students being screened know about print or literacy, how reading and spelling are taught.

Tasks and processes

Tasks included in the screening battery were those that were thought to assess important processes involved in literacy acquisition without being reading/spelling tasks themselves, and that discriminated well at the lower third of the distribution in pilot studies. In addition, tasks were similar if not identical to tasks that had been found by other researchers to distinguish good from poor readers.

Described below are the tasks that comprised the screening battery and the reading-related processes (bold) that each task was thought to assess. (For more about the rationale, see Skowronek/Marx 1989).

A. **Rudimentary Phonological Awareness**:
(1) Judging whether two words rhyme
(2) Segmenting words into syllables
(3) Judging whether a vowel sound occurs at the beginning of a spoken word
(4) Blending onset and rime units to form a word and then selecting from four choices either the picture named by the blend or the picture having the same rime but a different onset.

B. **Phonetic Recoding in Working Memory**: Repeating multisyllabic pseudowords.

C. **Attention to Visual Letter Sequences**: Picking from four spellings the one that matches a visible target word spelling; both accuracy and latency were measured.

(The following processes all involved naming the prototypic colors of four objects: lettuce - green, plum - blue, lemon - yellow, tomato - red.)

D. **Memory for Attributes of Visual Stimuli**: Accurately naming the colors of objects unaided by uncolored line drawings.

E. **Lexical Access/Recoding Speed**: Rapidly naming the colors of a sequence of objects from their uncolored line drawings.

F. **Attention: Susceptibility to Distraction**: Rapidly naming the colors of objects depicted in conflicting colors (type of Stroop task); the measure was the time difference between Tasks E and F.

Tasks A, B, and E assessed three types of phonological processes identified by Wagner/Torgesen (1987) as important for learning to read: phonological awareness, phonetic recoding in working memory, and phonological recoding in lexical access, respectively.

Regarding the choice of phonological awareness tasks, it is interesting to note that several more phonological awareness tasks were tried than were retained in the screening battery. Those rejected because they were too hard for students included four tasks measuring more advanced phonemic analysis skills: deleting phonemes in words, blending phonemes into words orally without picture prompts, detecting specified vowels in the middle or ends of words, and segmenting words into phonemes. These findings bear on the issue of the relationship between phonemic awareness and reading/spelling acquisition. The fact that the Bielefeld preschoolers who were non-readers failed these tasks, plus the fact that once students moved into reading and spelling they became able to perform these tasks, indicate that these phonological skills do not emerge until literacy acquisition is underway and children have learned about alphabetic representations of speech. In studies where these tasks have predicted reading achievement successfully, it is likely that the subjects were further along in their knowledge about print and reading.

In the Bielefeld study, more rudimentary levels of phonological awareness proved within the capability of non-reading preschoolers and were effective at predicting subsequent reading failure: detecting rhyming words and first sounds in words, segmenting words into syllables. It is noteworthy that the units within non-readers' scope of awareness were initial vowel sounds and syllables rather than phoneme-size units which apparently do not come within reach until reading instruction is underway.

One rudimentary phonological awareness task proved more difficult, that requiring preschoolers to blend onsets and rimes into words and select one of four pictures depicting the word. However, this task was retained in the battery and made easier by accepting either correct blends or blends that included the correct rime. Whether these results challenge claims of Goswami (1986) and Treiman (1985) that onsets and rimes are natural subsyllabic units of speech that are within the reach of prereaders needs further study.

The Bielefeld measure of "phonetic recoding in working memory" required subjects to repeat multisyllabic nonwords. Although others have used this same type of task successfully to predict beginning reading (Mann 1984), the task does not quite live up to its name but rather is a simpler memory span task. Wagner/Torgesen (1987) acknowledge that repeating a series of spoken items really only assesses the storage component of working memory. A more complete task would be one that assessed storage and processing operations simultaneously (e.g., selecting the odd item from an array of 3 or 4 items being held in memory). Perhaps the predictive success of the two types of tasks should be compared in future research.

The task to measure "phonological recoding in lexical access" is the most unique and least explored to my knowledge. According to Wagner/Torgesen (1987), this process involves "getting from a written word to its lexical referent by recoding the written symbols into a sound-based representational system" (p. 198). The Bielefeld measure appears to be an analog of this reading task that is within the reach of non-readers. The analog might be described as "getting from a visually depicted object to its color by recoding the drawing into a semantically-based representation." Although a non-automatic recoding operation is required, the phonological aspect of the process appears to be minimal. Nevertheless, the task makes an important contribution to prediction.

More commonly used measures of recoding/access simply require subjects to rapidly name a sequence of objects, colors, letters, or numbers (Denckla/Rudel 1976; Spring/Capps 1974; Wolf 1991). Catts (1991) complicated the task slightly by having subjects name the color and the object both of which were visually apparent (e.g., blue cow). The fact that performances on naming tasks are strong predictors of reading performance two years later raises curiosity about why, what underlying processes are tapped that are important for learning to read. Studies have shown that symbol naming speed contributes variance to reading quite independently of variance explained by phonological awareness and also by intelligence, so different aspects of reading are being predicted by these tasks (Blachman 1984; Bowers/Swanson 1991; Felton/Brown 1990; Mann 1984).

Bowers/Wolf (in press) propose an interesting hypothesis about why naming tasks predict reading. They do not regard the task as a measure of phonological ability. Rather they suggest that naming is an analog of the reading process. It is a simpler, earlier developing system that is less affected by knowledge of orthography and phonology but that shares many of the major processes that operate in learning to read. They propose that naming speed deficits reflect a disruption of precise timing mechanisms that are necessary for the automatic formation and unitization of orthographic and phonological representations in memory.

Another possibility is that naming speed is an indicator of letter name learning ability. There is evidence that the speed of color naming in kindergarten is correlated with how many letter names a child learns that year (Blachman 1984). We know that letter knowledge is as good a predictor of reading achievement as phonemic awareness (Share/Jorm/Maclean/Matthews 1984) and that reading acquisition cannot proceed without letter knowledge (Adams 1990). Perhaps the predictive success of naming speed tasks are linked to their relationship to letter learning.

A third hypothesis proposed by Spring/Davis (1988) is that the naming speed task taps a person's ability to process information in parallel. In naming a sequence of items rapidly, the eyes are ahead of the voice and each is processing different information. The eyes are viewing new stimuli and the visual system is registering the stimuli while the linguistic system is coding and transforming previously seen stimuli and the voice is articulating the earlier stimuli. All of these processes are happening and being coordinated concurrently. Deficits in the capacity to coordinate multiple concurrent processes may explain what is tapped by poor performance in the naming task and what predicts disabled reading.

The Bielefeld researchers believe that all of the tasks in their screening battery are successful in predicting reading failure because they measure processes that are causally involved in literacy acquisition and that if deficient make acquisition difficult or impossible. However, another possibility is that the tasks measure deficiencies that are correlates rather than causes of reading disability. Until we have a cohesive empirically supported theory of acquisition that explains the role of the processes, this alternative explanation cannot be dismissed. Presently there are theories of reading acquisition supported by evidence that clarify how phonemic awareness is involved in learning to decode words, to spell words, and to read words by sight (Adams 1990; Brady/Shankweiler 1991; Gough/Ehri/Treiman 1992). However, the involvement of the other processes is less certain and needs more research.

The Bielefeld researchers say little about whether the predictive success of the test battery might be influenced by the quality of instruction that students "at risk" receive. It may be that some processes are more susceptible to instructional effects than others. It would seem that with carefully planned instruction and sufficient practice to insure that learners master the alphabetic system and become able to use it automatically to decode new words and to acquire sight words, the predictive success of measures like phonological awareness and visual word matching might be *weakened* because good instruction should remediate any deficits and hence eliminate the influence of individual differences on the literacy acquisition process. However, whether good instruction would also weaken the predictive success of tasks like rapid naming is less clear. If the critical operations tapped in naming tasks involve timing mechanisms or parallel processing, it may not be possible for literacy instruction to touch and modify their operation. If this is true, then rapid naming tasks should remain successful in predicting reading difficulty regardless of instructional variation.

To what extent beginning instruction and also remedial instruction have the potential for creating normal readers and spellers out of preschoolers who are truly "at risk" for reading failure because they are deficient in one or several of the processes measured in the Bielefeld screening battery is a highly important question for future research. It may be that well designed instruction can remediate some deficits but not others.

True precursors and early criterion variables

One presumed strength of the Bielefeld study is that their subjects had little knowledge of letters, reading, or spelling so the success of the screening tests in predicting reading failure was not contaminated by differences in reading skill that already existed when the tests were given. In Germany, preschoolers are not taught about print by either teachers or parents. This contrasts with countries such as the U.S. where middle-class parents and preschool teachers spend lots of time reading stories to children and teaching the alphabet, letter-sound relations, and even simple forms of reading (Adams 1990). The Bielefeld researchers suggest that, as a result, preschool variables found effective for predicting subsequent reading achievement in the U.S. may be "early criterion variables" that result from this informal reading instruction rather than true precursors.

The fact that the Bielefeld study has gotten closer to "true precursors" of literacy acquisition than other studies is important theoretically. However, practically speaking, the value of a screening battery lies in its predictive success rather than what it measures. In cultures where informal reading is taught during the early years, the most effective screening tests may be ones that consist of measures more closely related to print and reading. An example of a successful test is the Early Reading Screening test developed by Uhry (in press) for kindergartners. Comparison of her tasks to the Bielefeld tests reveals that more phoneme manipulation is required. Also several print awareness tasks are included (e.g., writing one's name, fingerpoint reading a previously heard sentence, recognizing environmental print, spelling initial sounds of words).

Whether "early criterion" tests predict reading failure two years later more effectively than "true precursor" tests is an interesting question. One would expect that predictive measures which are closer to criterion behaviors would predict more accurately. However, if students taking early criterion tests have not had equal access to informal print instruction, then those identified "at risk" by tests such as letter naming would include students who lacked the opportunity to learn as well as students with information processing or learning deficits. The former students would be expected to catch up to other students by the end of the second year of formal instruction and hence to be incorrectly predicted as "at risk."

Are the performances of German preschoolers really untouched by literacy?

The Bielefeld researchers suggest that their battery measures "phonological precursors" of reading and spelling acquisition that emerge in children "with almost no literacy experience." However, I question whether this is true. Even though German kindergartners lack knowledge about print, they may receive print-specific informal literacy instruction of a different sort from parents and teachers.

The instruction I have in mind involves teaching preschoolers "Hochdeutsch," (translated writing German) which is a spoken form of German that corresponds closely to the written form, in contrast to other dialects of spoken German that differ markedly from the pronunciations of words symbolized in print. Hochdeutsch is considered good German and has higher status than other dialects. It is possible that parents who teach their children to speak Hochdeutsch are more attentive to the accuracy of their children's speech at the lexical/phonological level. They pronounce words carefully, particularly new words that their children might not know, they listen to their children's speech and help them articulate all the syllables and consonants in less familiar words.

This type of informal literacy-based instruction should benefit students in phonological awareness tasks and also pseudoword repetition tasks. Also it should help students learn to read and spell, because students' speech bears a close correspondence to print. In contrast, students having more difficulty on the phonological screening tests as well as in acquiring literacy might be those who speak a dialect of German that deviates from print and whose parents did not direct their attention to phonological properties of language as they learned to speak. This hypothesis is worth investigating.

In English, there is no term to designate a dialect that resembles written language. However, I have observed the influence of spellings upon parents and teachers when they tutor children in the correct pronunciations of words: saying February as "feb-*rue*-air-ee," not "feb-*you*-air-ee;" saying interesting as "in-*ter*-es-ting," not "in-*tres*-ting;" saying museum as "myou-zee-*um*," not "myou-zee-*im*." Because the correspondences between spellings and pronunciations are more transparent in German than in English, with a letter for almost every sound, the compulsion to speak words as they are spelled may be even stronger. Also because teachers and parents possess clear phonological representations of words supported by the spelling system, their compulsion to teach spelling-based pronunciations to children may be especially strong. Having spellings that specify phonemes in mind should make mispronunciations of words more obvious and easier to detect.

What leads me to the above hypothesis? My research on learning to read words has led me to the view that readers retain the spellings of words in memory as symbols for phonemes in pronunciations of words when they acquire reading and spelling skill. Spellings clarify how to pronounce words and which phonemes are in the words when there is uncertainty (i.e., "rue" in February and "ter" in interesting). At the outset of acquisition, orthography and phonology are totally separate stimulus modalities. What happens during the course of development is that they become intertwined and function as one system in which spellings become phonology made visible. In disabled readers, this does not happen; orthography and phonology do not merge into one system. (For a fuller explanation of this research and theory, see Drake/Ehri 1984; Ehri 1980, 1984, 1987, 1991, 1992; Ehri/Wilce 1979, 1980, 1982, 1983, 1986; Ehri/Wilce/Taylor 1987).

It is noteworthy that a number of preschoolers in the Bielefeld study performed at ceiling on the phonological awareness tasks despite minimal knowledge about print. Of those judged to be "not at risk," 24%-38% attained perfect scores on both administrations of the phonological awareness tasks; of those judged to be "at risk," only 6%-9% attained maximum scores (Skowronek/Marx 1989). These high scores suggest that despite their lack of print knowledge, many preschoolers had strong phonological awareness. We need more research to investigate how preschoolers acquire rudimentary forms of phonological awareness, whether literacy-based processes such as those outlined above are at all influential, and whether "at risk" students might lack these experiences and as a result have greater difficulty learning to read and spell.

References

Adams, M.J. (1990). Beginning to read. Cambridge, MA: The MIT Press.

Badian, N. (1988). Predicting dyslexia in a preschool population. In R. Masland & M. Masland (Eds.), Preschool prevention of reading failure. 78-103. Parkton, MD: York Press.

Blachman, B.A. (1984). Relationship of rapid naming ability and language analysis skills to kindergarten and first-grade reading achievement. Journal of Educational Psychology, 76, 610-622.

Brady, S.A. & Shankweiler, D.P. (Eds.) (1991). Phonological processes in literacy. Hillsdale, NJ: Erlbaum Associates.

Bowers, P.G. & Swanson, L.B. (1991). Naming speed deficits in reading disability: Multiple measures of a singular process. Journal of Experimental Child Psychology, 51, 195-219.

Bowers, P.G. & Wolf, M. (in press). Theoretical links among naming speed, precise timing mechanisms and orthographic skill in dyslexia. Reading and Writing.

Catts, H.W. (1991). Early identification of dyslexia: Evidence from a follow-up study of speech-language impaired children. Annals of Dyslexia, 41, 163-177.

Denckla, M. & Rudel, R.G. (1976). Rapid "automatized" naming (R.A.N.): Dyslexia differentiated from other learning disabilities. Neuropsychologia, 14, 471-479.

Drake, D.A. & Ehri, L.C. (1984). Spelling acquisition: Effects of pronouncing words on memory for their spellings. Cognition and Instruction, 1, 297-320.

Ehri, L.C. (1979). Linguistic insight: Threshold of reading acquisition. In T.G. Waller & G. MacKinnon (Eds.), Reading research: Advances in theory and practice Volume 1. 63-114. New York: Academic Press.

Ehri, L.C. (1980). The development of orthographic images. In U. Frith (Ed.), Cognitive processes in spelling. 311-338. London, England: Academic Press.

Ehri, L.C. (1984). How orthography alters spoken language competencies in children learning to read and spell. In J. Downing & R. Valtin (Eds.), Language awareness and learning to read. 119-147. New York: Springer Verlag.

Ehri, L.C. (1987). Learning to read and spell words. Journal of Reading Behavior, 19, 5-31.

Ehri, L.C. (1989). The development of spelling knowledge and its role in reading acquisition and reading disability. Journal of Learning Disabilities, 22, 356-365.

Ehri, L.C. (1991). Development of the ability to read words. In R. Barr, M. Kamil, P. Mosenthal & P. Pearson (Eds.), Handbook of reading research Volume II. 383-417. New York: Longman.

Ehri, L.C. (1992). Reconceptualizing the development of sight word reading and its relationship to recoding. In P.B. Gough, L.C. Ehri, & R. Treiman (Eds.), Reading acquisition. 107-143. Hillsdale, NJ: Erlbaum Associates.

Ehri, L.C. & Wilce, L.S. (1979). The mnemonic value of orthography among beginning readers. Journal of Educational Psychology, 71, 26-40.

Ehri, L.C. & Wilce, L.S. (1980). The influence of orthography on readers' conceptualization of the phonemic structure of words. Applied Psycholinguistics, 1, 371-385.

Ehri, L.C. & Wilce, L.S. (1982). The salience of silent letters in children's memory for word spellings. Memory and Cognition, 10, 155-166.

Ehri, L.C. & Wilce, L.S. (1983). Development of word identification speed in skilled and less skilled beginning readers. Journal of Educational Psychology, 75, 3-18.

Ehri, L.C. & Wilce, L.S. (1986). The influence of spellings on speech: Are alveolar flaps /d/ or /t/? In D. Yaden & S. Templeton (Eds.), Metalinguistic awareness and beginning literacy. 101-114. Exeter, New Hampshire: Heinemann.

Ehri, L.C., Wilce, L.S., & Taylor, B.B. (1987). Children's categorization of short vowels in words and the influence of spellings. Merrill Palmer Quarterly, 33, 393-421.

Felton, R. & Brown, I.S. (1990). Phonological processes as predictors of specific reading skills in children at risk for reading failure. Reading and Writing, 2, 39-59.

Goswami, U. (1986). Children's use of analogy in learning to read: A developmental study. Journal of Experimental Child Psychology, 42, 73-83.

Gough, P.B., Ehri, L.C., & Treiman, R. (Eds.) (1992). Reading acquisition. Hillsdale, NJ: Erlbaum Associates.

Jansky, J., Hoffman, M., Layton, J., Sugar, F., & Davies, M. (1989). Prediction: A six-year follow-up. Annals of Dyslexia, 39, 227-246.

Mann, V. (1984). Review: Reading skill and language skill. Developmental Review, 4, 1-15.

Morais, J., Cary, L., Alegria, J., & Bertelson, P. (1979). Does awareness of speech as a sequence of phones arise spontaneously? Cognition, 7, 323-331.

Read, C., Zhang, Y., Nie, H., & Ding, B. (1986). The ability to manipulate speech sounds depends on knowing alphabetic spelling. Cognition, 24, 31-44.

Share, D., Jorm, A., Maclean, R., & Matthews, R. (1984). Sources of individual differences in reading acquisition. Journal of Educational Psychology, 76, 1309-1324.

Skowronek, H. & Marx, H. (1989). The Bielefeld longitudinal study on early identification of risks in learning to read and write: Theoretical background and first results. In M. Brambring, F. Losel, & H. Skowronek (Eds.), Children at risk: Assessment, longitudinal research, and intervention. 268-294. Berlin: Walter de Gruyter.

Spring, C. & Capps, C. (1974). Encoding speed, rehearsal, and probed recall of dyslexic boys. Journal of Educational Psychology, 66, 780-786.

Spring, C. & Davis, J.M. (1988). Relations of digit naming speed with three components of reading. Applied Psycholinguistics, 9, 315-334.

Treiman, R. (1985). Onsets and rimes as units of spoken syllables: Evidence from children. Journal of Experimental Child Psychology, 39, 161-181.

Uhry, J.K. (in press). Predicting reading from print awareness and phonological awareness skills: An early reading screening. Educational Assessment.

Wagner, R. & Torgesen, J. (1987). The nature of phonological processing and its causal role in the acquisition of reading skills. Psychological Bulletin, 101, 192-212.

Wolf, M. (1991). Naming speed and reading: The contribution of the cognitive neurosciences. Reading Research Quarterly, 26, 123-141.

Two small longitudinal studies:
I. Developmental dyslexia
II. Early reading development

Nick Ellis

Introduction

This paper describes two small longitudinal studies of aspects of reading development that I have undertaken in North Wales. The first, with Barbara Large, concerns a 'broad brush' characterisation of early developmental dyslexia. The second, with Suzanne Cataldo, is a finer-grained analysis of early interactions in the early acquisition of reading, spelling and phonological awareness. It is true that these studies are 'small' with respect to sample size - a constraint imposed by the fact that we had no funding for these studies. We hope that they are more significant in their conception - thoughts which cost less but seemed harder won.

The studies demonstrate

(1) the most general information processing deficit in developmental dyslexia lies in phonological processing,

(2) an understanding of the development of reading can only come from longitudinal investigations of development itself, and such studies demonstrate typical sequences of interactive growth of related skills,

(3) a key stage in the development of reading is the acquisition of an alphabetic strategy and we can trace the evolution of this skill from implicit phonological awareness through explicit phonological awareness to spelling and hence to reading itself.

(1) Phonological processing in developmental dyslexia

Our research into developmental dyslexia began with cross-sectional studies which compared the skills of developmental dyslexics with those of age-matched controls. We showed, for example, that when two letters of the same case were presented simultaneously and the child had to report whether they are the same (OO) or different (OB), dyslexic and control children did not differ either in the speed or in the accuracy with which they could perform this task. Nor were the dyslexic children slower than age matched controls when the letters, though different, were visually confusable (OQ, RP, EF, CG) (Ellis 1981a, b). It seems unlikely, therefore, that dyslexic children have difficulty in dealing with the visual characteristics of letters as such. In contrast, when two letters of different case had to be adjudged same (Gg) or different (Gw, Gd) on the basis of name characteristics, the dyslexic children were reliably slower and more error prone than age-matched controls. Thus dyslexic children have no extra difficulty in dealing with the visual aspects of letters as such, but they show an impairment when the task demands the access and analysis of phonological features. This deficit in phonological access was confirmed in the wide range of demonstrations of dyslexic children being slow in naming letters, objects, colours, digits, pictures, non-words and words and their difficulties in verbal short-term memory which are often taken as symptomatic of the syndrome (Ellis/Miles 1981).

These findings underpin what is now the modal view of developmental dyslexia as a deficiency in phonological processing: developmental dyslexics are specifically impaired on tasks requiring perception, access, or analysis of phonological material and they evidence no dramatic disability to function with concrete or visual material (Ellis/Miles 1981; Frith 1981; Miles/Ellis 1981; Vellutino 1979, 182ff).

(2) Longitudinal study I

The development of reading disability

However, there are problems with cross-sectional studies and their meta-analysis. In 1979 we recognised that the then-current knowledge of reading, reflected in reviews of thousands of individual studies of reading (e.g. Gibson/Levin 1975; Vellutino 1979), predominantly arose from studies using ex post facto bivalent designs with little or no attempt to look for differential abilities. They had been performed by different investigators, with children of different cultures, education, age, socio-economic background and intelligence and they had involved radically different numbers of subjects. They had taken place over the last 50 years when educational practices had been changing. It was quite possible therefore that these reviews constituted a nomothetic generality which, from a heterogeneous population, reflected none of the individuals studied. Furthermore they potentially failed to lead to an understanding of the *development* of reading, since, if we want to study development we must do so directly.

Only when the same persons are tested repeatedly over time does it become possible to identify developmental changes and processes of organisation within the individual. Cross-sectional studies which compare different groups of people at different stages of acquisition must always come a poor second when small but reliable changes with age are to be detected, where teaching methods and teachers change with time, and where we do not wish to make the false assumption that the abilities of a younger cross-section were necessarily present in the older cross-section at a previous time. They also fail us with regard to the determination of causality: a cross-sectional study may show an association between two phenomena, but only a longitudinal investigation can determine which came first.

The membership of this symposium recognise these problems - it is this realisation, common to us all, which has led us independently to initiate our various longitudinal studies throughout the world, and which brings us together today.

Our particular response in 1979 was to embark on a study of the first three years of reading development in the same children using a longitudinal differential design (Ellis/Large 1987, 1988). The longitudinal nature of the study allowed a meaningful analysis of the changing nature of individual children's reading skill and the determination of which skills promote reading development and which benefit from it. The differential design allowed not only the determination of which skills are associated with reading, but also their relative importance.

A cohort of 40 children was assessed for their abilities on 44 variables which measured as wide a range of information-processing skills as was practically possible. These measures are briefly described in Appendix 1.

Besides the full WISC there were a variety of measures of reading, spelling, vocabulary, STM, visual skills, auditory-visual integration ability, auditory/ language abilities, language knowledge, and rote knowledge and ordering ability. The children were assessed on these measures each year, from 5 to 8 years old. In the first of our reports (Ellis/Large 1987) we extracted three groups at age 8 on the basis of reading and IQ scores. Group A showed a specific reading disability (high IQ, low reading), Group B were good readers of similarly high IQ, Group C showed a more generalised reading deficit in that they were at the same level as Group A in reading but their IQ scores were low. The specific reading disability of Group A is somewhat mild following the common usage of the term - their reading age is only a few months below age level. However, as is shown in Table 1, they are of above average intelligence: Reading achievement ratios (100*Reading age/ Mental Age) are 86% for Group A, 102% Group B, and 104% Group C.

Tab. 1: Reading characteristics of the three groups at 8 years old

	Reading Age yr.mo.
Group A. Low Reading, High IQ	
Reading Achievement Ratio	86%
WISC at 7 years old	116
Schonell Reading	7.5
Neale Rate	7.6
Neale Comprehension	8.10
Neale Accuracy	9.5
Group B. High Reading, High IQ	
Reading Achievement Ratio	102%
WISC at 7 years old	117
Schonell Reading	9.7
Neale Rate	8.9
Neale Comprehension	9.6
Neale Accuracy	10.10
Group C. Low Reading, Low IQ	
Reading Achievement Ratio	104%
WISC at 7 years old	93
Schonell Reading	7.4
Neale Rate	7.2
Neale Comprehension	7.10
Neale Accuracy	9.4

The data was then searched retrospectively to describe the development of these patterns of ability from the very beginnings of reading acquisition.

Table 2 shows these groups' WISC and reading scores over three years of development.

Tab. 2: Reading age and WISC scores of the three groups at 5, 6 and 7 years old

	5 years old	6 years old	7 years old
Group A. Low Reading, High IQ			
Schonell Reading Age	5.0 (0.0)	5.5 (0.0)	6.5 (0.0)
WISC Full	96.4 (5.1)	114.6 (12.3)	115.6 (9.8)
WISC Verbal	98.6 (8.3)	112.0 (8.9)	109.6 (7.2)
WISC Performance	95.6 (8.0)	115.2 (16.6)	119.2 (10.8)
Group B. High Reading, High IQ			
Schonell Reading Age	5.1 (0.0)	6.6 (0.1)	8.3 (0.0)
WISC Full	94.8 (12.4)	120.0 (6.9)	117.0 (7.5)
WISC Verbal	100.0 (8.0)	123.8 (10.6)	121.4 (6.0)
WISC Performance	93.4 (14.7)	111.4 (3.9)	108.8 (8.7)
Group C. Low Reading, Low IQ			
Schonell Reading Age	5.0 (0.0)	5.2 (0.0)	6.2 (0.0)
WISC Full	72.2 (5.2)	90.0 (5.2)	93.4 (6.8)
WISC Verbal	83.0 (6.7)	96.6 (6.4)	94.0 (1.7)
WISC Performance	63.3 (9.9)	84.4 (13.0)	92.8 (14.4)

Groups A and B are well matched for full IQ at all years of testing but this results from Group B scoring higher on the WISC Verbal items than on the Performance scales, whereas Group A develop more on the Performance items than on the Verbal scales. This follows the characteristic WISC profile of children with specific reading disability where there are consistent reports of difficulties on the Information, Arithmetic, Digit Span and Coding subtests (Miles/Ellis 1981; Spache 1976, 88ff).

The reading abilities of Groups A and B diverge from age five where performance is at floor level on the Schonell. Over the next three years Group B make 4.6 norm-years' worth of progress whilst Group A make a mere 2.5. Group C is consistently over 20 points behind the other two Groups on the WISC. The Schonell scores for Groups A and C are well-matched over the years.

For each year's set of data the scores for all 40 children on these 44 variables were normalised by conversion to stanines, a 9 point scale with mean 5.0 and s.d. 1.96. The child who had performed best on a particular variable would thus be given the score 9, the worst would score 1. This procedure allows the scores for different tests to become comparable and a child's profile of abilities can thus be produced in the same way as is done on standard attainment tests such as the WISC. It has the additional advantage of ensuring normally distributed scores with equal variances.

ANOVA demonstrated significant effects of group and a group x test interaction (see Ellis/Large 1987, 6ff for details). To summarise the effects we averaged the three Groups test stanine scores over years 5 - 7 and assessed pairwise comparisons between the Groups. The stanine differences (ordered by importance) are shown in Tables 3, 4, and 5.

a) *How do children with specific reading problems differ in development from their reading-skilled peers?*

Tab. 3: Longitudinal Study 1: Stanine differences between Group A Low reading, High IQ and Group B High reading, High IQ.

Rhyme - odd one out	2.73
Rhyme generation	2.67
Carver spoken-printed vocab	2.34
D&D picture-printed vocab	2.13
Auditory digit span	2.07
Schonell Reading	2.00
Colour naming rate	1.87
Sound blending	1.86
Letter recognition	1.73
Schonell spelling	1.73
Phonically simple D&D A	1.53
Nonsense words D&D H	1.53
Phonically complex D&D F	1.53
Sentence comprehension D&D R	1.46
Auditory sentence span	1.40
Reversible words D&D G	1.40
Auditory word span	1.34

From the wide and varied test battery there were few tests which discriminated between the children with specific reading disability and their age- and IQ-matched controls and they all concerned phonological processing, STM, or some aspects of accessing the articulatory equivalents of visual material. The most important discriminators were the rhyming tasks which require implicit use of phoneme segmentation and which had previously been demonstrated to be reliable discriminators between dyslexics and adequate readers in group studies (Snowling/Stackhouse/Rack 1985), and to be reliable predictors of later reading difficulty (Bradley/Bryant 1983). The next most strong discriminator was auditory digit span, a most common finding in the developmental dyslexia literature (see Ellis/Miles 1981 for reviews). Next came other tests of STM for verbal material (auditory sentence span, auditory word span), and of phonological processing (sound blending, phoneme segmentation). We additionally found that the rate at which children can access the articulatory equivalents for colours discriminated between the groups, and we confirmed the typical WISC profile of dyslexic children where they had problems with the Digit Span, Comprehension, Information and Coding subtests. The only discriminator which was not of a phonological type was visual serial ordering which squeezed in at the bottom of the list, a suitable placement because of the dispute over whether visual encoding problems fall out of group studies as being associated with dyslexia: some affirm this to be the case (Benton 1962; Ingram 1971), some deny (Ellis 1981; Yule/Rutter 1976), some find it to be dependent on spatial frequency with the deficiency only in the transient subsystem (Lovegrove/Martin/Slaghuis 1986), and some reinterpret the 'visual' tasks to involve implicit verbalisation strategies (Vellutino 1979, 182ff), but most would agree that such problems are negligible when compared with STM and phonological processing deficiencies.

None of the other tests, the larger part of the battery, significantly discriminated between these groups - the children with specific reading problems did not seem to show reliable patterns of developmental problems of visual processing (on tests of visual closure, picture completion, letter search, coding, block design, object assembly or picture arrangement), nor syntactic skills, nor rote knowledge and ordering. It is only by means of longitudinal and differential designs such as this that we can assess the relative importance of developmental deficits associated with dyslexia.

In summary, the children with specific reading retardation differed from their better-reading peers in terms of the relatively few variables which concerned phonological segmentation, STM and naming.

The data also address two further questions.

b) *How do children with generalised reading disability ('garden variety' poor readers) differ from their better-reading peers?*

Tab. 4: Longitudinal Study 1: Stanine differences between Group B High reading, High IQ and Group C Low reading, Low IQ

Rhyme - odd one out	3.93
Sound blending	3.60
Knowledge of syntax	3.54
D&D picture-printed vocab	3.40
WISC comprehension	3.40
Carver spoken-printed vocab	3.34
Colour naming rate	3.20
Visual digit span	3.20
WISC picture arrangement	3.20
Auditory sentence span	3.14
Token test	3.14
Visual serial ordering	3.13
Letter search	3.07
Visual digit span & A.S.	3.00
Syllable segmentation	3.00
Rhyme generation	2.94
WISC arithmetic	2.93
WISC information	2.87
Letter recognition	2.73
Phoneme segmentation	2.60
Auditory digit span	2.53
WISC spoken-spoken vocab	2.53
WISC coding	2.47
WISC similarities	2.46
Schonell spelling	2.46
Schonell reading	2.40
WISC picture completion	2.40
Grammatical closure	2.34
Peabody spoken-picture vocab	2.34
'Reversible' words D&D G	2.26
Nonsense words D&D H	2.20
Auditory word span	2.14
Phonically complex D&D F	2.13
Phonically simple D&D A	2.13
WISC object assembly	2.07
Sentence comprehension D&D R	1.93
Visual closure	1.87
WISC block design	1.87
Days backwards	1.74
Symbol>sound learning	1.67

Of course they do so in almost every respect because these children differ both in terms of reading-related abilities and general intellectual factors. However, as in the case of contrast a, the strong discriminators again concern phonological processing.

c) How do children with specific reading disability differ from those with generalised reading disability?

Tab. 5: Longitudinal Study 1: Stanine differences between Group A Low reading, High IQ and Group C Low reading, Low IQ

Peabody spoken-picture vocab	3.74
Object assembly WISC	3.47
Picture assembly WISC	3.27
Picture completion WISC	3.20
Visual digit span & A.S.	2.54
Knowledge of syntax	2.54
Block design WISC	2.54
Token test	2.40
Letter search	2.40
Coding WISC	2.33
WISC comprehension	2.27
WISC spoken-spoken vocab	2.20
Visual digit span	2.20
Syllable segmentation	2.00
Visual serial ordering	1.93
WISC Arithmetic	1.93
Grammatical closure	1.80
WISC information	1.80
Auditory sentence span	1.74
Sound blending	1.74
Visual closure	1.60
Phoneme segmentation	1.53
WISC similarities	1.46

They do so in terms of intelligence and abilities which involve visual processing. These are differences which more reflect different levels of general intellectual ability than different levels of reading skill (see Ellis/ Large 1981 for further discussion).

The 'BROAD-BRUSH' Longitudinal Study

We further analysed this first longitudinal study of the early reading development over all forty children in several ways. At each year the patterns of associates of reading skill were determined (with and without control for IQ); the abilities at one point in time which were associated with later reading skill were ascertained for the whole group, for a subset of children who at 5 years old started with no reading skill, and for another group of children who were progressing rapidly at 7 years old; cross-lagged correlation comparisons were made to investigate causal paths. These analyses allowed us to broadly chart the course of reading development and the interactive ways in which associated skills such as spelling, reading, phonological awareness and syntactic knowledge grow from each other differentially at different stages of development.

There is insufficient space to discuss this in detail here; the interested reader is referred to Ellis/Large (1988). However, in summary the analyses confirmed that the nature of reading skill changed rapidly in the first three years of acquisition. In information processing terms it began as an undifferentiated skill associated with knowledge of the letters of the alphabet, phonological awareness, and visual symbolic short-term memory processes. It then changed in character, being associated with holistic visual pattern recognition skills. By 6 years old phonological awareness and verbal short-term memory processes were by far the strongest associates. By 7 years old the better readers' skills were associated with analytic visual perceptual analysis, the learning of new symbol<>sound associations, and sound blending skill. Reading had become a multi-faceted ability tapping a wide range of different skills - from language comprehension to analysis of the order of elements in a visual array - and different strategic blends of these abilities were now being used in different reading situations.

The different patterns of skills associated with reading development at different stages are broadly in line with the developmental sequences of reading as described by Marsh/Friedman/Welch/Desberg (1981) and Frith (1985):

Stage 1: Logographic Reading. The child typically centres on one visual aspect of the stimulus such as the first letter and associates that with the oral response. Their natural strategy is congruent with the 'whole word' approach to teaching reading. If the child does not know the word she may guess on the basis of contextual cues. Marsh et al. suggest that the child next progresses to a stage of discrimination net substitution where "the number of graphemic features a young child can process is limited initially to the first letter, and it is only later that additional features such as word length, final letter etc. are added. The child at this stage appears to be operating according to a 'discrimination net' mechanism in which graphemic cues are processed only to the extent necessary to discriminate one printed word from another." (Marsh et al. 1981, 203).

Stage 2: Alphabetic Reading is characterized by the use of individual graphemes and phonemes and their correspondences. "It is an analytic skill involving a systematic approach, namely decoding grapheme by grapheme. Letter order and phonological factors play a crucial role. This strategy enables the reader to pronounce novel and nonsense words" (Frith 1985, 308).

Stage 3: Orthographic Reading - an extension to the simple decoding strategy (which was based on one-to-one correspondence) where the child now learns more complex rules of orthographic structure - the units are letter groups and higher order conditional rules (like the magic *e* rule) are used.

This first longitudinal study thus allowed us to chart the interactions between different skills in the first three year's development of reading, to identify the very different types of reading at different stages of development, and to clarify the prior skills which promoted reading development and the skills which themselves grow from practice in reading.

We also identified some powerful reciprocal interactions in development, for example those between reading and STM where we found from the *pre-reading* analyses that phonological skills promoted the acquisition of letter knowledge and that these two abilities, together with visual STM, led the development of reading and yet, from the *post-reading* analyses, reading promoted the acquisition of phonological skills and Auditory STM, and that the phonological skills in turn led to the development of visual STM (Ellis 1990). The literature on this topic thus far had tended to ask which direction of causality applies (e.g. Bradley/Bryant 1983; Bryant/Bradley 1985; Ehri 1979). The answer is that both directions apply because a new skill invariably initially builds on whatever relevant abilities are already present, then, as it is used, it may well legitimatize and make more relevant (Istomina 1975) those prior skills and so in turn cause their further development. Stanovich has persuasively argued the case for reciprocal relationships and bootstrapping effects: "In short, many things that facilitate further growth in reading comprehension ability - general knowledge, vocabulary, syntactic knowledge - are developed by reading itself" (Stanovich 1986, 364), "interrelationships between the various subskills of reading and intelligence increase with age, *probably due to mutual facilitation*" (Stanovich/Cunningham/Feeman 1984, 278, my emphasis). In the evolution of our research we have used three metaphors for skill development: river and delta formation, pace-makers and followers, and symbiosis. They are all images of reciprocal interactions of elements over time. Such is the growth and development of skill.

The study also provided details about the move from early whole-word reading to a strategy which capitalises on grapheme-phoneme associations. We have shown in sections 1 and 2 that developmental dyslexics are particularly deficient in their phonological abilities, the very skills which are needed for learning these grapheme-phoneme associations. Therefore a finer-grained longitudinal study was needed to identify how phonological skills grow and become incorporated into the reading process.

(3) The 'finer-grained' Longitudinal Study II

Although the importance of phonological awareness (PA) in the acquisition of reading had been established, causal pathways between the two abilities eluded clear definition (Bryant/Goswami 1987) since there are many and various factors which might influence studies of the co-development of phonological awareness and reading, viz., (i) the range of phonological awareness skills tapped by different tasks, (ii) the range of different types of reading tapped by different reading tasks and the child's ability to relate sound to graphic information, (iii) short term and working memory, and (iv) different methods of reading instruction. Research that examines the relationship of phonological awareness to the emergence of literacy had often neglected spelling as a bona fide agent that independently influences and is influenced by phonological awareness and reading. Whilst it had been acknowledged that use of a phonological strategy plays a fundamental role in spelling before it becomes important in reading (e.g. Bryant/Bradley 1980; Frith 1980), comparatively little attention had been focused on the possible routes of interaction among reading, spelling and phonological skills. Correlational studies provided evidence of a strong relationship between early reading and spelling and between spelling and phoneme awareness. However, the form of causal connections could not be determined from correlations alone.

Theoretical analyses which assign spelling a major role in the development of phonological as well as reading skills include Chomsky (1977), Ehri/Wilce (1987), Elkonin (1973), and Lewkowicz (1980). In a three-phase model of reading acquisition Frith (1985) proposes that an alphabetic or sound strategy is first utilized in spelling practice and later carried over to reading, which the child has previously approached using a logographic or visual strategy. Yet only a few studies have been designed to explore the manner in which spelling contributes to or benefits from phonological and reading skills, although Ehri/Wilce (1987) have recently demonstrated transfer of phonological strategy from spelling to reading.

We needed a broader and more detailed description of the interactive development of all three components: reading, spelling and phonological awareness. Cataldo/Ellis (1988, 1990) therefore adopted a longitudinal design to identify the early sequences of interactive development in reading, spelling and phonological awareness skills. We elucidated the early causal relations among these three variables by following the development of each skill in a group of children as they move from preliteracy through the beginning stages of learning to read and spell.

In this study the early interactive development of reading, spelling and phonological awareness were charted in a group of 28 children during their first three years in school. During this time the children were tested at four intervals in reading and spelling real and nonsense words, phoneme segmentation and auditory categorization. The Wechsler Preschool Primary Scale of Intelligence was included in the set of initial assessments. A test of phoneme segmentation was given as a measure of explicit phonemic awareness and a test of auditory categorization was taken as a measure of implicit phonological awareness. The majority of the sample had only begun to attend school when the initial assessments were taken at the beginning of the school year when their mean age was 4 years 6 months. The children were retested at the end of their first school year, at the beginning of the second year and finally at the beginning of the third school year.

As is shown in Figure 1, there were three measured phases of development. Phase One spans the children's first year in school. Phase Two charts the development from spring of the first school year to autumn of the second year. Phase Three looks at development from the beginning of the second year in school to the beginning of the third year.

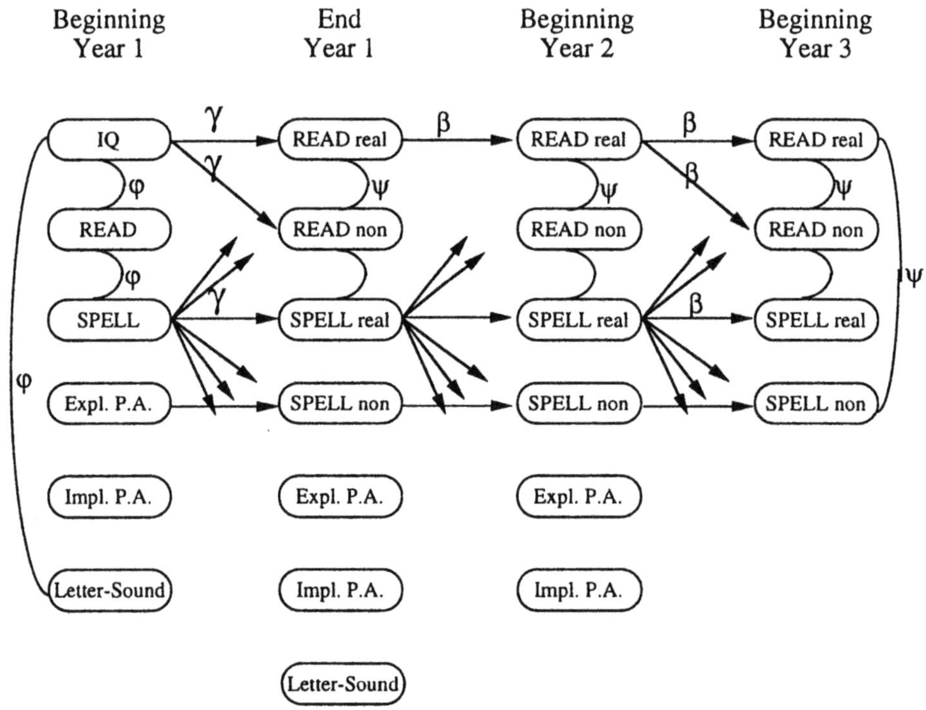

Fig. 1: *An illustration of the LISREL model used. All possible paths were allowed between adjacent time periods, thus allowing each variable to potentially contribute to the development of every other variable at the next time-point. However, in order not to clutter the diagram, we have not illustrated all the paths between stages - we have only shown this for spelling in the Figure. See text for further details.*

LISREL (Jöreskog/Sörbom 1984; Saris/Stronkhorst 1984) was used to formulate a descriptive model that identifies significant contributors to the early growth of literacy. With small samples LISREL is appropriate only for exploratory purposes (Crano/Mendoza 1987). The limited number of subjects in this study restricts us to a preliminary structural equation model which needs further validation with a larger number of subjects. We fitted exploratory low constraint time-interval type models (Cataldo/Ellis 1988; Ellis 1989) where each ability could result from an effect of any ability measured at the previous time (Figure 1). This type of model allows us to compare the effects of two different abilities on a third ability. Table 6 gives the pathweight coefficients indicating the contribution of each ability to the development of later abilities. With standardized data, pathweights represent the amount of change in a variable (in standard deviation (sd) units) caused by one sd of change in another variable. In Table 2 the column headers represent the abilities measured at the prior time, the rows the effect variable measured at the later time; thus we can see that an increase of one sd in spelling ability at the beginning of the first school year was associated with an increase of 0.31 sds in ability to read real words at the end of that year; in contrast, an increase of one sd of reading at the beginning of year one is only associated with an increase of 0.10 sds in later spelling ability.

The Phase One pathweights from spelling to reading real words and nonsense words identify spelling as an important contributor to the early formation of reading. This pattern of influence is repeated much more strongly in the second phase with high pathweights from spelling to reading real words and nonsense words. The pronounced influence of spelling on reading contrasts with a negligible contribution of reading to spelling in both Phases 1 and 2. Implicit PA initially predicts early attempts to read as well as to spell but loses its influence on both reading and spelling in the following two phases. In contrast to the diminishing predictive power of implicit PA, explicit PA consistently predicts spelling in all three phases, this influence increasing with phase. Explicit PA only emerges as a strong predictor of reading in Phase Three.

The early transfer between reading and spelling appears to be unidirectional: knowledge gleaned from spelling is contributing to reading. Similarly, both implicit and explicit PA affect spelling development with explicit PA increasing its influence as the contribution of implicit PA diminishes. Later in the developmental sequence, explicit PA begins to contribute directly to reading. The pattern of interactions among abilities in Phase One clarifies the different roles of implicit and explicit PA in the early formation of reading skill. Implicit information about the sound properties of words directly affects early reading attempts: explicit knowledge of phonemic content influences reading via spelling experience. Beginners may be using implicit PA both to help them detect acoustic properties that define a word by its sound boundaries and to detect sounds with salient qualities, and their use of these rudimentary sound strategies allows them to form associations between sounds in spoken words and pronunciations and to call upon these

Tab. 6: *LISREL path coefficients* indicating contributions of early ability to development of later ablities

Reading-Spelling Model

Phase One: Beginning first school year to end of first school year

GAMMA	READ	SPELL	EXPL.PA	IMPL.PA	LS
READ (real)	**0.37**	**0.31**	0.08	**0.36**	0.06
READ (non)	0.18	0.23	0.17	**0.41**	0.08
SPELL (real)	0.10	0.35	**0.32**	**0.38**	0.07
SPELL (non)	0.06	0.24	**0.31**	**0.31**	0.21
EXPL.PA	-0.04	0.13	**0.42**	**0.36**	0.11
IMPL.PA	0.15	**0.53**	0.06	**0.49**	-0.20

Phase Two: End of first year to Autumn of second year

BETA	READ REAL	READ NON	SPELL REAL	SPELL NON	EXPL. PA	IMPL. PA
READ (real)	**0.66**	-0.34	0.64	-0.10	0.21	-0.25
READ (non)	0.31	0.07	**0.60**	-0.09	0.18	-0.09
SPELL (real)	0.14	-0.33	**0.76**	-0.02	**0.34**	0.07
SPELL (non)	0.00	-0.04	**0.77**	-0.22	**0.45**	0.05
EXPL. PA	0.34	-0.10	-0.02	0.20	**0.50**	0.03
IMPL. PA	0.27	0.37	-0.22	-0.19	0.35	0.12
LS	0.36	0.24	-0.20	-0.14	0.26	-0.08

Phase Three: Beginning of second year to beginning of third year

BETA	READ REAL	READ NON	SPELL REAL	SPELL NON	EXPL. PA	IMPL. PA	LS
READ (real)	0.20	0.24	0.00	-0.12	0.30	0.08	**0.38**
READ (non)	0.03	0.22	-0.00	-0.05	**0.53**	0.01	**0.30**
SPELL (real)	0.03	0.01	0.04	-0.10	**0.63**	0.09	0.09
SPELL (non)	0.21	0.43	-0.32	0.13	**0.49**	0.27	0.17

Path coefficients in bold are significant at $p<.05$.
(READ: Reading; SPELL: Spelling; EXPL.PA: Explicit Phonological Awareness; IMPL.PA: Implicit Phonological Awareness; LS: Letter Sound)

associations to perform phonetic-cue reading (Ehri/Wilce 1985). The use of implicit awareness of rhyming components in words may also help beginners to generalize from an unknown word to a word that contains a similar spelling (Bryant/Goswami 1987), but this strategy is more likely to be employed at later stages of reading development when children have enough lexical entries from which to generalize. The first evidence of the direct influence of explicit PA on reading occurs in Phase Three, when explicit PA predicts ability to read nonwords. In earlier phases explicit PA does not influence reading directly but acts as the strongest predictor of spelling both real and nonsense words. In turn, spelling is the most consistent predictor of reading.

This early interactive sequence describes the pattern of growth from prealphabetic to alphabetic stage reading (Frith 1985). While implicit knowledge of the sound properties of words helps children forge initial connections between the printed word and its pronunciation, spelling acts as a mediator for the use of explicit PA until the child begins alphabetic stage reading by directly applying explicit PA to reading. Our data suggest that as children practise spelling they develop proficiency in the use of the alphabetic principle and apply this knowledge to the task of reading. The emergence of explicit PA as a significant predictor of reading marks the entry into the alphabetic stage of reading.

Models of reading and spelling must describe development, the movement from one stage to the next. Our results describe the ways in which spelling acts as a mediator for the influence of explicit phonological awareness on reading. Children's very first efforts at reading are characterized by a visual or logographic strategy where letters are analyzed for salient graphic cues to rapid word recognition; this is the PreAlphabetic Stage. When a small number of pronunciations can be accessed in this manner, the child may embark upon a more advanced strategy of using associations between partial phonetic cues in the spoken word with letters in the printed version and subsequently utilize these associations to recognize the words. Children appear to use implicit PA to help them make these rudimentary sound analyses of pronunciation. In addition, spelling practice may contribute to the store of associations between the spoken words and letter-sound constituents in printed words. At first, spelling may encourage children to focus on the first letter of printed words and to begin to analyse this first letter, in the reading task, for phonetic cues to pronunciations. Thus, the practice of turning attention to the first letter-sound unit in spelling may influence children to discriminate between stored pronunciations on the basis of the first letter of the printed word, the 'discrimination net substitution' of Marsh et al. (1981). As visual and phonetic cue strategies make increasing demands on the child's memory, the efficiency of this strategy decreases. Conversely, as the source of knowledge about letter-sound associates, and the relationships between letters in printed words and sounds in spoken words swells, the child is discovering that s/he can rely on the use of this knowledge for successful word recognition. Our studies support the idea that the transition from pre-alphabetic stage reading to alphabetic stage reading is facilitated by spelling. By employing explicit PA in spelling practice, the child gains familiarity with the alphabetic nature of writing and builds a reliable fund of information about letter-sound correspondences and explicit phonemic content in words. Spelling affords the opportunity to forge a meaningful link between phonological awareness and letter-sound knowledge. This connection is a prerequisite to the development of phonological strategies in reading.

Conclusions

These studies have confirmed the phonological deficits in developmental dyslexia. They show how reading changes in nature as it is learned and that an important early stage in its development is the adoption of an alphabetic reading strategy. We trace the precursors of the phonological knowledge that forms the foundations of grapheme-phoneme reading back through spelling, through explicit phonological awareness and in turn to its source in implicit phonological awareness. We confirm that the reading and spelling development of developmental dyslexics is limited by their prior failures to acquire this knowledge, as Frith (1985, 324) says: "Classic developmental dyslexia is the failure of alphabetic skills". We discuss the educational implications of these findings in Ellis/Cataldo (1990) where we also suggest that phonological awareness would be a useful screening measure for the early identification of children at risk of later reading problems.

There remains the need for further longitudinal studies which go back even further into early development. One promising example is that of MacLean/Bryant/Bradley (1987) who demonstrate the role of children's early experience of nursery rhymes in their gaining initial implicit phonological awareness. The question that then arises is why, assuming developmental dyslexics receive equal such early exposure, they do not assimilate this knowledge. We must determine the neurological and genetic reasons which underlie this constitutional disability.

References

Benton, A.L. (1962). Dyslexia in relation to form perception and directional sense. In J. Money (Ed.), Reading disability. 81-102. Baltimore: John Hopkins Press.

Bradley, L. (1980). Assessing reading difficulties: A diagnostic and remedial approach. London: Macmillan Education.

Bradley, L. & Bryant, P.E. (1983). Categorizing sounds and learning to read - a causal connection. Nature, 301, 419-421.

Bryant, P.E. & Bradley, L. (1980). Why children sometimes write words which they do not read. In U. Frith (Ed.), Cognitive processes in spelling. 355-370. London: Academic Press.

Bryant, P.E. & Bradley, L. (1985). Children's reading problems. Oxford: Blackwell.

Bryant, L. & Goswami, U. (1987). Phonological awareness and learning to read. In J.R. Beech & A.M. Coley (Eds.), Cognitive approaches to reading. 213-244. Chichester: Wiley.

Cataldo, S. & Ellis, N.C. (1988). Spelling, reading and phonological skills in interactive development. Journal of Research in Reading, 11(2), 86-109.

Cataldo, S. & Ellis, N.C. (1990). Learning to spell, learning to read. In P.D. Pumphrey & C.D. Elliott (Eds.), Children's difficulties in reading, writing and spelling: Challenges and responses. 101-125. Baisingstoke: Falmer Press.

Chomsky, C. (1977). Approaching reading through invented spelling. In L.B. Resnick & P.A. Weaver (Eds.), The theory and practice of early reading, Vol. 2. 43-65. Hillsdale, N.J.: Erlbaum.

Crano, W.D. & Mendoza, J.L. (1987). Maternal factors that influence children's positive behaviour: Demonstration of a structural equation analysis of selected data from the Berkeley Growth Study. Child Development, 58, 38-48.

Ehri, L.C. (1979). Linguistic insights: Threshold of reading acquisition. In T.G. Waller & G.E. MacKinnon (Eds.), Reading research: Advances in theory and practice, Vol. 1. 63-114. New York: Academic Press.

Ehri, L.C. & Wilce, L.S. (1985). Movement into reading: Is the first stage of printed word learning visual or phonetic? Reading Research Quarterly, 20, 163-179.

Ehri, L.C. & Wilce, L.S. (1987). Does learning to spell help beginners learn to read words? Reading Research Quarterly, 22, 47-65.

Elkonin, D.B. (1973). U.S.S.R. In J. Downing (Ed.), Comparative reading. 73-89. New York: Macmillan.

Ellis, N.C. (1981a). Information processing views of developmental dyslexia I-IV. Dyslexia Review, 4(1), 5-17.

Ellis, N.C. (1981b). Visual and name coding in dyslexic children. Psychological Research, 43, 201-218.

Ellis, N.C. (1989). Reading development, dyslexia and phonological skills. The Irish Journal of Psychology, 10(4), 551-567.

Ellis, N.C. (1990). Reading, phonological processing and STM: Interactive tributaries of development. Journal of Research in Reading, 13, 107-122.

Ellis, N.C. & Cataldo, S. (1990). The role of spelling in learning to read. Language and Education, 4, 1-28.

Ellis, N.C. & Large, B. (1987). The development of reading: As you seek so shall you find. British Journal of Psychology, 78, 1-28.

Ellis, N.C. & Large, B. (1988). The early stages of reading. A longitudinal study. Applied Cognitive Psychology, 2, 47-76.

Ellis, N.C. & Miles, T.R. (1981). A lexical encoding deficiency I: experimental evidence. In G.Th. Pavlidis & T.R. Miles (Eds.), Dyslexia research and its applications to education. 177-216. Chichester: Wiley.

Frith, U. (1981). Experimental approaches to developmental dyslexia: An introduction. Psychological Research, 43, 97-110.

Frith, U. (1985). Beneath the surface of developmental dyslexia. In K. Patterson, M. Coltheart, & J. Marshall (Eds.), Surface dyslexia. 301-330. London: Erlbaum.

Gibson, E. & Levin, H. (1975). The psychology of reading. Cambridge Mass.: MIT Press.

Gleitman, L.R., Gleitman, H., & Shipley, E. (1972). The emergence of the child as a grammarian. Cognition, 1, 137-164.

Ingram, T.T.S. (1971). Specific learning difficulties in childhood: A medical point of view. British Journal of Educational Psychology, 41(1), 6-13.

Istomina, Z.M. (1975). The development of involuntary memory in preschool age children. Soviet Psychology, 13, 5-64.

Jöreskog, KG. & Sörbom, D. (1984). Lisrel VI User's Guide. Uppsala: Department of Statistics.

Lewkowicz, N.K. (1980). Phonemic awareness training: What it is and how to teach it. Journal of Educational Psychology, 72, 686-700.

Liberman, I.Y., Shankweiler, D., Liberman, A.M., Fowler, C., & Fisher, F.W. (1977). Phonemic segmentation and recoding in the beginning reader. In A.S. Reber & D. Scarborough (Eds.), Towards a psychology of reading. 297-225. Hillsdale, N.J.: Erlbaum.

Lovegrove, W., Martin, F., & Slaghuis, W. (1986). A theoretical and experimental case for a visual deficit in specific reading disability. Cognitive Neuropsychology, 3, 225-267.

MacLean, M., Bryant, P., & Bradley, L. (1987). Rhymes, nursery rhymes and reading in early childhood. Merrill-Palmer Quarterly, 33, 255-281.

Marsh, G., Friedman, M.P., Welch, V., & Desberg, P. (1981). A cognitive-developmental theory of reading acquisition. In T.G. Waller & G.E. Mackinnon (Eds.), Reading research: Advances in theory and practice, Vol. 3. 199-221. New York: Academic Press.

Miles, T.R. & Ellis, N.C. (1981). A lexical encoding deficiency II: Clinical observations. In G.Th. Pavlidis & T.R. Miles (Eds.), Dyslexia research and its applications to education. 217-244. Chichester: Wiley.

Saris, W.E. & Stronkhorst, H.L. (1984). Causal modelling in nonexperimental research. Amsterdam: Sociometric Research Foundation.

Snowling, M.J., Stackhouse, J., & Rack, J. (1985). Phonological dyslexia and dysgraphia: Developmental aspects. Cognitive Neuropsychology, 3, 309-339.

Spache, G.D. (1976). Investigating the issues of reading disabilities. Boston: Allyn and Bacon.

Stanovich, K.E. (1986). Matthew effects in reading: Some consequences of individual differences in the acquisition of literacy. Reading Research Quarterly, XXI, 360-407.

Stanovich, K.E., Cunningham, A.E., & Feeman, D.J. (1984). Intelligence, cognitive skills, and early reading progress. Reading Research Quarterly, XIX, 278-303.

Vellutino, F.R. (1979). Dyslexia: Theory and research. Cambridge, Mass.: MIT Press.

Warrington, E.K., Logue, V., & Pratt, R.T.C. (1971). The anatomical localization of selective impairment of auditory short-term memory. Neuropsychologica, 9, 377-387.

Yule, W. & Rutter, M. (1976). Epidemiology and social implications of specific reading retardation. In R.M. Knight & D.J. Bakker (Eds.), The neuropsychology of learning disorders. 135-157. Baltimore: University Park Press.

Appendix 1: Summary of tests used in Longitudinal Study 1

Reading

1 Phonically Simple D&DA
Daniels and Dyack subtest 7a. A word recognition test involving phonically regular 2 and 3 letter words.
2 Phonically Complex D&DF
Daniels & Dyack subtest 7F. A word recognition test involving irregular words like 'who','any'. Extra items were added to this test and D&DA from Coltheart's (1979) Exception and Regular words to overcome ceiling effects.
3 Nonsense Words D&DH
Daniels & Dyack subtest 7H. A test of the pronunciation of phonically simple nonwords like 'bim'.
4 'Reversible' Words D&DG
Daniels & Dyack subtest 7G. A test of the recognition of words which can be read backwards like 'saw', 'net' and words high in content of 'reversible' letterslike 'b/d'.
5 Sentence Comprehension D&DR
Daniels & Dyack Standard Test of Reading Skill. A series of 36 questions like 'Can a dog run'. The order of difficulty of the sentences reflects phonic complexity. The child must comprehend the sentence in order to answer the question.
6 Schonell Reading
A word recognition test for ages 5 to 15. It is composed of 100 words, 10 for each year. The words are arranged in continuous order of difficulty.

Spelling

7 Schonell Spelling
A spelling test comprising 100 words, 10 for each year from 5 to 15. The first 10 are regular 3 letter words. Thereafter there are both regular and irregular words ordered according to difficulty.

Vocabulary

8 WISC Spoken-Spoken
The WISC R vocabulary test where the child has to describe the meaning of words spoken to him.
9 Peabody Spoken-Picture
Lloyd Dunn's Peabody Picture Vocabulary Test Form A. This tests the child's comprehension of spoken single nouns, verbs and adverbs. No reading is involved, the child being asked to select from among 4 pictures the one which he feels represents the word spoken by the investigator.
10 D&D Picture-Printed
Daniels & Dyack subtest 9. The printed word which matches a picture must be chosen from 5 alternatives.
11 Carver Spoken-Printed
This requires the child to choose from a set of 5 or 6 alternatives the printed word which represents that spoken by the examiner.

STM

12 Token Test
Warrington et al. (1971) shortened form of the Token test. The child is given 3 shapes each in four colours and is asked to perform 15 instructions such as 'Put the red circle on the green square'.
13 Auditory Sentence Span
The child is asked to repeat 20 sentences ranging in length from 2 to 11 words.
14 Auditory Word Span
The child is asked to repeat a series of words ranging in length from 2 to 5 syllables.
15 Auditory Digit Span
The child is asked to repeat a string of numbers after the experimenter has said them. The initial sequence comprises 2 digits. The length is stepped up until there are 2 successive errors at the same length.
16 Visual Digit Span
Cards containing a series of digits are presented for the same number of seconds as there are digits on the card. The child has to recall the digits in the correct order once the card has been removed. There are 3 trials per length from 2 up to 8 digits.
17 Visual Digit Span & Articulatory Suppression
As visual digit span except that the child was to say 'hello, hello, hello, ...' all the time when studying the card. This was to suppress articulatory rehearsal.
18 Visual Serial Ordering
VSO from the Illinois Test of Psycholinguistic Abilities. Sequences of from 2 to 6 chips bearing graphic designs must be duplicated from memory having just seen the test series in a booklet.

Visual

19 Visual Closure
ITPA visual closure test. The child must find 'hidden' objects in a picture strip.
20 Picture Completion WISC
WISC R subtest of picture completion. The child must detect and name the missing elements from simple line drawings.
21 Letter Search
Two visual search tasks. 1) find the 10 instances of the target letter among a page of random letters. 2) the same for word targets and foils. A rate of search score is calculated.
22 Coding WISC
WISC R coding subtest. The child must remember paired associates of geometric symbols and use these to decode a passage.
23 Block Design WISC
WISC Block Design subtest. The childs must arrange small geometric blocks to copy geometric shapes shown in the booklet.
24 Object Assembly WISC
WISC Object Assembly subtest. The child is to assemble the parts of a jigsaw like puzzle.
25 Picture Arrangement WISC
The child must arrange a set of still pictures so that they relate a sequential story.

Auditory-Visual

26 Letter Recognition
The child is asked to name the letters indicated one by one.
27 Symbol>Sound Learning
Nonsense names must be learnt for nonsense shapes.The shapes were presented and the child had to name them. Scores were the inverse of the number of trials taken to learn the complete set.
28 Sound>Symbol Learning
As Symbol>Sound learning except that here the names were given and the child was to point to the corresponding shape.
29 Colour Naming Rate
The child was to name the color patches on a card of 40 random instances of 8 colours as quickly as possible. A mean rate score was calculated over 4 trials.

Auditory

30 Syllable Segmentation
Liberman et al. (1977). The child was to tap out with a stick the number of syllables which he could hear in each word of a list.
31 Phoneme Segmentation
As Syllable Segmentation but tap out the number of phonemes.
32 Rhyme - Odd One Out
Bradley (1980). Sets of 4 monosyllabic words were spoken to the child. Three of the words had a sound in common which the other did not share. In one series the odd sound was the final phoneme, in the other it was the middle phoneme. The child was to say the 'odd one out'.
33 Rhyme Generation
Ten words were spoken to the child and he was to give more words rhyming with each.
34 Sound Blending
ITPA Sound Blending Task. Words and nonwords are spoken to the child as successive, separate sounds and the child must blend them into whole words.

Language Knowledge

35 Grammatical Closure
ITPA subtest. 33 orally presented items are accompanied by pictures portraying the content of the verbal expressions. Each statement consists of a complete statement followed by one that the child must complete - 'Here is a bed, here are two ....'. The items test syntax and grammatical inflection.
36 Knowledge of Syntax
Gleitman et al. (1972). A glove puppet is used and the child is required to say whether the sentences spoken by the puppet are 'all right' or silly. There is then a request to help him say it properly. The sentences tap a wide range of syntactic rules.

Rote & Ordering

37 Days Forwards
Time taken to say the days of the week forwards. This is then converted into a rate score (accuracy only at 5 and 6 years old).
38 Days Backwards
As above, but backwards.
39 Count Forwards
As days forwards but 1 to 10.
40 Count Backwards
As above but 10 to 0.

Oddments

41 WISC Information
WISC R subtest. "What is the main material used to make glass" etc.
42 WISC Similarities
WISC R subtest. "In what way are an apple and a pear alike" etc.
43 WISC Comprehension
WISC R subtest. "Why do people pay bills by check instead of cash" etc.
44 WISC Arithmetic
WISC R subtest. Counting trees, and mental arithmetic. A fairly mixed bag.

Commentary on Ellis:
Two conceptually-rich longitudinal studies

Keith E. Stanovich

It is relatively easy to comment on the studies Nick Ellis has presented because they can be interpreted quite easily within the framework of current theories of reading disability. This is actually a major compliment, for it is quite common for longitudinal studies of reading to be outdated by the time they are reported. Between the time a longitudinal study is conceived and finally reported, theories - and their associated tasks, methods, and paradigms - often change, leaving the study, in a conceptual no-man's land, to be dismissed as historical curiosity. This has most definitely not been the fate of Nick Ellis' studies. He has shown extraordinarily good scientific judgment in picking tasks and measures for his longitudinal studies that are still of intense interest to reading researchers over ten years after he began.

Another reason that it is easy to comment on Ellis' studies is that he anticipated my major criticism in his paper. It is, of course, the sample sizes - particularly as regards the LISREL analyses conducted on the data from his second study. But I am prone to be generous here and at least attempt to look past this flaw because of the extraordinary importance of the reading-related variables in Ellis' study and because his design directly addresses some of the most important conceptual issues in current research in reading disabilities.

The focus for my comments will be the continuing controversies over whether dyslexia - conceived in terms of aptitude/achievement discrepancy - is a useful scientific and service-delivery concept (Rispens/van Yeren/van Duijn 1991; Siegel 1989, in press; Stanovich 1991). Ellis' first study contains a comparison of much interest to those investigators who are concerned with exploring the conceptual underpinnings of the term dyslexia: a comparison between two groups of children underachieving in reading, one high in IQ and one low.

As is well known, the initial formulation of research professional, and legal definitions of reading disability in a variety of different countries emphasized the existence of discrepancies between actual school achievement and assumed intellectual capacity (see Frankenberger/Fronzaglio 1991; Hammill 1990; Stanovich 1991). All of these professional and legal definitions highlighted the same salient feature: The fact that a dyslexic child has an "unexpected" disability in the domain of reading, one not predicted by their general intellectual competence and socioeducational opportunities. Practically, this has meant a statistical assessment of the difference between their objectively measured reading ability and general intelligence (Frankenberger/Fronzaglio 1991; Kavale 1987).

The critical assumption that has fueled theoretical interest in the dyslexia concept from the beginning - and that has justified differential educational classification and treatment - has been that the degree of discrepancy from IQ is meaningful: That the reading difficulties of the dyslexic (I am here using the term dyslexic to signify a discrepancy-defined child) stem from problems different from those characterizing the poor reader without IQ discrepancy - what Gough/Tunmer (1986) have termed the "garden variety" poor reader.

The operationalization of this assumption for purposes of empirical tests has been dominated by two different research designs. One is the reading-level match design where an older group of dyslexic children is matched on reading level with a younger group of nondyslexic children. The logic here is that if the reading-related cognitive subskills of the two groups do not match, then it would seem that they are arriving at their similar reading levels via different routes. In contrast, if dyslexic children are reading just like any other child who happens to be at their reading level, they become much less interesting from a theoretical point of view.

The second major design - one pertinent not only to theoretical issues but also one quite relevant to the educational politics of reading disability - is to compare dyslexic children with children of the same age who are reading at the same level, but who are not labeled dyslexic and who of course have lower IQs. Adapting the terminology of Gough/Tunmer (1986), I have termed this design the garden-variety control design (see Stanovich 1991). Again, the inferences drawn are relatively straightforward. If the reading subskill profiles of the two groups do not match, then this is at least consistent with the assumption that they are arriving at their similar reading levels via different routes. In contrast, if the reading subskill profiles of the two groups are identical, this would certainly undermine the rationale for the differential educational treatment of dyslexic children and would again make dyslexic children considerably less interesting theoretically. Nick Ellis' study contains this critical comparison of poor readers high and low in IQ.

Before discussing Ellis' evidence, I will outline what patterns, given our current conceptions of dyslexia, our data should show, in the best of all possible worlds. I have summarized the idealized situation in a model that has been termed the phonological-core variable-difference framework (Stanovich 1988, 1991) - a modal model of current theory. The model rests on a clear understanding of the assumption of specificity in definitions of dyslexia (see Stanovich 1986). This assumption underlies all discussions of the concept of dyslexia, even if it is not explicitly stated. It is the idea that a child with this type of learning disability has a brain/cognitive deficit that is reasonably specific to the reading task. That is, the concept of dyslexia requires that the deficits displayed by such children do not extend too far into other domains of cognitive functioning. If they did, this would depress the constellation of abilities we call intelligence and thus reduce the reading/intelligence discrepancy that is central to all current definitions.

In short, the key deficit in dyslexia must be a domain-specific process rather than a process that operates across a wide variety of domains. For this, and other reasons, many investigators have located the proximal locus of dyslexia at the word recognition level and have been searching for the processing flaw in the word recognition module (e.g., Bruck 1990; Morrison 1987; Perfetti 1985; Siegel 1985; Stanovich 1986, 1988). Research in the last ten years has focused intensively on phonological processing abilities. It is now well established that dyslexic children display deficits in various aspects of phonological processing. Children having difficulty in reading also have difficulty making explicit reports about sound segments at the phoneme level, they display naming difficulties, their utilization of phonological codes in short-term memory is inefficient, their categorical perception of certain phonemes may be other than normal, and they may have speech production difficulties (e.g., Catts 1991; Kamhi/Catts 1989; Olson/Wise/Conners/Rack 1990; Pennington 1986; Perfetti 1985; Snowling 1987; Vellutino/Scanlon 1987; Wagner/Torgesen 1987; Werker/Tees 1987; Wolf 1991). Importantly, there is increasing evidence that the linkage from phonological processing ability to reading skill is a causal one (e.g., Bryant/Bradley/Maclean/Crossland 1989; Cunningham 1990; Lie 1991; Lundberg/Frost/Peterson 1988; Maclean/Bryant/Bradley 1987; Perfetti/Beck/Bell/Hughes 1987; Rack/Snowling/Olson 1992). Whether all of these phonologically related deficits are reflective of a single underlying processing problem and whether all of them can be considered causal or are instead correlates is a matter for future research, but some important progress is being made on this issue (e.g., Pennington/Van Orden/Smith et al. 1990).

In the phonological-core variable-difference model, the term variable difference refers to the performance contrasts between the garden-variety and the dyslexic poor reader outside the phonological domain. The idealized data pattern predicted by this model is that the cognitive status of the garden-variety poor reader should be well described by a developmental lag model. Cognitively, they should be similar to younger children reading at the same level. A logical corollary of this pattern is that the garden-variety reader will have a wide variety of cognitive deficits when compared to chronological age controls who are reading at normal levels. This is precisely what Nick Ellis reports. However, it is important to understand that the garden-variety poor reader should also share the phonological problems of the dyslexic reader (probably to an equal extent, see Beech/Awaida 1992; Felton/Wood 1992; Fredman/Stevenson 1988; Siegel 1988; Stanovich in press). This pattern is again clearly present in Ellis' data.

However, the model predicts that for the garden-variety reader the deficits - relative to CA controls - should extend into a variety of domains and some of these (e.g., vocabulary, language comprehension) may also be causally linked to reading comprehension. Such a pattern should not characterize the dyslexic, who should have a deficit localized in the phonological core. Again, this is essentially what Nick Ellis has shown us with his data. Ellis' data then, fit well within the phonological-core variable-difference model which is a model that preserves at least some of the conceptual integrity of the classical notion of dyslexia. How does his data fit in with the rest of the literature? In order to consider the pattern of results from the two designs I have mentioned, we must make one final distinction: the distinction concerns what particular measure of reading that we use to match the groups. A certain fuzziness on this point confused the literature on the reading-level match in the mid-1980s (see Stanovich/Nathan/Zolman 1988). In particular, it must be specified whether the groups are to be matched on reading comprehension or on word recognition, for to use one or the other of these two matches means that one is asking somewhat different questions.

The simplest case involves the reading comprehension match. The phonological-core model predicts that, when compared to reading-level controls, discrepancy-defined dyslexic children should display a pattern that I have characterized as macro-compensation - tradeoffs among global processes that result in equivalent reading comprehension. The predicted pattern derives for the following reasons: First, the two groups will presumably be close in intelligence, IQ being a matching variable in most reading level studies. Of course, similar intelligence test scores at different ages mean different things in terms of the raw score or absolute level of performance on a given test or index of ability. Thus, when older dyslexics are matched with younger children progressing normally in reading, the former will have higher raw scores on the intelligence measure. It should then also be the case that the dyslexics will score higher on any cognitive task that is correlated with the raw score on the intelligence test, and of course there are a host of such tasks. Thus, the psychometric constraints imposed by the matching in a comprehension level investigation should result in a pattern that I have characterized as global, or macro-compensation. The constraints dictate that a rigorously-defined sample of reading-disabled children should display performance inferior to the younger comprehension-matched children on phonological analysis and phonological coding skills and thus on word recognition, but should simultaneously display superior vocabulary, real-word knowledge, and/or strategic abilities (i.e., superior performance on other reading-related variables that should be correlated with the raw score on the IQ test). The similar overall level of comprehension ability in the two groups presumably obtains because the dyslexic children use these other skills and knowledge sources to compensate for seriously deficient phonological processing and word recognition skills. The same pattern macro-compensation should characterize comparisons of discrepancy-defined dyslexics and garden variety poor readers of the same age, for exactly the same reasons. In short, the interrelations of the processes that determine reading comprehension should be different when dyslexics are compared to either garden variety or comprehension level equated younger children.

Ellis' study is also indirectly relevant to this issue. This is because a word recognition match study can serve as an indirect test of macro-compensation if a reading comprehension test is included in the study. Dyslexics, matched with garden-variety poor readers on word recognition skills, should display superior reading comprehension. Nick Ellis' low and high IQ poor readers are matched on Neale accuracy and on the Schonell and the high IQ readers do have higher Neale comprehension scores, thus confirming the pattern of macro-compensation in the literature (see Stanovich in press).

However, it is important to note that even if compensatory processing does characterize the comprehension patterns of dyslexic children, this does not necessarily guarantee the applicability of an analogous explanation of similar levels of decoding in a word recognition match. That is, it is perfectly possible that the comprehension ability of disabled readers is determined by compensatory processing (relative to younger comprehension controls), but that the operation of their word recognition modules is similar (in terms of regularity effects, orthographic processing, context effects, etc.) when compared to younger word recognition controls. Note that from the macro-compensatory hypothesis it follows that the word recognition match controls for an older disabled group of readers are logically precluded from completely overlapping with the disabled group's comprehension controls.

In studies employing word level matches to study the organization of word recognition processes, the phonological-core model predicts another tradeoff among relative strengths of processes - what we might call a micro-compensation. Specifically, for the majority of dyslexics with a phonological deficit, a word recognition match with a younger group of nondyslexic controls should reveal another pattern of ability tradeoffs: deficits in phonological sensitivity and in the phonological mechanisms that mediate lexical access - but superior orthographic processing and storage mechanisms. A similar pattern should hold when dyslexics are compared to a same-age garden-variety group.

Turning first to the results from word-level designs. Not too many years ago, when I first reviewed this literature (Stanovich/Nathan/Zolman 1988), it was a confusing mass of contradictions. However, in just the last couple of years things here have become considerably clarified. Rack/Snowling/Olson (1992) have recently completed an extremely important meta-analysis of this research that clarifies this literature considerably and explains many discrepancies between studies that have heretofore been puzzling. My own reading of literature, aided greatly by their meta-analysis, is that there is now a consensus in the literature indicating that samples of dyslexic children, when matched with younger children on word recognition ability will display inferior phonological coding skills, particularly so in the case of pseudoword naming. This conclusion is based on data from dozens of subjects collected by numerous investigators from several different continents. It is true that there are some exceptions to the pattern, but most of these can be explained by a variety of factors that Rack/Snowling/Olson (1992) discuss in their meta-analysis, for example, the nature of the words on the word recognition test must be carefully considered, as must the pseudowords used in the nonword naming tests.

When we turn to studies employing garden-variety matches, where we would expect a similar type of micro-compensation - if that is, the concept of discrepancy-defined dyslexia has construct validity - we find something very puzzling. The literature provides no strong support for a differential organization of cognitive subskills within the word recognition module among readers of different IQ levels. Several different studies have failed to find such differences (Felton/Wood 1992; Fredman/Stevenson 1988; Siegel 1988). Nick Ellis' data provide further negative evidence. There is no indication of microcompensation in the performance on the phonological tasks in his study. Indeed, his trends are in the opposite direction. We thus have a convergence of findings against the hypothesis of micro-compensation. The paradox here is that dyslexics appear to be mismatched on phonological processing skills with reading level-controls but not with garden-variety controls. Age thus appears to be a better predictor than IQ of the reorganization of cognitive skills in word recognition which compensates for poor phonological skills.

Or, rather than age, one might say that it is reading failure which is a better predictor because, of course, reading failure is something that the dyslexics and the garden variety poor readers also have in common. And here might be the key to the apparent puzzle. Whether low phonological sensitivity is due to developmental lag, neurological insult, or whatever, the key fact is that the necessity of confronting the demands of reading triggers the reorganization of skills we see in dyslexic and garden-variety poor readers when either are compared to RL controls. This interpretation --and the finding it seeks to explain - non-differentiability of dyslexic and garden-variety poor readers-- is, however, a bit of a threat to the construct validity of IQ-based discrepancy measurement. This is because, when we look at the macro-level of comprehension processes we find a different organization of subskills among dyslexic and garden-variety poor readers, but when it comes to the critical locus of dyslexia - word recognition - the structure of processing looks remarkably similar.

Finally, I will turn to Ellis' second, more fine-grained, longitudinal study of reading, spelling, and phonological awareness. The results here must, as I have indicated, be interpreted weakly because the LISREL analyses are compromised by low sample size. Nevertheless, the results are very consistent with two important theoretical speculations in the literature. First, the data are supportive of Frith's (1985) stage model of reading acquisition that involves reciprocal relationships between reading and spelling. Ellis' interpretation of Frith's hypothesis is that spelling acts as a mediator for the use of explicit phonological awareness until the child begins the alphabetic stage of reading by directly applying explicit phonological awareness to reading.

Secondly, Ellis' results with the implicit and explicit PA tasks presents us with one way of resolving the long-running controversy between the Brussels group and the Oxford group (e.g., Bertelson/Morais/Alegria/Content 1985; Bryant/Bradley 1985) regarding whether phonological awareness is a prerequisite for alphabetic reading. Ellis' results suggest that a shallow phonological sensitivity (what he terms implicit phonological awareness) may well serve some sort of prerequisite function in early reading development and that the deeper forms of phonological awareness (what Ellis terms explicit phonological awareness) might be largely a consequence of reading acquisition (see Stanovich 1987, 1992). However, Ellis' analysis suggests the important conclusion that this more explicit phonological awareness can feed back to affect stages of alphabetic literacy that are still quite early.

In summary, what I hope I have demonstrated is that Ellis' studies speak to an extraordinarily wide range of issues in reading and reading disability research. Ellis takes pains to warn about the small sample sizes in his studies. However, I think that if one looks at the range of variables in Ellis' studies and considers carefully their relevance to issues in current reading theory, we must conclude that these studies contain a conceptual richness which more than compensates for their modest scale.

Note

Preparation of this chapter was assisted by a grant from the Social Sciences and Humanities Research Council of Canada.

References

Beech, J.R. & Awaida, M. (1992). Lexical and nonlexical routes: A comparison between normally achieving and poor readers. Journal of Learning Disabilities, 25, 196-206.

Bertelson, P., Morais, J., Alegria, J., & Content, A. (1985). Phonetic analysis capacity and learning to read. Nature, 313, 73-74.

Bruck, M. (1990). Word-recognition skills of adults with childhood diagnoses of dyslexia. Developmental Psychology, 26, 439-454.

Bryant, P.E., & Bradley, L. (1985). Reply to Bertelson et al. Nature, 313, 74.

Bryant, P.E., Bradley, L., Maclean, M., & Crossland, D. (1989). Nursery rhymes, phonological skills and reading. Journal of Child Language, 16, 407-428.

Catts, H.W. (1991). Early identification of reading disabilities. Topics in Language Disorders, 12(1), 1-16.

Cunningham, A.E. (1990). Explicit versus implicit instruction in phonemic awareness. Journal of Experimental Child Psychology, 50, 429-444.

Felton, R.H. & Wood, F.R. (1992). A reading level match study of nonword reading skills in poor readers with varying IQs. Journal of Learning Disabilities, 25, 318-326.

Frankenberger, W. & Fronzaglio, K. (1991). A review of states' criteria and procedures for identifying children with learning disabilities. Journal of Learning Disabilities, 24, 495-500.

Fredman, G. & Stevenson, J. (1988). Reading processes in specific reading retarded and reading backward 13-year-olds. British Journal of Developmental Psychology, 6, 97-108.

Frith, U. (1985). Beneath the surface of developmental dyslexia. In K. Patterson, J. Marshall, & M. Coltheart (Eds.), Surface dyslexia. 301-330. London: Erlbaum.

Gough, P.B. & Tunmer, W.E. (1986). Decoding, reading, and reading disability. Remedial and Special Education, 7, 6-10.

Hammill, D.D. (1990). On defining learning disabilities: An emerging consensus. Journal of Learning Disabilities, 23, 74-84.

Kamhi, A. & Catts, H. (1989). Reading disabilities: A developmental language perspective. Boston: College-Hill Press.

Kavale, K.A. (1987). Theoretical issues surrounding severe discrepancy. Learning Disabilities Research, 3, 12-20.

Lie, A. (1991). Effects of a training program for stimulating skills in word analysis in first-grade children. Reading Research Quarterly, 26, 234-250.

Lundberg, I., Frost, J., & Peterson, O. (1988). Effects of an extensive program for stimulating phonological awareness in preschool children. Reading Research Quarterly, 23, 263-284.

Maclean, M., Bryant, P., & Bradley, L. (1987). Rhymes, nursery rhymes, and reading in early childhood. Merrill-Palmer Quarterly, 33, 255-281.

Morrison, F.J. (1987). The nature of reading disability: Toward an integrative framework. In S. Ceci (Ed.), Handbook of cognitive, social, and neiropsychological aspects of learning disabilities. 33-62. Hillsdale, NJ: Erlbaum.

Olson, R., Wise, B., Conners, F., & Rack, J. (1990). Organization, heritability, and remediation of component word recognition and language skills in disabled readers. In T. Carr & B. Levy (Eds.), Reading and its development: Component skills approaches. 261-322. San Diego: Academic Press.

Pennington, B.F. (1986). Issues in the diagnosis and phenotype analysis of dyslexia: Implications for family studies. In S.D. Smith (Ed.), Genetics and learning disabilities. 69-96. San Diego: College-Hill Press.

Pennington, B.F., Van Orden, G.C., Smith, S.D., Green, P.A., & Haith, M. M. (1990). Phonological processing skills and deficits in adult dyslexics. Child Development, 61, 1753-1778.

Perfetti, C.A. (1985). Reading ability. New York: Oxford University Press.

Perfetti, C.A., Beck, I., Bell, L., & Hughes, C. (1987). Phonemic knowledge and learning to read are reciprocal: A longitudinal study of first grade children. Merrill-Palmer Quarterly, 33, 283-319.

Rack, J.P., Snowling, M.J., & Olson, R.K. (1992). The nonword reading deficit in developmental dyslexia: A review. Reading Research Quarterly, 27, 28-53.

Rispens, J., van Yeren, T., & van Duijn, G. (1991). The irrelevance of IQ to the definition of learning disabilities: Some empirical evidence. Journal of Learning Disabilities, 24, 434-438.

Siegel, L.S. (1985). Psycholinguistic aspects of reading disabilities. In L. Siegel & F. Morrison (Eds.), Cognitive development in atypical children. 45-65. New York: Springer-Verlag.

Siegel, L.S. (1988). Evidence that IQ scores are irrelevant to the definition and analysis of reading disability. Canadian Journal of Psychology, 42, 201-215.

Siegel, L.S. (1989). IQ is irrelevant to the definition of learning disabilities. Journal of Learning Disabilities, 22, 469-479.

Siegel, L.S. (in press). Alice in IQ land or why IQ is still irrelevant to learning disabilities. In M. Joshi & C. K. Leong (Eds.), Reading disabilities: Diagnosis and component processes. Dordrecht, The Netherlands: Kluwer Academic.

Snowling, M. (1987). Dyslexia. Oxford: Basil Blackwell.

Stanovich, K. E. (1986). Cognitive processes and the reading problems of learning disabled children: Evaluating the assumption of specificity. In J. Torgesen & B. Wong (Eds.), Psychological and educational perspectives on learning disabilities. 87-131. New York: Academic Press.

Stanovich, K.E. (1987). Perspectives on segmental analysis and alphabetic literacy. European Bulletin of Cognitive Psychology, 7, 514-519.

Stanovich, K.E. (1988). Explaining the differences between the dyslexic and the garden-variety poor reader: The phonological-core variable-difference model. Journal of Learning Disabilities, 21, 590-612.

Stanovich, K.E. (1991). Discrepancy definitions of reading disability: Has intelligence led us astray?. Reading Research Quarterly, 26, 7-29.

Stanovich, K.E. (1992). Speculations on the causes and consequences of individual differences in early reading acquisition. In P. Gough, L. Ehri, & R. Treiman (Eds.), Reading Acquisition. 307-342. Hillsdale, N.J.: Erlbaum Associates.

Stanovich, K.E. (in press). Problems in the differential diagnosis of reading disabilities. In M. Joshi & C.K. Leong (Eds.), Reading disabilities: Diagnosis and component processes. Dordrecht, The Netherlands: Kluwer Academic.

Stanovich, K.E., Nathan, R.G., & Zolman, J. E. (1988). The developmental lag hypothesis in reading: Longitudinal and matched reading-level comparisons. Child Development, 59, 71-86.

Vellutino, F. & Scanlon, D. (1987). Phonological coding, phonological awareness, and reading ability: Evidence from a longitudinal and experimental study. Merrill-Palmer Quarterly, 33, 321-363.

Wagner, R.K. & Torgesen, J.K. (1987). The nature of phonological processing and its causal role in the acquisition of reading skills. Psychological Bulletin, 101, 192-212.

Werker, J.F. & Tees, R.C. (1987). Speech perception in severely disabled and average reading children. Canadian Journal of Psychology, 41, 48-61.

Wolf, M. (1991). Naming speed and reading: The contribution of the cognitive neurosciences. Reading Research Quarterly, 26, 123-141.

Emerging literacy from kindergarten to second grade: Evidence from the Munich Longitudinal Study on the Genesis of Individual Competencies

Jan Carol Näslund
Wolfgang Schneider

The opportunity to closely study children's cognitive and affective development longitudinally for five years rarely presents itself. When this opportunity does arise, careful planning for exact methods and content of data collection weighs heavily on researchers' minds. However, at the same time, such an undertaking necessarily requires the flexibility to alter, and sometimes change direction in order to keep up-to-date with new findings found in the literature and (most often) as a result of personal insights and innovations. The Munich Longitudinal Study for the Genesis of Individual Competencies (Weinert/Schneider 1987, 1991, 1992) provided the team of researchers at the Max Planck Institute for Psychological Research in Munich such an opportunity.

The collection of data in the area of cognitive development for this project provided the foundation on which the study of later emergent literacy was based. This paper will focus only on a subset of cognitive factors which affect reading acquisition. These cognitive areas are: 1) memory development, 2) general and verbal intelligence, and 3) metalinguistic competencies. Memory and intelligence were first assessed at about age four (at the beginning of kindergarten), and again with metalinguistic competencies, and early letter knowledge at age six (in the last year of kindergarten). After children entered first grade, and began to learn to read formally, memory, intelligence, and metalinguistic skills were assessed again in addition to reading performance.

Other longitudinal studies assessing the influence of preschool cognitive factors on later reading performance have been completed recently (Juel 1988; Lundberg/Frost/Peterson 1988; Maclean/Bryant/Bradley 1987). These studies indicate preschool metalinguistic awareness to be a major factor in emerging literacy and later reading performance in school. However, there is some indication that metalinguistic awareness at the level of phonological segmentation covaries with children's learning the alphabetic principle (Foorman/Francis/Novy/Liberman 1991; Perfetti/Beck/Bell/Hughes 1987). Ehri (1989), Morais/Cary/Alegria/Bertelson (1979), and Read/Zhang/Nie/ Ding (1986) provide evidence that phonological segmentation skills do not arise in the absence of some formal instruction in the alphabetical principle. However, Lundberg et al.'s (1988) longitudinal training study of Scandinavian children demonstrates that phonological segmentation skills can develop independently of specific literacy instruction. Some forms of metalinguistic awareness may actually be necessary to learn the alphabetic principle (an hypothesis supported by Tunmer/Rohl 1991).

German and Scandinavian school children similarly begin formal training in reading at later ages than in other industrialized countries. Whereas children in the British system begin reading instruction at about age four, the age for Scandinavian and German children is about age six and a half or seven. This difference may be responsible for some of the recent inconsistent findings pertaining to possible causal influences of phonological segmentation and alphabetic knowledge. Results of the study reported here with German children adds to the evidence in favor of preliterate phonological awareness development, and differentiates phonological awareness tasks as to their relative dependency on alphabetic knowledge.

Pioneering research beginning about fifteen years ago and conducted at the Haskin Laboratories under the direction of Isabelle Liberman has led to breakthroughs in discovering cognitive factors which specifically affect reading development (Brady/Shankweiler/Mann 1983; Liberman/Shankweiler/Liberman et al. 1977; Mann/Liberman/Shankweiler 1980; Mark/ Shankweiler/Liberman/Fowler 1977). These researchers provide convincing evidence that reading performance is related to working memory via phonological recoding of text. Memory span alone does not explain differences in performance among poor and better readers. Better readers appear to phonologically recode verbal information, increasing the efficiency of their working memory. Poorer readers phonologically recoded verbal information to a lesser extent than better readers, and this is believed to explain in part their less efficient working memory while reading. The evidence for this phonological recoding effect came from findings that better readers were adversely affected in their recall of verbal information if this information contained phonologically similar items (letters, words, sentences) in comparison to recall for phonologically dissimilar items. Poorer readers were less adversely affected in recall by phonologically similar lists of information in comparison with phonologically dissimilar lists of information. The observed phonological interference effect for better readers was the basis for proposing that phonological recoding in working memory was likely a significant cognitive component in reading. Better readers appeared to spontaneously and automatically phonologically recode information, whereas poorer readers did this less so. The developmental relationship between memory and phonological awareness is also a focus of this paper. If phonological awareness arises independently of alphabetic knowledge, then one would expect that the relationship between phonological awareness and memory would also arise independently of alphabetic knowledge.

Stanovich/Cunningham/Feeman (1984) have shown that phonological awareness influences reading comprehension indirectly through its direct effect on text decoding. The finding that both pseudoword and word reading predicted reading comprehension suggested that a child's facility with phonological recoding of text was in large part responsible for their reading performance. This result, in addition to those found by Isabelle Liberman and colleagues suggests that better readers cognitively process phonological components of text as they read, whereas poorer readers process phonological components less so.

In a review and critique of whole-language and code-oriented approaches to reading instruction, Vellutino (1991) has argued that good readers use phonological recoding more than poorer readers, and that poorer readers tend more than good readers to use less efficient context strategies. Whole-language refers to an instructional approach with the major premise being that reading is a "psychological guessing game" (Goodman 1967). Teachers are discouraged from teaching phonetics of any kind. (Phonetics refers to any teaching of phonemic properties of letters and letter clusters, such as syllabic or onset/rime units. Traditional phonics refers to teaching that each letter corresponds to one, or sometimes two - in the case of some languages - individual sounds.) Children are encouraged to use contextual cues in "guessing" the meaning of text. The major goal is to teach reading without disturbing the "whole-ness" of language. Contemporary code-oriented approaches make use of more phonetic approaches in teaching decoding of text. In the more accepted phonetic techniques, perceptual phonological units are preserved. For example, /b/ is only an abstract phoneme, given that it can only be detected in combination with a vowel, such as when comparing the difference heard in /bi/ and /i/. Recent attempts to advocate a mixture of whole-language and code-oriented teaching ignores the basic tenet of whole-language. As soon as any decoding is taught, the approach ceases to be whole-language. Findings from longitudinal studies of reading acquisition are pertinent to the conflict surrounding whole-language and code-oriented approaches. Such studies can help reveal the cognitive development of children as they enter into reading instruction, especially if the early stages of the study take place before most children are taught the alphabet. Vellutino's (1991) argument concerning the importance of code-based instruction would be supported by longitudinal findings showing that preliterate children's level of phonological awareness, independent of alphabetic knowledge and verbal aptitude, explained a significant proportion of their later reading performance. If better readers spontaneously develop phonological awareness, and use this to become proficient readers, this would suggest that reading instruction encouraging attention to phonological properties of language should be encouraged.

In summary, this paper focuses on several specific concerns in emerging literacy. First, we compare the predictive relationship of preschool verbal and general intelligence, verbal memory, metalinguistic skills, and decoding on reading comprehension in the early grades. Second, the relationship between memory and phonological awareness is assessed developmentally. Third, the relative independence of metalinguistic awareness and alphabetic knowledge is assessed.

Method

The original sample included 220 children from Munich and surrounding suburbs. Beginning at about age four, children visited one of two test sites two or three times during the school year (one in Munich and one in a nearby suburb). The major goal of the LOGIC project was to assess intraindividual changes in a variety of cognitive and social skills, and to explore the pattern of change in these interrelationships over time (cf. Weinert/Schneider 1987). One of the subgoals of the study concerned the prediction of reading acquisition, which is the topic of the present paper. The analyses reported below include the first five years of the study, ending when most children were in the second grade. Not all 220 children are included in the analyses presented here. Due to organizational problems, a subgroup of children were not tested on the word and nonword decoding speed tests and the reading comprehension tests to be described below. For various reasons, 21 subjects were not promoted to first grade at the time most other children were, and were omitted from analyses concerning school-related tasks. There were absentees on some of the testing days, and some children chose to discontinue their participation in the study. As a consequence, the following analyses are based on those 133 subjects with complete data sets.

Description of assessments

As noted above, several cognitive measures of the LOGIC study that were assessed at different points in time seemed suitable as predictors of reading acquisition. These measures are summarized below.

Age four:
Columbia Mental Maturity Scale (CMMS). The American version of the CMMS (Burgemeister/Blum/Lorge 1972) was adopted for the LOGIC study because the German version of the test cannot be used with kindergarten children. Children were presented with pictorial and figural classification items. Each item consisted of three to five drawings. The children's task was to look at all the pictures on the card, select the one that was different from or unrelated to the others, and to indicate their choice by pointing to it. The number of correct choices was taken as a measure of children's nonverbal intellectual ability.

Word Span. An German adaptation of the word span task given by Case/Kurland/Goldberg (1982) was administered to assess children's memory capacity. The items to be recalled in the word lists were all concrete nouns. The lists to be recalled ranges in length from three to seven words. Children were first given a list of three words to recall. If children recalled two sets of three words each correctly, two lists of four words each were presented. Children were given successively more words to recall only if they recalled at least one set at the previous level.

A second word span was also devised. The lists were so constructed that words in each list would sound similar, either by rhyming, or by having the same first sound.

Assessments at age five:
Hannover-Wechsler Intelligence Scale for Kindergarten Children (HAWIVA, Eggert 1978). This test represents the German adaptation of the Wechsler Intelligence Test for Children (WISC) for four- to six-year-old children. The verbal section (verbal comprehension, word usage and vocabulary, and general knowledge) of this inventory was used in these analyses, yielding a sum score that represented children's verbal intelligence.

Assessments at age six:

Battery of metalinguistic tasks. A battery of meta-linguistic tasks for preschool children devised by Jansen/Knorn/Mannhaupt et al. (1986; see also Skowronek/Marx 1989) and Brügelmann (1986) was adopted for the LOGIC study. In addition to these, a German version of Bradley/Bryant's (1985) phonological oddity (rhyming) task was also administered in the last kindergarten year. In the second grade, children received a phonological awareness and segmentation inventory devised by the first author. Tasks taken from the Jansen et al. (1986) battery were: *repetition of nonsense words, detecting word pairs that rhyme, syllable counting, blending two syllables to make a word,* and *detecting particular sounds within words.* The tasks used from Brügelmann's (1986) inventory were *syllable segmenting of words* and *syllable synthesizing* (identifying words which were pronounced with elongated vowels). The Bradley/Bryant (1985) tasks consisted of identifying which word of four either differed in initial consonant, or in the middle vowel, or did not rhyme with the other three.

Word span. The word span test developed by Case et al. (1982) and described above was administered again. The second memory span test was also repeated at this measurement point.

Sentence span. A German version of the listening span test developed by Daneman/Blennerhassett (1984) was additionally used to assess children's memory capacity. Groups of sentences (ranging from one to seven sentences) were presented to children. The total number of sentences correctly recalled was used for children's score on this measure.

Columbia Mental Maturity Scale (CMMS, Burgemeister/Blum/Large 1972). This test was identical to the one presented at age four and was given as a non-verbal intelligence measure.

Alphabetic knowledge. This was an assessment also taken from the Jansen et al. (1986) inventory of preschool predictors of reading performance. Children were shown letters in a fixed random order and asked if they recognized any of them, and if so, to name them. For purposes of this paper, answers were considered correct if either the letter name or sound were correctly identified.

Assessments at age seven:

Hamburg Wechsler-Intelligence Scale for School Children (HAWIK, Tewes 1985). This is the age-corrected form of the HAWIVA described above. Again, the verbal part was used for purposes of this study and taken as an indicator of verbal intelligence.

The **Sentence span** given at age five was repeated at age seven.

Word Discrimination. Whereas the previous measures were used as predictors of reading skills, the word discrimination test given at the end of the first year in elementary school was chosen to assess children's early reading skills. Children were presented with four sets of pictures of familiar objects (i.e., an eye, house, cow, etc.). After correctly identifying the pictures, children were then asked to watch the screen of a table-top slide projector very carefully. The pictures remained in front of the child during each set of trials. They were to read the word flashed on the screen (shown for 1 second) and indicate if the word corresponded to one of the pictures that was in front of them, and if so, to point to the picture. Distractor words were phonologically and visually similar to the target words (i.e., for the target "Apfel", "Ampel" was one of the distractor words).

Assessments at age eight:
The **CMMS, Word span**, and **Sentence span** tasks described previously were repeated at age eight.
Phonological awareness and segmentation. An inventory of phonological awareness and segmentation tasks was devised by the first author. These tasks were more difficult than those administered in the preschool metalinguistic awareness inventory. The first task required *identifying altered phonemes* between sets of pseudowords. The second task required *replacing phonemes* in pseudowords, and third task required *switching phonemes* within pseudowords. The scores of all of these tasks are combined for the second grade phonological awareness variable.
Word and non-word decoding speed. This task was administered at the beginning and end of second grade. Children were presented with one-syllable real words and pseudowords on a computer screen. Letters were about four inches high. A computer timer was activated as soon as each word or pseudoword appeared on the screen. Speed of decoding was recorded when the research assistant pressed the space bar as the child was pronouncing the last sound in each target. Onset speed was not used in this case given that pilot work indicated that many children pronounced the first sound of the words presented whether or not they recognized the word. Serial pronunciation of letters is possible in German, and therefore onset time does not necessarily indicate word recognition or decoding.
Reading comprehension. The reading comprehension test devised by the first author was administered at the beginning and end of second grade. 18 items were intended to measure word identification within the context of a sentence. Close-type multiple choice format was used. The second part of the test consisted of reading five short stories and responding to a total of 12 multiple choice comprehension items, intended to require inferences based on the text.

Predicting later reading performance

Kindergarten and second grade predictors

A first aim of this study was to estimate and test a structural (causal) model describing and explaining individual differences in reading acquisition. In order to increase the reliability of findings, a latent variable structural equation model using multiple indicators of particular factors was specified. In the case of predicting reading comprehension, the four proposed predictive factors are verbal ability, memory capacity, phonological awareness, and decoding speed. Decoding speed is also believed to be predicted by phonological awareness. In addition, both decoding speed and phonological awareness are themselves proposed as being predicted by memory capacity and verbal ability.

At least two separate measures were administered for each of the factors proposed to influence reading performance. The same predictive factors (memory capacity, phonological awareness, and verbal ability) were measured by several tasks each in kindergarten and in early elementary school (see Näslund/Schneider 1991). The latent memory capacity factor comprised the word span tasks (phonologically similar and dissimilar word lists). The latent phonological awareness variable consisted of the first and last sound oddity tasks, and the syllable blending task. The verbal ability factor consisted of the vocabulary and verbal comprehension subtests of the HAWIVA and HAWIK inventories. The purpose of two measurement points, one before and one after the start of formal reading instruction, was to assess the viability of the proposed structural model and the persistence of influence of the predictive factors before and after the start of formal reading instruction.

Linear Structural Relationships modelling (LISREL VI, Jöreskog/Sörbom 1984) was used to test these and some alternate hypotheses about the likely causal relationships among these factors and reading comprehension. LISREL analyses are specifically designed to directly test hypotheses (for details see Näslund/Schneider 1991; Schneider/Näslund 1992). The proposed structural model for each time period is found in Figure 1.

Models tested. Verbal ability and memory capacity were conceived of as primary sources of influence on the rest of the latent predictive and criterion variables. Preliminary analyses revealed that phonological awareness was

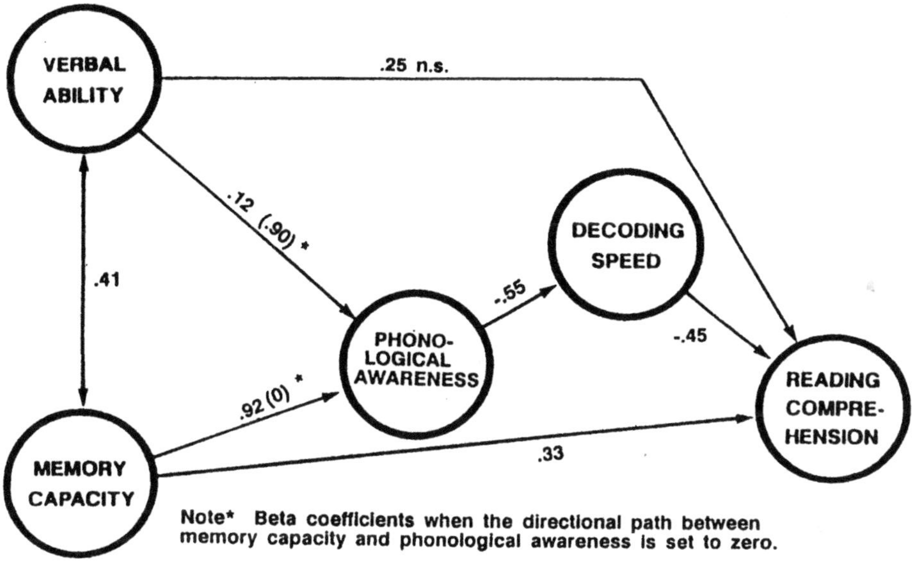

Fig. 1: *LISREL model for preschool predictors of second grade decoding speed and reading comprehension*

likely to be significantly influenced by memory capacity, and possibly verbal ability. Although memory capacity was strongly correlated to all other factors in the model, the direct connections between memory capacity and decoding speed were not significant in this particular model. The directionality between memory capacity and phonological awareness developed into an issue in this study, and will be addressed more directly in the next section of this paper. Decoding speed, as demonstrated in the literature, was proposed to be directly influenced by phonological awareness, and in turn decoding speed was proposed to have a direct influence on reading comprehension. Verbal memory capacity has repeatedly been shown to have a strong relationship with reading comprehension. Therefore, this direct influence is also tested in the model, and compared with the direct effects of verbal ability on reading comprehension.

This particular model fitted the observed measured variables acceptably when it included the kindergarten factors (χ^2 = 37.86, p = .15). However, the influence of verbal ability on both phonological awareness and reading comprehension were not strong enough to be significant (see Figure 1). The rest of the proposed relationships were significant. In order to test the strength of memory as an influence on phonological awareness and reading, the proposed relationship between memory capacity and phonological awareness was set to be zero. This one change caused the model to have unacceptable fit ($\chi^2 = 49.51$, $p < .05$). This result attests to the importance of memory as a preschool factor in development of skills related to success in reading.

The same procedure was applied to the model containing the elementary school predictive factors (see Figure 2). This analysis included reading comprehension and decoding measures administered at the end of second grade. The same results emerged, except that there was no significant direct effect of memory capacity on reading comprehension as found for preschool memory capacity ($\chi^2 = 29.60$, $p = .13$). Deleting the proposed connection between memory capacity and phonological awareness also had the effect of reducing the acceptability of the model significantly ($\chi^2 = 42.46$, $p < .01$). Each of the alternative models, which deleted the connection between memory capacity and phonological awareness, was found to have a significantly

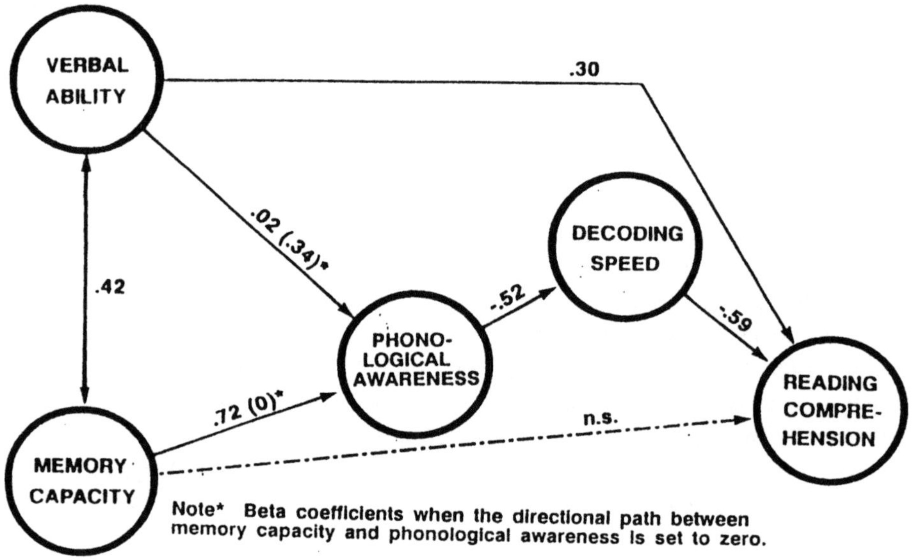

Fig. 2: *LISREL model for second grade predictors of second grade decoding speed and reading comprehension*

lower fit than the actual proposed models when applying χ^2 analyses for estimating significant differences in model fit.

These analyses would appear to demonstrate the primacy of memory in predicting phonological awareness and reading performance, and the direct effects of phonological awareness on decoding speed. However, in second grade, the influence of memory on reading comprehension would appear to be only indirect through its direct influence on phonological awareness and decoding speed. Decoding speed was not directly influenced by memory capacity in any model, but taking memory capacity out of the models resulted in an unacceptable model fit, indicating that memory capacity was a necessary factor in explaining the structure of relationships among the factors.

The results of these LISREL analyses are somewhat unsettling given the evidence that phonological recoding is likely a primary source of influence on working memory in reading (Brady et al., 1983; Liberman et al., 1977; Mann et al., 1980; Mark et al., 1977; Siegel/Linder 1984; Siegel/Ryan 1989). Our results appear to show the primacy of memory span in predicting performance on phonological awareness tasks. The following section assesses the relationship between phonological awareness and memory capacity beginning at an earlier age than the LISREL analyses just described.

Phonological recoding and verbal memory

Hitch/Woodin/Baker (1989) found differences in performance of preschoolers (6-7 years of age) and older children (10-11 years of age) on tasks used to measure phonological recoding in memory retrieval. Younger children recalled groups of objects with similar shapes less well than groups of objects with similar sounding labels, but of varying shape. In contrast, older children recalled the names of less objects in groups with similar sounding labels than compared with groups of similar shaped objects. Hitch et al. (1989) interpreted these results as indicating that older children were more likely than younger children to spontaneously phonologically recode information to be recalled. Younger children appeared to recode other information, such as the shape of the objects, in their recall processes.

The results reported in this section provide further information concerning the development of phonological recoding in working memory. Word span was measured at three ages (4, 6, and 8 years of age), and phonological awareness was measured twice (at 6 and 8 years of age). Phonological awareness usually does not develop until the age of five or older. The phonological awareness measures chosen for these analyses were the first and last sound oddity tasks from the Bradley/Bryant oddity tasks, given that these tasks are not dependent on alphabetic knowledge (Näslund 1992). Partial cross-lag correlations among these measures were performed. All partial cross-lag correlations are shown controlling for preschool letter knowledge. The pattern of results suggest developmental differences in the relationship between phonological awareness and verbal memory.

In Figure 3, there is surprisingly no significant correlation between verbal memory at age 4 and at age 6. However, there is a significant correlation between verbal memory at age 4 and phonological awareness at age 6. This implies that although verbal memory at age 4 is not a stable predictor of verbal memory at age 6, verbal memory does predict later phonological awareness. In addition, verbal memory at age 4 does predict verbal memory and phonological awareness at age 8 (controlling for verbal memory and letter knowledge at age 6). Verbal memory would appear to be a relatively stable factor in the long run (over a four year period), but not between the ages of 6 and 8. The partial cross-lag correlations among the verbal memory and phonological awareness measures between the ages of 6 and 8 demonstrate an interesting pattern. Although phonological awareness predicts memory span at age 6 more so than memory span at age 4 does, phonological awareness at age 6 does not predict verbal memory at age 8. Instead, verbal memory at age 6 predicts phonological awareness at age 8. This direction of influence is also suggested by the partial cross-lag correlations at age 8 between verbal memory and phonological awareness. An additional analysis supports the hypothesis that phonological recoding in verbal memory is present in some children at the age of six independent of letter knowledge. The correlation between intra-individual differences in verbal memory and the combined phonological oddity task in kindergarten was significant controlling for preschool letter knowledge ($r = .57$, $p < 0.0001$). This reflects the findings in other studies concerned with phonological awareness and its relationship to verbal memory. Larger discrepancies in recall of phonologically similar and dissimilar lists of verbal information most likely reflects interference due to spontaneous phonological recoding of information.

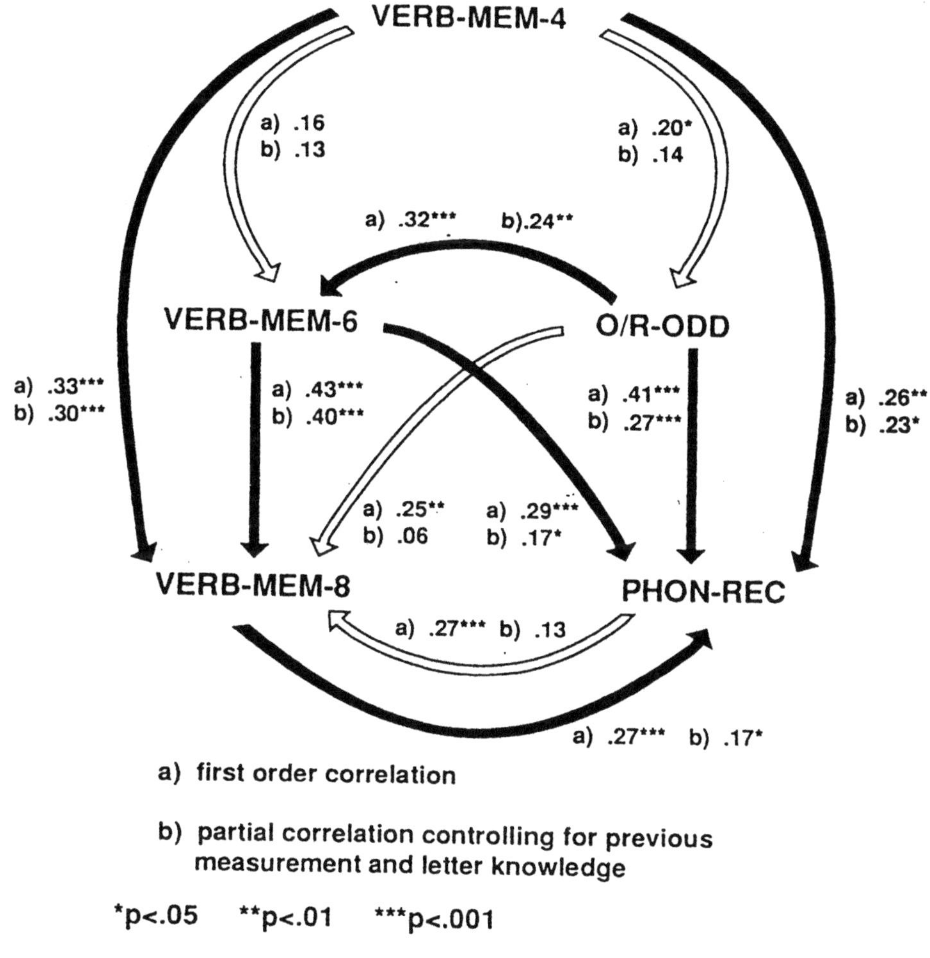

Fig. 3: *Partial cross-lag correlations among word span (VERB-MEM), onset & rhyme oddity (O/R-ODD), and phonological recoding (PHON-REC) variables*

To summarize these results and their implications, it would appear that verbal memory at all ages predicts children's performance on phonological awareness tasks at both testing times. However, the lack of significant correlation between verbal memory at age 4 and age 6 together with the significant correlation of phonological awareness at age 6 with verbal memory at age six would suggest that at about age six, phonological awareness may elicit phonological recoding of verbal information in some children. Development of phonological awareness around the age of six may actually explain the lack of significant correlation of verbal memory from ages four to six, given that children differentially develop phonological awareness at around age five to seven.

Children also varied in their letter knowledge at the time of testing at age 6. This prompted including letter knowledge in the analyses. The next section addresses the issue of the influence of early alphabetic knowledge on the development of phonological awareness. Specifically, does phonological awareness predict reading performance independently of early alphabet knowledge?

Is letter knowledge necessary for the development of phonological awareness?

Lundberg (1987) has responded directly to this question. Children in Scandinavia begin formal instruction in reading at the age of about seven, two years later than in the U.S., and one year later than in Germany. Letter knowledge is therefore very minimal for Scandinavian and German children in the kindergarten years. In our own sample, the average number of letter or letter sounds correctly identified by children was 5.8. The median number was even lower than this (3 letter or letter sounds correctly identified). Results with our German sample concerning preliterate phonological awareness development reflect the same findings as Lundberg's studies (1987; see also Lundberg/Høien 1991; Lundberg/Olofsson/Wall 1980). However, the large variation in tasks used to assess metalinguistic and phonological awareness elicit varying results.

The means and medians of all metalinguistic tasks and their correlations with the early grade school tasks are found in Table 1. Tasks pertaining to analysis or synthesis of onset/rime units, and the segmenting of syllables were found to be the most difficult for our sample of children in the last month of kindergarten. Vowel and rhyme detection tasks, syllable blending and counting, and repeating nonsense words displayed a ceiling effect.

Not all of the phonological awareness tasks administered in this study predicted later reading skills (see correlations on Table 2). Syllable counting and segmenting in prereaders have been highly predictive of reading in other, mainly English-speaking, studies. Almost all of the German children

Tab. 1: Means and medians for metalinguistic tasks given in kindergarten

Preschool Tasks	Mean	Median
Onset-Oddity	34%	44%
Onset/Rime-Blend	54%	50%
Syllable Segmenting	64%	65%
Rhyme-Oddity	68%	78%
Pseudoword Repetition	69%	70%
Mid-Vowel-Oddity	70%	78%
Syllable Blending	75%	80%
Syllable Counting	84%	80%
Sound-in-Word	88%	100%
Rhyme Detection	92%	100%

Tab. 2: Correlations of preschool psycholinguistic tasks and letter knowledge with grammar school measures

	EARLY GRADE SCHOOL TASKS				
Preschool Tasks	COMP	WORD-DEC	PWORD-DEC	W-DISC	PHON-REC
Onset & Rhyme-Oddity (Combined Tasks)	.54	-.43	-.38	.41	.50
Onset-oddity	.43	-.38	-.33	.33	.35
Onset/Rime-Blend	.25	-.26	-.19	.16*	.22
Syllable Segmenting	-.02*	.01*	.06*	.01*	.01*
Rhyme-Oddity	.48	-.32	-.28	.36	.49
Pseudoword-Repeat	.19	-.27	-.28	.17	.26
Middle Vowel-Oddity	.22	-.09*	-.13*	.20	.34
Syllable Blending	.14*	-.28	-.24	.16*	.07*
Syllable Counting	.09*	-.11*	-.16*	.03*	.10*
Sound in Word	.31	-.16*	-.12*	.17	.35
Rhyme Detection	.35	-.13*	-.17	.17	.26
Letter Knowledge	.36	-.37	-.32	.30	.35

COMP=Reading Comprehension, WORD-DEC= Word Decoding Speed
PWORD-DEC=Pseudoword Decoding Speed, W-DISC= Word Discrimination
PHON-REC=Phonological Recoding (Awareness)
* $p > 0.05$, nonsignificant

in this study were prereaders in the last month of kindergarten. Given that most English speaking kindergartens teach formal reading skills, prereaders in English and American studies are younger, and likely less cognitively mature than the German children in this study. The advanced age, and low level of alphabetic knowledge in our sample provided an opportunity to test whether Lundberg's or Morais' and Ehri's hypotheses were correct: Is letter knowledge necessary or not for developing phonological awareness? In addition, and more importantly, does preschool phonological awareness predict later reading performance independent of alphabetic knowledge? In order to answer this question, regression analyses were performed for each metalinguistic task that correlated significantly with either reading comprehension, word decoding or pseudoword decoding speed. The scores of onset and rhyme oddity are combined for these regressions as a phonological awareness variable. The first set of regression analyses (see Table 3) have verbal ability, verbal memory, and letter knowledge as the first three regressors, and enter the various metalinguistic measures as the fourth step. As shown, only the onset/rhyme oddity, onset/rime blending, and rhyme recognition tasks were significant in at least one reading measure after controlling for letter knowledge.

These results reflect Bryant/Bradley/Maclean/Crossland's (1989) findings that sensitivity to rhyme is a likely first step toward metalinguistic awareness. Bryant et al. (1989) found that early knowledge of nursery rhymes (at ages 3 and 4) predicted later linguistic analysis skills. These analysis skills allow a preliterate child to detect sounds and sound changes within syllabic word components, which is reflected in the oddity and blend tasks.

This first set of regression analyses revealed that only a subset of the metalinguistic awareness skills assessed in kindergarten predict later reading performance independently from alphabet knowledge. In order to test whether some forms of metalinguistic awareness may actually be necessary to learn the alphabetic principle (see Tunmer/Rohl 1991), a second set of regression analyses were performed. For these analyses, letter knowledge was placed last in the models. Only the metalinguistic tasks which demonstrated significance in the amount of variance explained in at least one of the reading measure.

Results in Table 4 show that letter knowledge still explains a significant proportion of the variance in the reading measures after accounting for the variance in onset/rime blending and rhyme detection, but not after accounting for the variance explained by onset/rhyme oddity. These results suggest

Tab. 3: *Hierarchical regression models for comparing the effects of O/R-ODD (Onset & Rhyme Oddity), O/R-BLEND (Onset/Rime-Blend), and PWORD-REP (Pseudoword-Repeat) tasks with LETT-KNOW (Letter Knowledge), VERB-MEM (Word Span), and VERB-IQ (Verbal Ability) on early elementary school reading and phonological awareness measures*

	EARLY ELEMENTARY SCHOOL MEASURES				
ORDER OF ENTRY	COMP	WORD-DEC	PWORD-DEC	W-DISC	PHON-REC
1. VERB-IQ	.16***	.03*	.05**	.08***	.09***
2. VERB-MEM	.01	.06***	.09***	.03*	.04**
3. LETT-KNOW	.04**	.11***	.04*	.05**	.08***
-------------					
4. O/R-ODD	.09***	.08***	.04*	.05**	.09***
4. O/R-BLEND	.03*	.02	.00	.01	.01
4. PWORD-REP	.00	.01	.01	.00	.00

* $p < 0.05$ ** $p < 0.01$ *** $p < 0.001$

Tab. 4: *Hierarchical regression models for comparing the effects of LETT-KNOW with O/R-ODD and O/R-BLEND on early elementary school reading and phonological awareness measures*

	EARLY ELEMENTARY SCHOOL MEASURES				
ORDER OF ENTRY	COMP	WORD-DEC	PWORD-DEC	W-DISC	PHON-REC
1. VERB-IQ	.16***	.03*	.05**	.08***	.09***
2. VERB-MEM	.01	.06***	.09***	.03*	.04**
-------------					
3. O/R-ODD	.13***	.17***	.07**	.06***	.15***
3. O/R-BLEND					
-------------					
4. LETT-KNOW	.01	.01	.01	.02	.03**
4. LETT-KNOW					

* $p < 0.05$ ** $p < 0.01$ *** $p < 0.001$

that onset/rhyme oddity measures may be tapping a primary cognitive factor in emergent literacy, which is independent of formal instruction in reading. Rhyme detection is likely a precursor to phonological awareness, as results from Bryant et al. (1989) would suggest. Facility with rhyme detection does not necessarily indicate presence of phonological segmentation ability. The onset/rime blending task does require phonological segmentation, and performance on this task is likely to be enhanced by the ability to represent sounds orthographically. It is therefore not surprising that a significant proportion of reading comprehension and word decoding would be explained by both letter knowledge and onset/rime blending. According to Tunmer/Rohl (1991), this type of task may be more a measure of instruction in phonics than of actual phonological awareness.

In contrast, letter knowledge did not explain a significant proportion of the variance in any of the reading tasks when placed in the regression model after onset/rhyme oddity. According to the results found in this study, this task requires phonological analysis and segmentation, but not Letter Knowledge. The results found here support Bradley/Bryant's (1985), Lundberg's (1987), and Tunmer/Rohl's (1991) claim that phonological awareness can precede formal reading instruction, and even predict to a large extent future success in reading performance.

General discussion

This study supports evidence found in other longitudinal studies that metalinguistic (especially phonological) awareness, verbal memory, and general verbal ability (but to a lesser extent) as measured in kindergarten and early elementary school contribute to explaining later reading performance. Our results suggest that this finding is a fairly universal one, not only applying to the (irregular) English and (regular) Scandinavian language systems but also to the German langage system which is in between, as far as regularity is concerned. The structural equation models used in testing the most likely pattern of causal relations among these variables supported the hypothesis that memory span and phonological awareness as measured in kindergarten and in second grade are pivotal factors in predicting reading performance in second grade. Verbal ability was found to be of less importance in comparison with the other factors. In addition, results indicated that early alphabetic knowledge is not necessary for the development of phonological awareness. This does not support claims made by Ehri (1989), Morais et al.

(1979), and Read et al. (1986) that phonological awareness does not arise spontaneously in the absence of familiarity with an alphabetic system and some instruction in phonetics. This result does support the position taken by Lundberg (1987), Lundberg/Høien (1991), and Tunmer/Rohl (1991) that phonological awareness can and does arise spontaneously before formal reading instruction, and that perhaps phonological awareness is a necessary precursor to acquiring the alphabetic principle.

In addition, it would appear that phonological awareness and verbal memory interact developmentally. Testing children in verbal memory span at ages four, six, and eight and phonological awareness at ages six and eight, indicates that emergent phonological awareness likely begins to influence verbal memory span of some children at some time between the ages of four and six. However, caution must be exercised in drawing conclusions based on these analyses. This investigation did not systematically rule out all possible intervening factors, besides preschool letter knowledge and literacy, to explain the longitudinal relationships found between verbal memory span and phonological awareness. Supporting evidence that some children in our sample were developing phonological recoding in working memory was found in comparing differential performance on word span tasks that used phonologically similar and dissimilar words.

Some researchers have argued that larger discrepancies between recall of phonologically similar and dissimilar lists of words is evidence for phonological recoding in working memory (Brady et al. 1983; Liberman et al. 1977; Mann et al. 1980; Mark et al. 1977; Shankweiler/Liberman/Mark et al. 1979). It is still difficult to definitively substantiate this claim, given that children with larger discrepancies are also usually those who perform better overall on memory tasks and are usually better readers. Evidence thus far in the literature certainly is convincing that a causal relationship between phonological awareness and memory development is highly likely. Although verbal memory and reading are strongly correlated, more proof is needed to substantiate claims that the developmental of phonological awareness is responsible for changes in a child's heuristic for storing verbal information, which in turn increases reading performance.

Another caution is Ehri's (1989) criticism of the claim that phonological awareness is a causal facilitating factor in reading acquisition that necessarily precedes literacy instruction. Not all children who demonstrate early phonological awareness deficits become dyslexic or poor readers. Stanovich (1989) has countered this argument by citing evidence that very few children who are phonologically aware in preschool or kindergarten develop reading problems. Phonological awareness may arise spontaneously for some children in the absence of reading instruction (Lundberg 1987). On the other hand, it may not be exclusively developmental. Other children may develop these skills after they enter formal instruction and begin learning reading skills. Direct learning about letter-sound relationships may trigger phonological awareness for those who were not phonemically aware in preschool. Others may not fully develop phonological awareness, and may need to rely on some other heuristic for holding verbal information in working memory while reading. For this last group of children, reading is going to be a difficult task. Their reading skills will be far below those children who phonologically recode information while reading. For dyslexics, this does not represent a cognitive deficit in the traditional sense. Intelligence, verbal comprehension, and even working memory may all be average or above average. It's the presence of spontaneous phonological recoding of verbal information in average and good readers that actually seems to define dyslexia in some groups of poor readers. Dyslexia would then be defined as lack of a certain ability to segment speech sounds that arises spontaneously in many children. This condition may actually be somewhat historical in nature. As literacy in humans emerges, changes in cognition are likely, especially in the literacy "revolutions" throughout history. The spread of literacy in the Sudan during the spread of Islam in the tenth century is a case in point for the sudden emergence of a new skill revolutionizing human thought and cognition.

More research needs to be done on linguistic environments that hinder or facilitate spontaneous phonological awareness in individuals. We may be coming closer to understanding the cognitive mechanisms and environments that are responsible for phonological awareness, especially in the most recent research on infants' phonemic discrimination during the first year of life. Babies begin life with the ability to distinguish between phonemes that adults no longer discriminate. As time passes, they build classes of phonemes in their own languages. Losing this sound discrimination and building classes of phonemes helps us understand speech spoken by the many individuals in our language group. At six months, they can still distinguish phonemes of non-native languages, but perform almost as adults in not being able to distinguish phonemes within certain linguistic classes. At ten to twelve months, babies perform like adults in their inability to distinguish phonemes within the same class in native and non-native languages. This also corresponds to the time when first words are learned. It is after this time that whole words become children's linguistic realities, and children do not segment or distinguish among phonemes until just about the time they begin to learn to read (Smith 1986). Perhaps Maclean/Bryant/Bradley's (1987) findings indicate that learning and reciting nursery rhymes at an early age is helping to trigger this lost discrimination skill. Children cannot segment speech consciously yet at the age of three or four years, but some phonological awareness may be triggered by such exposure and recitation practice.

Results of this study appear to support findings of other studies that show the importance of metalinguistic skills in emergent reading. There were also differences found in comparison with some of the other studies mentioned earlier (Ehri 1989; Morais et al. 1979; Read et al., 1986). The German findings were similar to the Swedish results (Lundberg et al. 1988) in terms of letter knowledge not being necessary for the development of phonological awareness. Differences likely reflected the fact that German and Swedish children are older when they learn to read in comparison to other industrial nations. Their psycholinguistic development at about age six is therefore not shaped by early literacy skills. Despite a lack of rudimentary literacy ability, psycholinguistic development does not appear to be hindered, as evidenced by ceiling level performance in easier metalinguistic tasks. In addition, phonological awareness also develops despite lack of letter knowledge in German (as well as Swedish) children. This suggests that phonological awareness is a more naturally occurring developmental stage which can (as possibly should) precede learning to read.

References

Bradley, L. & Bryant, P. (1985). Rhyme and reason in reading and spelling. Ann Arbor, MI: University of Michigan Press.

Brady, S., Shankweiler, D., & Mann, V. (1983). Speech perception and memory coding in relation to reading ability. Journal of Experimental Child Psychology, 35, 345-367.

Burgemeister, B., Blum, L., & Lorge, J. (1972). Columbia Mental Maturity Scale. New York: Harcourt Brace.

Brügelmann, H. (1986). Lese- und Schreibaufgaben für Schulanfänger. Universität Bremen: Studiengang Primarstufe.

Bryant, P., Bradley, L., Maclean, M., & Crossland, J. (1989). Nursery rhymes, phonological skills and reading. Journal of Child Language, 16, 407-428.

Case, R., Kurland, D.M., & Goldberg, J. (1982). Operational efficiency and the growth of short-term memory span. Journal of Experimental Child Psychology, 33, 386-404.

Daneman, M. & Blennerhassett, A. (1984). How to assess the listening comprehension skills of prereaders. Journal of Educational Psychology, 76, 1372-1381.

Eggert, D. (Ed.) (1978). Hannover-Wechsler-Intelligenztest für Vorschulkinder (HAWIVA). Bern: Huber.

Ehri, L. (1989). The development of spelling knowledge and its role in reading acquisition and reading disability. Journal of Learning Disabilities, 22(6), 356-365.

Foorman, B.R., Francis, D.J., Novy, D.M., & Liberman, D. (1991). How letter-sound instruction mediates progress in first grade reading and spelling. Journal of Educational Psychology, 83(4), 456-469.

Goodman, K.S. (1967). Reading: A psycholinguistic guessing game. Journal of the Reading Specialist, 4, 126-135.

Hitch, G.J., Woodin, M.E., & Baker, S. (1989). Visual and phonological components of working memory in children. Memory and Cognition, 17(2), 175-185.

Jansen, H., Knorn, P., Mannhaupt, G., Marx, H., Beck, M., & Skowronek, H. (1986). Bielefelder Screening zur Vorhersage von Lese-Rechtschreibschwierigkeiten. Universität Bielefeld, SFB 227, F.R.G.

Jöreskog, K.G., & Sörbom, D. (1984). LISREL VI: Analysis of structural relationships by the method of maximum likelihood. Mooresville, IN: Scientific Software, Inc.

Juel, C. (1988). Learning to read and write: A longitudinal study of 54 children from first through fourth grades. Journal of Educational Psychology, 80, 437-447.

Liberman, I.Y., Shankweiler, D., Liberman, A.M., Fowler, C., & Fischer, F.W. (1977). Phonetic segmentation and coding in the beginning reader. In A.S. Reber & D.L. Scarborough (Eds.), Toward a psychology of reading: The proceedings of the CUNY conferences. 297-225. Hillsdale, NJ: Erlbaum.

Lundberg, I. (1987). Are letters necessary for the development of phonological awareness? Cahiers de Psychologie, 7, 472-475.

Lundberg, I., Frost, J., & Petersen, O.-P. (1988). Effects of an extensive program for stimulating phonological awareness in preschool children. Reading Research Quarterly, 23, 263-284.

Lundberg, I., Olofsson, Å., & Wall, S. (1980). Reading and spelling skills in the first school years predicted from phonemic awareness skills in kindergarten. Scandinavian Journal of Psychology, 21, 159-173.

Lundberg, I. & Høien, T. (1991). Initial enabling knowledge and skills in reading acquisition: Print awareness and phonological segmentation. In D.J. Sawyer & B.J. Fox (Eds.), Phonological awareness in reading: The evolution of current perspectives. 73-96. New York: Springer-Verlag.

Maclean, M., Bryant, P., & Bradley, L. (1987). Rhymes, nursery rhymes and reading in early childhood. Merrill-Palmer Quarterly, 33, 255-282.

Mann, V.A., Liberman, I.Y. & Shankweiler, D. (1980). Children's memory for sentences and word strings in relation to reading ability. Memory & Cognition, 8(4), 329-335.

Mark, L.S., Shankweiler, D., Liberman, I.Y., & Fowler, C.A. (1977). Phonetic recoding and reading difficulty in beginning readers. Memory & Cognition, 5(6), 623-629.

Morais, J., Cary, L., Alegria, J., & Bertelson, P. (1979). Does awareness of speech as a sequence of phones arise spontaneously? Cognition, 7, 323-331.

Näslund, J.C. (1992). How do preschool letter knowledge and metalinguistic skills affect later reading and spelling performance? Manuscript submitted for publication.

Näslund, J.C. & Schneider, W. (1991). Longitudinal effects of verbal ability, memory capacity, and phonological awareness on reading performance. European Journal of Psychology of Education, 6(4), 375-392.

Perfetti, C., Beck, I., Bell, L., & Hughes, C. (1987). Phonemic knowledge and learning to read are reciprocal: A longitudinal study of first grade children. Merrill-Palmer Quarterly, 33, 283-319.

Read, C., Zhang, Y., Nie, H., & Ding, B. (1986). The ability to manipulate speech sounds depends on knowing alphabetic reading. Cognition, 24, 31-44.

Schneider, W. & Näslund, J. (1992). Cognitive prerequisites of reading and spelling: A longitudinal approach. In A. Demetriou, M. Shayer, & A. Efklides (Eds.), Neo-Piagetian theories of cognitive development: Implications and applications for education. 256-274. London: Routledge.

Shankweiler, D., Liberman, I.Y., Mark, L.M., Fowler, L.A., & Fischer, F.W. (1979). The speed code and learning to read. Journal of Experimental Psychology: Human learning and memory, 5, 531-545.

Siegel, L.S. & Linder, B.A. (1984). Short-term memory process in children with reading and arithmetic abilities. Developmental Psychology, 20, 200-207.

Siegel, L.S. & Ryan, E.B. (1989). The development of working memory in normally achieving and subtypes of learning disabled children. Child Development, 60, 973-980.

Skowronek, H. & Marx, H. (1989). The Bielefeld longitudinal study on early identification of risks in learning to read and write: Theoretical background and first results. In M. Brambring, F. Lösel, & H. Skowronek (Eds.), Children at risk: Assessment, longitudinal research, and intervention. 245-267. New York: De Gruyter.

Smith, P.T. (1986). The development of reading: The acquisition of a cognitive skill. In P. Fletcher & M. Garman (Eds.), Language acquisition: Studies in first language acquisition. 475-493. Cambridge, GB: Cambridge University Press.

Stanovich, K.E. (1989). Various varying views on variation. Journal of Learning Disabilities, 22(6), 366-369.

Stanovich, K.E., Cunningham, A.E, & Feeman, D.J. (1984). Intelligence, cognitive skills, and early reading progress. Reading Research Quarterly, 19, 278-303.

Tewes, U. (1985). Hamburg-Wechsler-Intelligenztest für Kinder (HAWIK). Bern: Huber.

Tunmer W.E. & Rohl, M. (1991). Phonological awareness and reading acquisition. In D.J. Sawyer & B.J. Fox (Eds.), Phonological awareness in reading: The evolution of current perspectives. 1-30. New York: Springer-Verlag.

Vellutino, F.R. (1991). Introduction to three studies on reading acquisition: Convergent findings on theoretical foundations of code-oriented versus whole-language approaches to reading instruction. Journal of Educational Psychology, 83(4), 437-443.

Weinert, F.E. & Schneider, W. (Eds.) (1987). The Munich Longitudinal Study on the Genesis of Individual Competencies (LOGIC). Report No. 2: Documentation of assessment procedures used in waves one to three. Munich, FRG: Max Planck Institute for Psychological Research.

Weinert, F.E. & Schneider, W. (Eds.) (1991). The Munich Longitudinal Study on the Genesis of Individual Competencies (LOGIC). Report No. 7: Results of wave 4. Munich, FRG: Max Planck Institute for Psychological Research.

Weinert, F.E. & Schneider, W. (Eds.) (1992). The Munich Longitudinal Study on the Genesis of Individual Competencies (LOGIC). Report No. 8: Results of wave 5. Munich, FRG: Max Planck Institute for Psychological Research.

Interventions in developmental reading and spelling disorders

Gerheid Scheerer-Neumann

Introduction

Considering the high quality research on the analysis of reading disabled children's abilities and cognitive processes (Snowling 1991 for review), one would expect comparable efforts also in the realm of intervention. However, this is not the case. There is a vast literature on very diverse methods which all claim to be helpful for reading and writing disabled children, but well designed evaluative studies are rare. The urgent need to help reading and writing disabled children stands in opposition to methodological problems in evaluative studies which are almost insurmountable:

- Consensus exists that reading disabled children need to be taught in an adaptive, individual manner. Yet in empirical designs all children should preferably be treated by the same method.
- Consensus again exists that reading and spelling disabled children need to be treated for an extended period of time in order to show substantial improvement; however, it is very difficult to control long-term treatment in a fashion necessary for empirical research.
- As in all intervention studies, control groups pose immense problems: For ethical reasons it is not possible to treat control children with any type of placebo over a longer period of time or simply leave them untreated. Yet, if no control group is employed, it is difficult to estimate the size of regression, the Hawthorne effect and 'normal' learning and development.
- There are also many variables which are difficult to control, although they basically can be controlled or at least documented. These include on the child's side the particular type of the reading and spelling problem and other cognitive variables, achievement motivation, and social background, and on the therapist's side enthusiasm, optimism and a positive relationship to the child. These variables can - positively or negatively - override any other effect of a training program.
- In many studies the experimental designs are not optimal, to say the least. In particular, the relationship between the contents of training and

the contents of the criterion test are often not clear. We need to spell and test according to whether improvement is expected exactly in the areas trained or on transfer tasks.

There are even more problems involved in evaluation studies. Yet those mentioned suffice to explain why most scientists working in the area prefer to analyse the cognitive problems involved in reading disability or choose to train unselected kindergardeners or first graders rather than reading disabled children. Yet remedial methods should not only be judged by their empirical evaluation; another important aspect is the plausibility and the consistency of the theories involved. Compatibility with well-established research findings and current theories of reading and spelling development should be further criteria in evaluating remedial approaches.

In 1973, Y. Liberman drew attention to young children's problems in analyzing phonemes in spoken words (see also Bosch 1937). Since then, poor reader's deficits in tasks demanding phonemic analysis and/or phoneme blending have been impressively confirmed and should be taken into account in any remedial reading or spelling program dealing particularly with younger children (cf. Wagner/Torgesen 1987 and Brady/Shankweiler 1991 for a review). There seem to be less problems with reading comprehension once basic decoding skills are acquired. In the area of spelling, difficulties often continue even if decoding is mastered. Teaching orthographically correct spelling is therefore an additional step which is required in remedial programs.

Remedial programs should acknowledge the progress which has been made in recent years in our understanding of the processes which are involved in reading, writing and their development. Unfortunately, there is too little contact between basic and applied research in the area. It may also be the case that some reading and spelling models are too complicated to be directly implemented in remedial programs; yet there are also theories which lend themselves very well to remedial instruction. I am referring particularly to Ehri's important research (Ehri 1987 for review) and to Frith's (1985) model of reading and writing development. The Frith model is rather coarse and could be refined in several ways (cf. Scheerer-Neumann 1989), but its message is very important. Frith proposes that children's predominant reading and writing strategies change during the acquisition of literacy; the stages she postulates are the logographic, the alphabetic and finally the orthographic stage. Particularly the assumption of an obligatory alphabetic stage as a transitory step to literacy has helped us both to understand poor readers' and spellers' problems and has influenced - or rather confirmed - certain approaches in remedial teaching.

While it can be expected that adequate models of reading and spelling and their development stimulate the development of efficient treatment methods, inadequate models can also lead to effective therapies. Orton (1937) had assumed that dyslexics' problems are mainly visual (he coined the term "strephosymbolia"), but this assumption has not been confirmed empirically for the majority of reading disabled children. Orton's coworkers Gillingham/Stillman (1969) developed a training program mainly based on phonics. Their idea was to teach children by their strengths and not by their weaknesses. Today we know that the program is effective, because most reading disabled children have problems in the phonological domain. The issue of phonological training will be covered later in the paper. The following section will give a survey on the impressively wide scope of remedial methods for reading and spelling disabled children.

Remedial methods for reading and writing disabled children: An overview

Although remedial teaching is required to be adaptive to the child's particular problems, no treatments have been found so far to be differentially effective for specifically reading disabled children as compared to generally backward readers (Reason 1990). Studies using samples from either population will therefore not be reported separately. There is further no other satisfactory classificatory scheme for disabled readers from which appropriate treatment programs could be deduced. Therefore the different approaches are classified only according to their theoretical origin. Table 1 gives the classificatory scheme on which the paper is structured.

Pharmacotherapy

After Gittelman/Klein/Feingold (1983) had shown rather convincingly that reading disabled children receiving both Ritalin and specific reading instruction performed no better on reading measures than a control group receiving specific reading instruction and a placebo, it is now Piracetam

Tab. 1: Classification of intervention methods for developmental reading and spelling disorders

---

* Pharmacotherapy (Ritalin, Piracetam)
* Ophtalmological intervention
  e.g. Eye occlusion
  Tinted lenses
* Methods related to laterality
  - motor training
  - direct projection of reading material to one hemisphere
* Psychotherapy
  - directed at primary symptoms
  - directed at secondary symptoms
* The training of perceptual and cognitive abilities ("Prescriptive Teaching")
  - motor and visual-motor
  - visual perceptual
  - auditory perceptual
  - attention
* Direct Instruction
  - the phonics approach
  - the structural-linguistic approach
  - the lexical approach
  - behavior modification
  - training of memory strategies
  - the 'Language Experience' approach

---

which is alleged to be "the reading pill". Piracetam is considered a "nootropic" drug, influencing specifically the "higher" functions of the brain, particularly those which normally reside in the left cerebral hemisphere. It has also been hypothesized that it influences transcallosal transfer, but apparently there is no sound evidence for this assumption. Some experimental studies show that Piracetam does improve verbal short-term memory in normal adults (i.e. college students) (e.g. Dimond/Brouwers 1976). Thus it is not very surprising that in several well designed double blind studies the drug has also been shown to improve reading in reading disabled children (e.g. Conners/Reader 1987). However, although significant improvement on some reading measures occurred in the experimental groups compared to placebo control groups, the amount of the effects seems to be rather small. This is a very general issue: The statistical significance of after-training achievement compared to a control group can only be taken as a first step in the evaluation of intervention programs. A remedial method can only be said to be effective, if substantial gains are achieved. What counts is not a statistically significant difference, but the size of the step towards a level of achievement expected on the basis of a child's chronological age.

Some other aspects are left open in the studies reported on Piracetam. It is surprising that most researchers use a simple pre-post-design. It would be important to know which *cognitive processes* are affected by the drug. It could be that children just *performed* better under the influence of pharmacotherapy; alternatively the effect could be attributable to more efficient learning at school.

Ophthalmological intervention

Reading disability was first conceptualized as a visual or visual-cognitive problem (Morgan 1896) and although we now have realized that it is mainly rooted in the verbal domain, the idea that there is something "wrong with the child's eyes" still remains. This should not be dismissed too easily, because it is probably true for some children. It is plausible that unstable binocular fixation might degrade the visual stimulus and thus interfere with reading. The argument that many good readers also show binocular instability (Newman/Karle/Wadsworth et al. 1985) does not necessarily disprove the point, because unstable fixation could be compensated by superior linguistic skills. Cornelissen/Bradley/Fowler/Stein (1991) have shown that reading disabled children with binocular instability are impeded mainly when using an alphabetic strategy which requires precise discrimination. The occlusion of one eye has been proposed for children with binocular instability. A positive effect of this treatment has been claimed by Stein/ Fowler (1985); however, the data are not entirely conclusive.

Another alleged "visual remedy" is the use of a tinted overlay or tinted lenses. Reports of improved reading with this method used to be mainly anecdotal or were based on poorly controlled data (e.g. Irlen 1983). However, there are two recent single case reports which demonstrate impressive changes of the quality of the percept with tinted lenses (Hannell/Gole/ Dibden et al. 1991). Under the instruction to "draw the pattern just as you see it" a 9-year-old dyslexic boy reproduced a pattern with micro zigzag outlines (corresponding to his introspective report of "furriness" in his perception of normal black and white print). When he wore blue tinted lenses his reproductions changed to normal. Similar observations were obtained from his brother. The mechanism why tinted lenses can be helpful for some children is not yet clear. It is hypothesized that they synchronize information from the transient and the sustained visual subsystems which are out of synchronization (for the hypothesis of a transient system deficit in retarded readers see Lovegrove/Martin/Slaghuis 1986).

Methods related to laterality

Delacato (1959) has been the main proponent of the idea that motor training - like throwing a ball - can promote a consistent lateral dominance and thereby improve reading and writing in dyslexic children. Although the relationship between laterality in the sense of the functional differentiation of the two hemispheres and reading disability is still under discussion (Kinsbourne/Hiscock 1987 for review) there has been no sound evidence that motor training has any influence on reading and spelling. A recent attempt to influence directly the two hemispheres' involvement in the reading task should be mentioned, though. Bakker/van Leeuwen/Spyer (1987) claim that they can accelerate slow readers' performance by flashing words to the left hemisphere and improve inaccurate but fast reading by flashing words to the right hemisphere. While the basic idea that the hemispheres contribute differentially to literacy is well taken, Bakker's study is not entirely conclusive due to the lack of convincing control groups.

Psychotherapy

Psychotherapy has been suggested by Axline (1947) and others as a treatment of reading disability. There may indeed be cases where reading disability should be mainly viewed as neurotic behavior and treated accordingly. However, in the majority of cases, emotional and behavioral problems in reading disabled children are secondary to their failure at school. Constant failure in important school subjects affects many children severely; psychotherapy is sometimes needed as a precondition for more direct instruction. Child guidance institutions usually offer integrated remedial programs including counseling and remedial instruction. Unfortunately, there are no acceptable data to document the influence of each line. It would be of interest to find out whether successful remedial instruction has in itself a positive effect on the child's emotional behavior, particularly when it includes stimulating tasks and materials as in the Language Experience Approach (see p. 342).

The training of perceptual and cognitive abilities ("Prescriptive Teaching")

The training of perceptual and cognitive abilities, which is known in English speaking countries as "Prescriptive Teaching", is still one of many remedial teachers' favourite methods. The basic idea is the following: Reading disabled children show deficits in certain perceptual and cognitive abilities and these should be compensated as a prerequisite for reading and writing. As evident in the expression "prescriptive teaching", training programs should be prescribed to children according to a differential diagnosis. (This is not true for Germany, where 'Funktionstrainings' are often just part of remedial instruction for all children). Training can be applied in the area of visual perception, auditory perception, in various aspects of language or in "attention". None of these areas is directly related to the partial processes of reading and writing. The materials used in these programs (e.g. Frostig/Horne 1964) are often nonverbal and are thus motivating for children who have failed in reading and writing tasks.

However, the approach has not been found to be effective. At best there is progress in the ability trained; yet there is no transfer to reading and writing. This is particularly true for the visual domain which is often favoured by teachers. Larsen/Hammill (1975) and Arter/Jenkins (1979) have reviewed a large number of studies; the majority of methodologically acceptable studies do not support the effectiveness of "Prescriptive Teaching".

I myself have conducted a study with students as trainers in which third class spelling disabled children were trained to use more effective problem solving strategies in visual tasks like matching figures (Edler/Ostrau/Schulze 1977; Scheerer-Neumann 1979). Appropriate strategies were modeled and taught by a method of verbal self-control (see Meichenbaum/Goodman 1969). After 12 one-hour training sessions the trained children showed better performance in most of the tasks used in training; yet there was no transfer to spelling (not even a Hawthorne effect). The children then participated in a spelling program. The rationale was the following: If training of cognitive abilities improves the prerequisites for learning to read and to spell, there should be no immediate effect on those skills, but the children should profit more from subsequent direct instruction. This hypothesis was also not supported: Although the trained children improved their spelling performance considerably after having taken part in the spelling program, they did not exceed a control group which had only received training in spelling. Incidentally, the spelling program was also modeled on the Meichenbaum/Goodman approach of verbal self-control; however, the strategies taught were adapted to the requirements of spelling.

Figure 1 shows some self-instructions from the initial training phase; the instructions were associated with visual symbols which were available to the children on cards and as stamps. The children were not only taught to carry out the steps demanded by the symbols, but also to make their own plans in advance using the symbol cards and stamps as cues. The success of this procedure was confirmed in another study with an increased group size (five to six children as opposed to two in the original study; Höreth 1977). Thus it seems that the acquisition of more efficient problem solving strategies does indeed improve children's spelling, but only when the strategies are directly related to spelling.

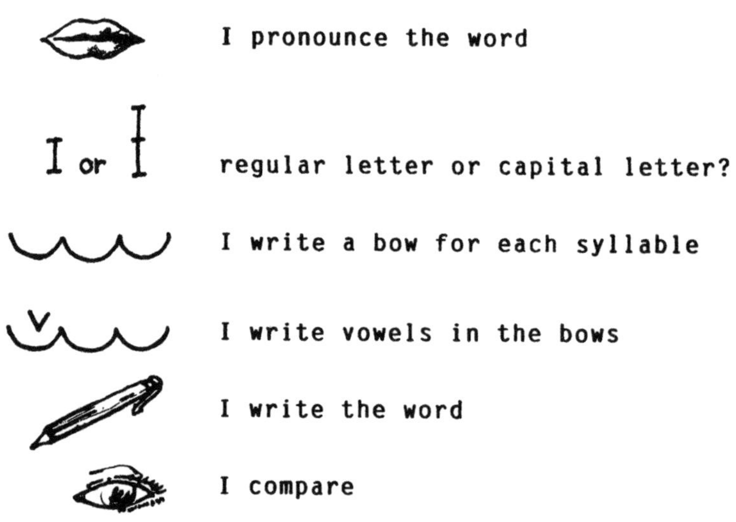

Fig. 1: *Symbols and verbal self instructions used in the spelling program (Edler/Ostrau/Schulze 1977; Scheerer-Neumann 1979, p. 109 cf.)*

There are several reasons why the "prescriptive teaching" approach has failed in our studies and in those cited above: Concepts like "visual perception" or "auditory perception" do not seem to be valid entities in the sense that they can be trained as such and manifest themselves in a variety of different tasks. We know from the information processing literature that the processes involved in visual tasks can be quite diverse depending on the stimulus material and the specific task requirements (Neisser 1967). Thus transfer of training between pictorial and verbal stimuli can hardly be expected. The child who mixes up <d> and <b> has to learn which visual stimulus to associate with the phoneme 'd'; sorting elefants according to the direction of their trunks does not help.

Direct Instruction

The term "Direct Instruction" is used here to refer to programs which basically implement reading and writing instruction, if necessary starting at a first grade level. Despite differences in detail, there are common elements in almost all remedial approaches using direct teaching: Consensus exists that, whatever the specific method, teaching should be adaptive, i.e. be tailored to the child's previous knowledge and progress (Hornsby/Miles 1980; Thomson 1988; Scheerer-Neumann 1989).

There are many studies which show improvement in reading disabled children's reading and writing with different types of direct instruction. Indeed, it seems rather difficult not to get at least a short-term effect in a treated group as compared to a reading disabled control group (Scheerer-Neumann 1979). The reason for this is rather obvious: Reading disabled children usually experience a "teaching deficit", because the instruction offered to them at school is far ahead of their actual needs. Thus any type of adaptive help is almost predestined to have some positive effect. However, if a program is really effective, it should not just lead to statistically significant improvement as compared to a control group, but show substantial effects with reference to the child's chronological age.

Promoting the alphabetic strategy: Phonics

A look at the predominant methods used in direct remedial instruction reveals that exercises directed at alphabetic processing are most often preferred in the initial stages of teaching. Indeed, phoneme-grapheme--correspondences, phoneme analysis and phoneme blending are at the core of effective remedial programs (Gillingham/Stillman 1969; Hornsby/Miles

1980; Kossow 1972). However, the programs and in particular the evaluative studies differ with respect to the actual methods used to promote alphabetic processing.

Comprehensive "phonics" approaches. The phonics approach usually includes the teaching of letter and sound correspondences, phoneme analysis tasks, phoneme blending tasks, and a thorough control of the reading material which increases slowly in difficulty on several dimensions. One of these dimensions is consonant-vowel-structure, another the number of syllables per word. Some programs which start with phonics include two additional features: The programs developed by Kossow (1972) and by Dummer/Hackethal (1984) teach the child to become conscious of the movements of his/her speech organs when pronouncing sounds (see also Skjelfjord 1976). Although there are no data on the effectiveness of this particular feature of the programs, it fits very well with observations on the actual processes involved in children's phonemic analysis: Children tend to analyze their own articulation (Schreuder/van Bon 1989; Skjelfjord 1976).

An additional feature of the programs developed by Kossow (1972) and Dummer/Hackethal (1984) is the introduction of hand signs corresponding to phonemes. This method is believed to be particularly helpful for children with severe reading problems. Again, we do not have any good data on the effectiveness of this method, nor is it theoretically clear, why hand signs could be effective. It could be that - due to their simple structure (there are e.g. no symmetrical hand signs) - they add to letter sound discriminability. It is also possible that the child is helped by the clear sequential order of signing which models the spoken word much better than the parallel visual input of the written word.

In a field study, Williams (1979) tested a comprehensive phonics program (The ABD of reading - Analyses, Blending, Decoding) with generally learning disabled children. The children (7-10 years of age) were trained daily for a period of two years. The author reports an outstanding progress in phonemic tasks as well as in reading and spelling in comparison to an untrained control group. A similarly impressive effect was found in a field study by Wallach/Wallach (1979). First grade low-income children were given daily additional training in phoneme analysis, letter-sound correspondences, decoding of simple regular words, and in reading regular classroom reading material. The differences in reading and writing achievement between the trained children and an untrained control group were not only statistically significant, but also "sufficiently large in their magnitude to be important in practical terms" (Wallach/Wallach 1979, 212).

Working with older children (M = 11 years), Lovett/Ransby/Barron (1988) studied the effect of training word recognition and decoding skills as compared to a more general language program which included comprehension of oral language, reading, and written composition. Although both groups scored higher on a word recognition task and in a reading test than a control group after 40 treatment sessions, it was the 'decoding' group which gained most.

In long-term studies with school-children a variety of phonological tasks is used and these are complemented rather early by a word training; it is thus difficult to isolate the effects of the different phonological tasks.

Training phoneme analysis and synthesis. Several investigations have looked into the effects of a phoneme analysis and/or blending training in a more controlled setting (Ball/Blachman 1988, 1991; Bradley/Bryant 1983; Fox/Routh 1984; Hohn/Ehri 1983; Kerstholt/van Bon/Schreuder 1991; Lie 1991; Mannhaupt 1990; Rosner 1971; Torneus 1984; Treiman/Baron 1983; Vellutino/Scanlon 1984). Unfortunately, most of these studies used unselected preschoolers as subjects; hence the results may not be directly transferable to reading disabled children. Still, some issues are probably of general relevance.

The main result of the cited studies is the finding that, while phonemic analysis does not seem to develop spontaneously in preschool children (in contrast e.g. to sensitivity to rhymes), it can be trained quite successfully (e.g. Ball/Blachman 1991; Bradley/Bryant 1983; Lundberg/Frost/Peterson 1988). Effects are visible even after a very short training period (e.g. Content/Kolinsky/Morais/Bertelson 1986). Secondly, the training of phonemic analysis and blending in kindergarten has been shown to directly improve reading and spelling skills (Ball/Blachman 1991; Fox/Routh 1984) or to accelerate the acquisition of reading and writing in the early school years (Bradley/Bryant 1983; Lundberg/Frost/Peterson 1988).

In a long-term setting training is also effective for children with low scores on pretest. In the Bradley/Bryant (1983) study the children trained in phoneme categorization tasks during preschool and first grade attained better scores in reading and writing as compared to an untrained control group even several years after training had ended. Torneus (1984) showed that training in phoneme segmentation and blending in first grade had a particularly strong effect on children with low pretest scores in phonological tasks. Lie (1991), who also trained first graders, found that children of lower intelligence profited most from phonological training in posttest reading and spelling.

What method of teaching phonological skills is most effective and shows optimal transfer for later reading and writing? In her review of training studies, Lewkowicz (1980) concluded that the most effective phonological tasks are those which are most closely related to reading and spelling, i.e. sequential phonemic analysis (as compared e.g. to a positional analysis of single phonemes) and blending. This conclusion has been confirmed empirically by Lie (1991), who studied the influence of a 'positional phoneme analysis' training (which sound do you hear at the beginning of a word? in the middle? at the end?) compared to a complete 'sequential analysis' training during kindergarten on later reading and writing. Whereas there was no differential effect on reading ability at the end of first grade, the children trained in complete sequential analysis reached better scores in spelling. However, the differential effect was reduced by the end of second grade.

Another important issue is the question whether phonemic analysis should be complemented by some kind of visual structure or even by letters. Lewkowicz/Low (1979) found a positive effect of visual squares representing the number of phonemes of a word early in training (see also Elkonin 1973). Hohn/Ehri (1983) showed that phoneme analysis can be promoted even more by introducing the corresponding letters. The authors argue that letters provide the children with a mental symbol system for representing phonemes.

The superiority of a letter condition in phoneme analysis tasks has not been supported unequivocally in studies using reading disabled children. Confirmative evidence comes from Bradley/Bryant (1983) who introduced plastic letters in their second year of training for one group of children. On the other hand, Mannhaupt (1990), who trained phonemic segmentation in low achievers in the second half of first grade, did not obtain differential effects between a letter and a blank tile condition. Working with older reading disabled children (7 - 10 years of age) Kerstholt/van Bon/Schreuder (1991) could not confirm the advantage of a training condition with letters and/or squares as visual support. Thus it seems that the introduction of letters within a phoneme training program is mainly effective for preschoolers who might not be aware of the structure of an alphabetic writing system prior to training. This interpretation can be supported by data from Cunningham

(1990), who found better transfer from a phoneme segmentation training to reading when the children (first graders) were explicitly introduced to the value and utility of phoneme awareness for the activity of reading. Older reading disabled children who have already learned the basics of an alphabetic orthography apparently do not profit as much from letters as support for phonemic analysis.

In future research, efforts definitely need to be directed at training phonological skills in reading disabled children; mere extrapolation from preschool studies is certainly not justified. What is also needed is an analysis of the microstructure of phoneme segmentation. First attempts indicate that 'onset' and 'rime' (e.g. c-at) might be possible functional units (Wise/Olson/Treiman 1990). It is also known that initial consonants are more difficult to isolate when they belong to a consonant cluster. Schreuder/van Bon (1989) also found an effect of word length on phoneme segmentation; it seems that a strictly serial model of phoneme segmentation cannot be adequate.

In conclusion of this section it should be mentioned that although phoneme analysis and blending are certainly important partial processes of reading and spelling, they need not necessarily be trained in isolation. Ehri (1987) and Morais/Alegria/Content (1987) argue that phonological skills are acquired while learning to read and to spell. Particularly in 'creative spelling' (Read 1986) children are constantly required to analyze words into their constituent phonemes.

Promoting the orthographic strategy

While phonological segmentation and the blending of phonemes seem to be necessary skills for attaining literacy in an alphabetic orthography like English or German, they do not suffice for advanced reading and writing. The competent reader and speller has to deal with many words which do not conform to simple phoneme-grapheme correspondences; these words either display higher order phonographic, graphotactic, or morphemic structure or are orthographically irregular. There are basically two different educational approaches to teach children how to cope with regular, but complex words: The 'structural linguistic approach' introduces the child to higher order regularities of the written language; the 'lexical' or 'word-specific' approach teaches strategies for directly learning the orthographic code of regular (and irregular) words. In long-term programs these approaches are usually combined.

Structural linguistic approaches

Basic research has provided overwhelming evidence that orthographic structure is used in mature reading and writing (Gibson/Shurcliff/Yonas 1970; Glushko 1979; Seidenberg 1987; Taft 1979, 1987; and others). Although evidence is emerging constantly (see Coltheart 1987 for review), the exact nature of the utilization and - particularly - the acquisition of orthographic structure is still open for further research. Gibson/Shurcliff/Yonas (1970) believed that invariant spelling patterns are being learnt; Goswami (1986) suggested that children may use analogies to extract rules. Connectionist models of reading acquisition (Seidenberg/ McClelland 1989) may be opening new research avenues.

There is evidence that reading and writing disabled children do not make as much use of orthographic structure as better readers and spellers (Guthrie/ Seifert 1977; Manis/Morrison 1985; Morrison/Manis 1982; Scheerer-Neumann 1981). While Guthrie/Seifert (1977) regard this deficit as a consequence of delayed reading acquisition rather than as a basic cause of reading retardation, Manis/Morrison (1985) believe that reading disabled children have general difficulties in learning complex and inconsistent rules.

In any case, the utilization of orthographic structure is basically teachable. Graphophonic regularities in reading can be taught by rules like "'i' before 'e'". Insight into the morphemic structure of words allows children to take advantage of building blocks like the <ed>-ending of the past tense in English. The Hornsby/Miles (1980) and Thomson (1988) programs make intensive use of these regularities. In Germany, this approach has been proposed by Kossow (1972) and Pilz/Schubenz (1979) among others. I myself have developed two programs which are relevant in this context: A reading program taught children to use syllables as a structural help to decode long words (Scheerer-Neumann 1981). In a spelling program, the children were mainly taught how to make use of morphemic structure (Scheerer-Neumann 1988).

The syllable training study. 30 third graders were selected according to their low performance in an oral reading test including both word list and paragraph reading (Zürcher Lesetest, Linder/Grissemann 1967). The children were quite proficient at phoneme blending, but had problems in decoding particularly long words. 15 children (11 boys, 4 girls) took part in 12 training sessions lasting between 30 and 45 minutes in groups of two or three (the 'experimental group'). 15 children, who were matched to the trained children according to sex, reading level and nonverbal intelligence, remained untrained as a control group. During the first four sessions the children in the experimental group had to segment spoken words into syllables; a variety of different responses and games (e.g. hand clapping, speaking 'like a robot' in syllables, writing bows for syllables, writing the vowels in the syllable bows) were used. In sessions 5 and 6 the children first segmented the spoken and then the corresponding written word. In sessions 7 and 8 the children were taught to use the vocalic center group in order to identify syllables. In session 9 to 12 the children were introduced to two formal syllable segmentation rules and explained the function of punctuation (as a help to structure sentences). The posttest used a parallel form of the reading test as well as tachistoscopical projected pseudowords which had also been included in the pretest. As can be seen in Figure 2, the trained children showed a (highly significant) decrease in oral reading errors after training, particularly for words with three or more syllables, while the control group exhibited even an insignificant increase in errors. The trained children also

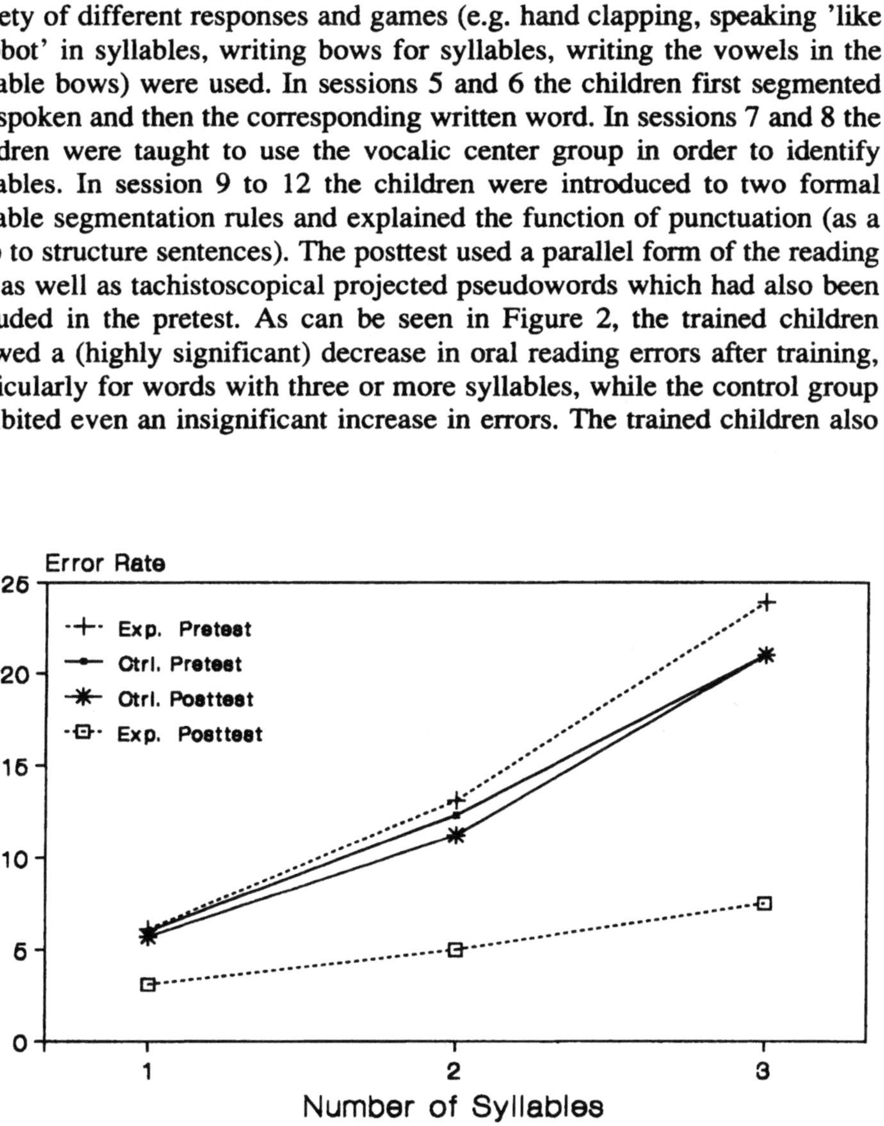

Fig. 2: Mean error rate as a function of the number of syllables in a word for experimental (trained) and control Ss before (pretest) and after (posttest) training (the 3-syllable condition also includes words of 4 syllables)

improved their performance on pseudowords indicating that it really was their decoding skill which had been trained. This interpretation is also backed by the fact that word list and paragraph reading profited equally from training. The rather large and specific training effect after only 12 training sessions is remarkable. Syllables seem to be very helpful as segments for children to structure words, probably because they are the units of spoken language and as such easily accessible (Liberman/Shankweiler/Liberman et al., 1977). In a recent paper Thomson (1990) also reported on the positive effect of a very similar syllable training program.

Teaching orthographic structures to fifth graders. In another study which illustrates the "structure" approach we trained 40 poor fifth grade spellers twice a week in groups of 3 to 5. The children attended the German 'Hauptschule' which is the second lowest level in our four level secondary school system (the lowest level offers special education for the mentally retarded); the 'Hauptschule' is comparable to the British secondary modern school. In order to get information on the trained children's relative position in class, whole classes were asked to take part in the spelling pretests and posttests. Two spelling tests were given: One had been designed by us for the purpose of the study and included words of the orthographic structures which were to be trained, the other was a standardized spelling test (DRT 4 and 5, Meis 1970). The control children were classmates matched to the trained children according to spelling level and nonverbal intelligence. Although all experimental and control children attained poor scores on the spelling test, almost all were basically proficient in the alphabetic strategy of writing.

As training contents we chose orthographic regularities which are not covered by the phonological principle of the German orthography or are even contrary to it. The selected topics included capitalization and morpheme constancy. Here is an example of morphemic constancy: The phoneme /e/ corresponds with the grapheme <e> as well as with <ä>, an ambiguity which leads to common spelling errors. In the word <Hände> (hands) the phoneme /e/ is represented by the grapheme <ä> indicating the morphemic relationship to the singular <Hand>. In the spelling program the students were introduced to the morphemic principle of the German orthography and also given algorithms to use it: In the above-mentioned example they were asked to find the singular of a noun (in case of verbs the infinitive) in order to disambiguate the phoneme grapheme correspondence. This as well as other rules were systematically trained and given to the children on algorithm cards. Some of the words used in rule training were additionally taught lexically by the look-cover-write-check method. The posttest included a subset of these trained words as well as untrained words of the same orthographic structure in order to investigate a possible transfer effect.

Figure 3 shows the results combined for both types of words after a total of 30 - 35 training sessions distributed over a four months period: There was a highly significant training effect for the experimental group as compared to the control group; the trained students did not quite reach the mean value of the entire class.

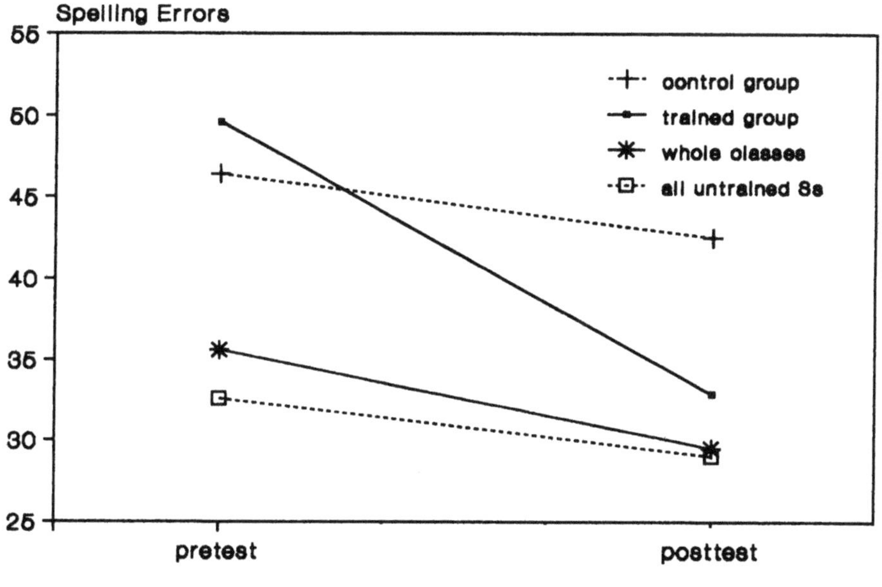

Fig. 3: *Error rates in the specially designed spelling test on pre- and posttest for trained Ss, control Ss, all Ss tested (whole classes), and all untrained Ss.*

Figures 4a and b present the results of the trained children individually. It can be seen that the trained children moved toward the mean of the total distribution. The three children who stayed at the low end were rather poor

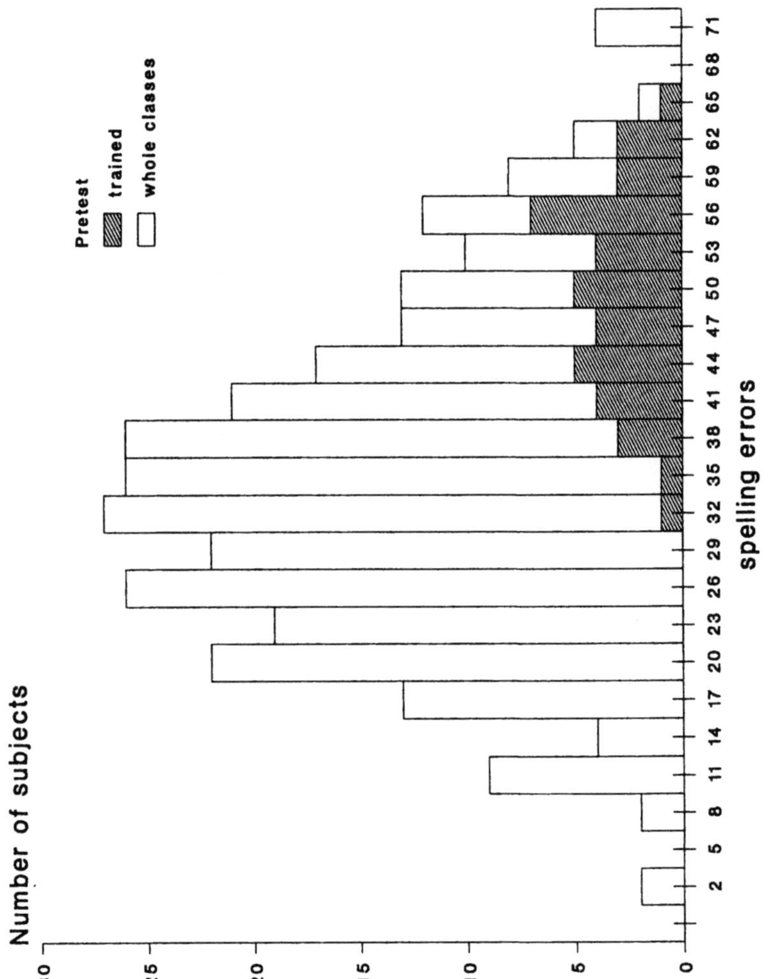
Number of subjects
30
25
20
15
10
5
0
2
5
8
11
14
17
20
23
26
29
32
35
38
41
44
47
50
53
56
59
62
65
68
71
spelling errors
Pretest
trained
whole classes

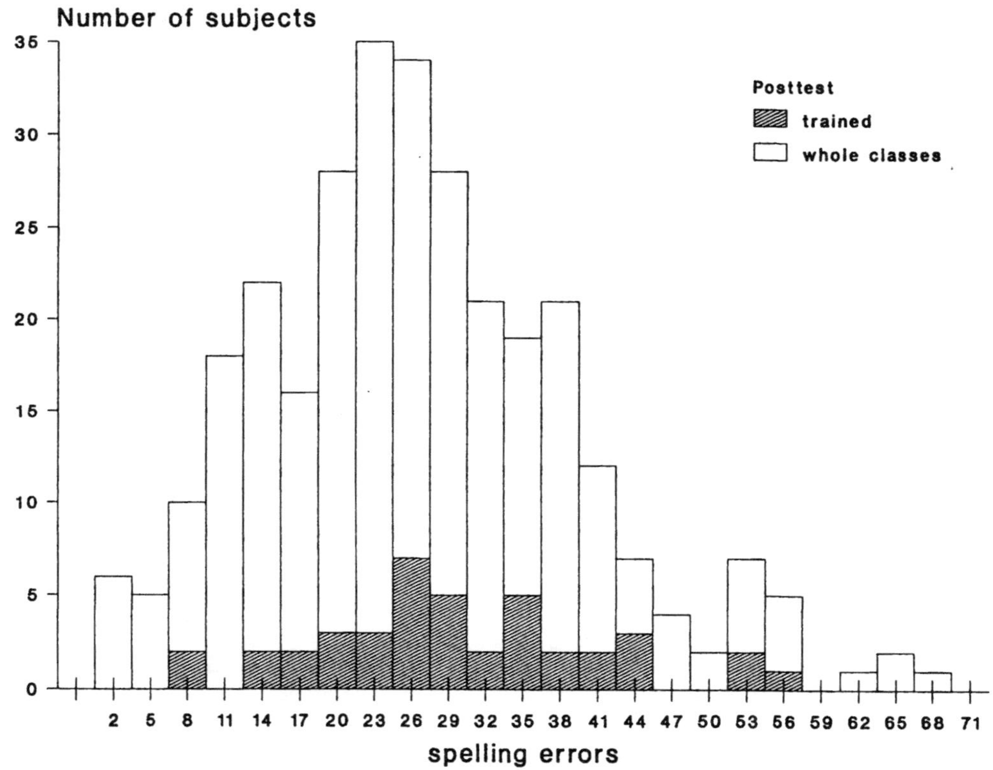

Fig. 4a & b: *Relative position of the trained Ss on the specially designed test within the distribution of all tested children (whole classes)*

on pretest. A qualitative analysis of their errors showed that they also progressed; however, they still did not get many words correct, which is what is counted in Figure 4. The corresponding diagram for control children has been omitted for reasons of space. On posttest they belonged to the very lowest end of the distribution.

Transfer of the trained regularities to new words was very high, though not perfect: We found a 45,4% reduction in spelling errors for words which had also been trained lexically, compared to 38% for transfer words. This result characterizes two tendencies: A very good transfer effect, indicating that the regularities really had been learned, but also an effect of word-specific training.

There is another interesting aspect of the data: the standardized spelling test included many words with orthographic regularities which were not part of the program (e.g. geminated consonants). The trained children significantly outscored the control group on posttest, but the effect was relatively small. Thus the data of the study can be summarized as follows: There is evidence of transfer of learned structures to new words of the same structure (though not perfect), but only little transfer to new words with new orthographic structures. An additional word specific training increases the effectiveness of a structural linguistic training program. The rationale of the word specific approach will be elaborated in the following section.

Lexical approaches

The basic idea of "word training" or the "lexical approach" is the acquisition of a reading and spelling vocabulary with single words as units. In terms of cognitive models (e.g. Coltheart 1989) training is directed at the orthographic lexicon. While their origin is probably rooted in educational practice, word training procedures have been influenced - or at least backed up - by two different theoretical traditions: behavioristic learning theory and cognitive developmental memory research.

Behavior modification. In behavior modification correct responses - here the correct reading or writing of a word - are positively reinforced; alternatively, errors are punished in a response-cost system. Apart from the look-cover-write-check procedure, which has been shown to be very effective (Murphy/Hern/Williams/McLaughlin 1990), no cues or strategies are given which might help the children to memorize the spellings. The words to be learned are repeated systematically according to a scheme derived from learning theory. Intervals between words are shorter for recently learned words than for words introduced earlier. This technique is rather powerful and has been shown to be effective empirically (Kerr/Lambert 1982; Machemer 1972). It is simple enough to be applied even by parents. When parents are the trainers, training can take place daily and a very high cumulative learning effect can be achieved. There are limitations to this approach, however: It is only appropriate for children who have overcome basic decoding difficulties, i.e. children who have reached the alphabetic stage in the Frith model (Frith 1985).

Training memory strategies. Whereas the behavior modification approach basically leaves it to the child *how* s/he memorizes the spelling of a word, cognitively oriented programs try to modify the memory strategies used. The vast literature on memory development has convincingly shown that younger children do not use as effective memory strategies as older children (e.g. Ornstein/Naus 1978; for review see Hagen/Jongeward/Kail 1975; and Ornstein 1978) and that here learning disabled children rather resemble younger children. When learning the spelling of new words reading disabled children often display impulsive behavior; they do not take enough time and make more errors than their peers (Kossow 1972).

There is also extensive literature showing that the use of more efficient memory strategies can be trained (Hagen/Hargrave/Ross 1973; for review see Bauer 1987; Hagen/Jongward/Kail 1975). The question then is which memory strategies are most effective for retaining the spelling of words. The 'copy, cover, write, compare' procedure mentioned in connection with the behavior modification approach is a first step in this direction. Yet the decisive step is to specify and train strategies which directly influence how orthographic information is retained. There are some short-term experimental studies on this question which are also relevant for comprehensive programs.

The main issue refers to the modality of the code used: This is the classic question, whether learning is most efficient using the visual, the auditory or the kinesthetic modality, or a combination of any two or three. Gillingham/Stillman (1969) proposed a strategy they called "simultaneous oral spelling"; the child first copies the word to be learned, naming each individual letter as s/he puts them down. Since this procedure involves a visual, an auditory and a motor component it is often referred to as 'multisensory training'. The importance of a motor component was also stressed by Fernald (1943) and of course by Montessori (1913).

Hulme (1981) tested the efficiency of different spelling codes experimentally and further studies followed. In a very convincing study Hulme/Bradley (1984) found that retarded spellers (M = 11 years) profited most from simultaneous oral spelling compared to a condition without letter naming and a condition in which letter cards were used instead of writing. Performance under the 'simultaneous oral spelling' condition was best after training and even four weeks later. The results were dissimilar for normal spellers who were chronologically younger (M = 6 years, 8 months) but of the same spelling age: They did not show any differential effects under the various conditions.

The result obtained from the retarded spellers is in accordance with basic memory research. Paivio (1971) demonstrated that items which can be coded both visually and verbally are better retained in memory. In my interpretation, 'multisensory' training is basically an instance of multiple code learning; thus additional codes need not necessarily be in yet another modality. A structural property of a word could also serve as an additional code (e.g. the morphemic structure of a word like "child/ish").

The interesting result in the Hulme/Bradley study that normal spellers did not profit from 'simultaneous oral spelling' could be due to their spontaneous use of some type of verbal code. Unfortunately, Hulme/Bradley do not report relevant data. Incidentally, in languages with more regular phoneme-grapheme correspondences like German, the verbal code used spontaneously by most children seems to be the 'overpronunciation' of the word with respect to its spelling rather than the letter names (Scheerer-Neumann 1986).

In any case, Hulme/Bradley's (1984) data fit the picture of inefficient memory strategies in poor spellers, which can be improved by training. This conclusion is supported by research showing that in spelling instruction particularly poor spellers need a memorization set for successful learning. Bosman/de Groot (1991) found that copying a stimulus word while it was still in view was totally ineffective in poor spellers (grade 1), while it had a small effect in good spellers. The low performance of the poor spellers probably has to do with their inability to spontaneously generate additional codes while copying. The finding that a memorization set is necessary for appreciable retention to occur conforms with the idea of the child as an active learner whose task it is to select and code information. This is very different from the conception of the orthographic lexicon as a store of "photographic word pictures", which is what many of our teachers still believe. There are some additional data which demonstrate active processes in spelling acquisition: Kaufmann/Hallahan/Haas et al. (1978) and Hasselbring (1982) found a higher improvement in spelling when the children were shown their errors together with the correct spellings instead of the correct spellings alone. This shows that children do not just store the correct spelling but rather selectively pay attention to the letters they missed before.

Word training programs can be implemented very well by a microcomputer. A computer program has the advantage of being easily adapted to a child's basic level and daily performance, a feature which is essential for spelling disabled children. Adaptive spelling programs for disabled spellers have been reported among others by Hasselbring (1982) and Breuninger/Betz (1989).

Comprehensive studies. Long term studies within the 'Direct Instruction' approach usually include phonological training as well as structural linguistic and word specific exercises. While it is difficult to partial out the effectiveness of each component in a comprehensive program, these studies are very valuable for a general evaluation of the effectiveness training programs. On the whole, empirical investigations show that training indeed can be very effective, a fact which was doubted not very long ago (Silberberg/Silberberg 1969).

Of particular interest are the comprehensive studies by Hornsby/Miles (1980) and by Thomson (1988). Both used phonics as well as a structural and a lexical approach; the program developed by Hornsby/Miles has a strong emphasis on phonological and linguistic structure. Hornsby/Miles (1980) observed the progress of reading disabled children who received individualized instruction for several hours each week. The data from 107 children show clearly that most children made considerable progress. Not only did they progress normally for their reading and spelling ages, but they also got closer to their age norm. On average the children gained 27 months in spelling and reading ages in a 20-month remedial period. 15% of the children did not reach the criterion of "keeping up with the clock", i.e. they fell further behind with regard to their chronological ages.

Impressive data are reported by Thomson (1988) from the East Court School for Dyslexic Children. The training offered at this school includes many building blocks from direct instruction. The children are residential and are taught daily. Results from children are reported in terms of an "improvement ratio", the ratio between the increase in reading and spelling age and chronological time passed. Over a three-year period the average improvement ratio was 1.46 for reading and 1.53 for spelling. In reading, the children almost approached their age norm on the average; there was also substantial improvement in spelling.

To complete this section: Comprehensive studies with favorable outcomes have also been reported by Balow/Fuchs/Kasbohm (1978), Branwhite (1983), and Lovett/Ransby/Barron (1988). All these studies basically show that with appropriate instruction reading disabled children can indeed substantially improve their reading and spelling.

Language Experience Approach

The 'Language Experience Approach' or 'Whole Language Approach' can be included in the section of 'Direct Instruction', because reading and writing activities are the center of teaching. However, in contrast to the programs discussed above, the child's attention is focussed on the functional aspect rather than on the structural properties of written language (e.g. Hildreth 1965). Instead of basal readers children's literature is used as reading material as early as possible. Children are encouraged to communicate by writing even at a stage where they cannot be expected to avoid errors. As a matter of fact, errors are not only tolerated but considered unavoidable signs of certain developmental stages (Spitta 1985). Stahl/Miller (1989) recently completed a meta-analysis of a large number of studies which compared the effectiveness of the language experience approach with a basal reader approach. Although they found in general that the approaches were similar in their effectiveness, there were differential results too. The language experience approach was more effective in teaching children concepts about print and reading at the kindergarten level. Unfortunately, the authors did not look specifically at slow learners; yet data are reported on disadvantaged children and a large overlap between the learning disabled and the "disadvantaged" population can be assumed. The disadvantaged children also profited from the language experience approach at the kindergarten level; however, at the first grade level the basal reader approach proved more effective. The authors conclude that - in Downing's (1979) terms - the language experience approach is more efficient in the cognitive phase, when children become aware of print and reading, but that the basal reader approach is more helpful during the mastering phase. The advantage of the basal reader approach in the skill acquisition phase fits a presupposition underlying most remedial approaches: Most of these explicitly demand a step-by-step procedure where nothing is left to chance and no transfer is expected from the child (Dummer/Hackethal 1984; Hornsby/Miles 1980; Thomson 1988). On the other hand, the language experience approach does rely upon learning which is not explicitly taught. In practice, both approaches can be combined to a certain extent. It is possible to use highly motivating elements from the language experience approach and have children read and write on their own very early and still introduce elements of the written language in a rather systematic form. Further, spontaneous, creative writing implies extensive practice in phoneme analysis because the children often want to write words whose spelling they are not familiar with. They have to construct these words using an alphabetic strategy. This practice effect also occurs when the words written are not yet correct orthographically. As a matter of fact, in a study which included kindergarten and first grade, Sawyer (1988) found best results for poor segmenters when a combination of a phonics and a language experience approach was used (see also Reason 1990).

Creative writing can be facilitated by a text processor (e.g. Levin/Boruta/Vasconcellos 1983) which can also be used for checking the spelling. Computers offer new possibilities to help reading disabled children; the possibilities have not yet been fully explored.

Future research

The basic question whether reading and spelling disabled children's achievements can be improved by appropriate intervention has been answered in this paper with slight optimism. But the effectiveness of remedial efforts could certainly be increased if we knew more about the microstructure of the learning processes involved. Although the basic dilemma between adaptive multifacetted remedial teaching and the strict methodological demands of empirical research cannot be conclusively resolved, promising research seems possible, if the gap between basic and applied research is diminished and interdisciplinary efforts are encouraged. We need detailed longitudinal studies which monitor and analyze the child's progress in a theory oriented way. Perhaps single cases could be a good starting point. Scientists should also take a look at 'good practice' and analyze teaching programs which appear helpful for children at school or in child guidance institutions; the relationship between theory and practice is definitely not a one way route.

References

Arter, J.A. & Jenkins, J.R. (1979). Differential diagnosis-prescriptive teaching: A critical appraisal. Review of Educational Research, 49, 517-555.

Axline, V. (1947). Nondirective therapy for poor readers. Journal of Consulting Psychology, 11, 61-69.

Bakker, D., van Leeuwen, H.M.P., & Spyer, G. (1987). Neuropsychological aspects of dyslexia. In D. Bakker, C. Wilsher, N. Debruyne, & N. Bertin (Eds.), Developmental dyslexia and learning disorders. 30-39. Basel: Karger.

Ball, E.W. & Blachman, B.A. (1988). Phoneme segmentation training: Effect on reading readiness. Annals of Dyslexia, 38, 208-225.

Ball, E.W. & Blachman, B.A. (1991). Does phoneme awareness training in kindergarten make a difference in early word recognition and developmental spelling? Reading Research Quarterly, 26, 50-66.

Balow, B., Fuchs, D., & Kasbohm, M. (1978). Teaching nonreaders to read: An evaluation of the Basic Skill Centers in Minneapolis. Journal of Learning Disabilities, 11, 351-354.

Bauer, R.H. (1987). Control processes as a way of understanding, diagnosing, and remediating learning disabilities. In H.L. Swanson (Ed.), Memory and learning disabilities: Suppl.2. Advances in learning and behavioral disabilities. 41-81. Greenwich, CT: JAI Press.

Bosch, B. (1937). Grundlagen des Erstleseunterrichts. Beiheft zur Zeitschrift für angewandte Psychologie und Charakterkunde, 76, 81-98.

Bosman, A. & de Groot, M.B. (1991). Differential effectiveness of reading and nonreading tasks in learning to spell. Paper presented at the 7th European Conference on Reading, Edinburgh, Scotland, August 1991.

Bradley, L. & Bryant, P.E. (1983). Categorizing sounds and learning to read: A causal connection. Nature, 301, 419-421.

Brady, S.A. & Shankweiler, D.P. (Eds.)(1991). Phonological processes in literacy. Hillsdale, N.J.: Lawrence Erlbaum.

Branwhite, A.B. (1983). Boosting reading skills by direct instruction. British Journal of Educational Psychology, 53, 291-298.

Breuninger, H. & Betz, D. (1989). Der Einsatz des Computers in der außerschulischen Lerntherapie. In I.M. Naegele & R. Valtin (Eds.), LRS in den Klassen 1-10. 113-118. Weinheim: Beltz.

Coltheart, M. (Ed.)(1987). The psychology of reading. Attention and performance XII. London: Lawrence Erlbaum.

Coltheart, M. (1989). Functional architecture of the language-processing system. In M. Coltheart, G. Sartori, & R. Job (Eds.), The cognitive neuropsychology of language. 1-25. London: Lawrence Erlbaum.

Conners, C.K. & Reader, M. (1987). The effects of piracetam on reading achievement and visual event-related potentials in dyslexic children. In D.J. Bakker, C. Wilsher, H. Debruyne, & N. Bertin (Eds.), Developmental dyslexia and learning disorders: Diagnosis and treatment. 75-90. Basel: Karger.

Content, A., Kolinsky, R., Morais, J., & Bertelson, P. (1986). Phonetic segmentation in prereaders: Effects of corrective information. Journal of Experimental Child Psychology, 42, 49-72.

Cornelissen, P., Bradley, L., Fowler, M.S., & Stein, J.F. (1991). What children see affects how they read. Developmental Medicine and Child Neurology, 33, 755-762.

Cunningham, A.E. (1990). Explicit versus implicit instruction in phonemic awareness. Journal of Experimental Child Psychology, 50, 429-444.

Delacato, C. (1959). The diagnosis and treatment of speech and reading problems. Springfield, Ill.: Thomas.

Dimond, S.J. & Brouwers, E.Y.M. (1976). Improvement of human memory through the use of drugs. Psychopharmacology, 49, 307-309.

Downing, J. (1979). Reading and reasoning. Edinburgh: Chambers, New York: Springer.

Dummer, L. & Hackethal, R. (1984). Handbuch zum Kieler Leseaufbau. Kiel: Veris.

Edler, M., Ostrau, R., & Schulze, K. (1977). Rechtschreibtraining mit Legasthenikern. Unpublished Diplom-Thesis, Ruhr-Universität Bochum.

Ehri, L. (1987). Learning to read and spell words. Journal of Reading Behavior, 19, 5-31.

Elkonin, D.B. (1973). The psychology of mastering the elements of reading. In B. Simon & J. Simon (Eds.), Educational psychology in the U.S.S.R. 165-179. London: Routledge & Kegan Paul.

Fernald, G. (1943). Remedial techniques in basic school subjects. New York: McGraw Hill.

Fox, B. & Routh, D.K. (1984). Phonemic analysis and synthesis as word attack skills: Revisited. Journal of Educational Psychology, 76, 1059-1061.

Frith, U. (1985). Beneath the surface of developmental dyslexia. In K.E. Patterson, J.C. Marshall, & M. Coltheart (Eds.), Surface dyslexia. 301-330. Hillsdale, N.J.: Lawrence Erlbaum.

Frostig, M. & Horne, D. (1964). The Frostig program for the development of visual perception: Teacher's guide. Chicago: Follett.

Gibson, E., Shurcliff, A., & Yonas, A. (1970). Utilization of spelling patterns by deaf and hearing subjects. In H. Levin & J. Williams (Eds.), Basic studies on reading. 57-73. New York: Basic Books.

Gillingham, A. & Stillman, B.W. (1969). Remedial training for children with specific disability in reading, spelling, and penmanship. Cambridge, Mass.: Educators Publishing Service.

Gittelmann, R., Klein, D.F., & Feingold, I. (1983). Children with reading disorders - II. Effects of methylpeniate in combination with reading remediation. Journal of Child Psychology and Psychiatry, 24, 193-212.

Glushko, R.J. (1979). The organization and activation of orthographic knowledge in reading aloud. Journal of Experimental Psychology: Human Perception and Performance, 5, 674-691.

Goswami, U. (1986). Children's use of analogy in learning to read: A developmental study. Journal of Experimental Child Psychology, 42, 73-83.

Guthrie, J.T. & Seifert, M. (1977). Letter-sound complexity in learning to identify words. Journal of Educational Psychology, 69, 686-696.

Hagen, J.W., Hargrave, S., & Ross, W. (1973). Prompting and rehearsal in short-term memory. Child Development, 44, 201-204.

Hagen, J.W., Jongward, R.H., & Kail, R.V. (1975). Cognitive perspective on the development of memory. In H.W. Reese (Ed.), Advances in Child Development and Behavior, 10, 57-101.

Hannell, G., Gole, G.A., Dibden, S.N., Rooney, K.F., Pidgeon, K.J. (1991). Reading improvement with tinted lenses: a report of two cases. Journal of Research in Reading, 14, 56-71.

Hasselbring, T.S. (1982). Remediating spelling problems of learning-handicapped students through the use of microcomputers. Educational Technology, 22(4), 31-32.

Hildreth, G.H. (1965). Experience related reading for school beginners. Elementary English, 42, 280-297.

Hohn, W. & Ehri, L. (1983). Do alphabet letters help prereaders acquire phonemic segmentation skills? Journal of Educational Psychology, 75, 751-762.

Höreth, G. (1977). Einfluß eines programmierten Selbstinstruktions-Rechtschreibtrainings auf die Rechtschreibleistung lese-rechtschreibschwacher Kinder des 3. Schuljahrs. Unpublished Diplom-Thesis. Ruhr Universität Bochum.

Hornsby, B. & Miles, T.R. (1980). The effects of a dyslexia-centered teaching programme. British Journal of Educational Psychology, 50, 236-242.

Hulme, C. (1981). Reading retardation and multi-sensory teaching. London: Routledge & Kegan Paul.

Hulme, C. & Bradley, L. (1984). An experimental study of multisensory teaching with normal and retarded readers. In R.N. Malatesha & H.A. Whitaker (Eds.), Dyslexia: A global issue. 431-443. The Hague: Martinus Nijhoff.

Irlen, H.L. (1983). Successful treatment of learning disabilities. Paper presented to American Psychological Association.

Kaufman, J.M., Hallahan, Haas, K., Brame, T., & Boren (1978). Imitating children's errors to improve their spelling performance. Journal of Learning Disabilities, 11, 217-222.

Kerr, M.M. & Lambert, D.L. (1982). Behavior modification of children's written language. Progress in Behavior Modification, 13, 79-108.

Kerstholt, M., van Bon, W., & Schreuder, R. (1991). Training in phonemic segmentation: The effect of alphabet letters as visual support. Paper presented at the 7th European Conference on Reading, August 1991, Edinburgh, Scotland.

Kinsbourne, M. & Hiscock, M. (1987). Language lateralization and disordered language development. In S. Rosenberg (Ed.), Advances in applied psycholinguistics. 220-263. Cambridge: Cambridge University Press.

Kossow, H.-J. (1972). Zur Therapie der Lese-Rechtschreibschwäche. Berlin: Deutscher Verlag der Wissenschaften.

Larsen, S.C. & Hammill, D.D. (1975). The relationship of selected visual-perceptual abilities to school learning. Journal of Special Education, 9, 281-291.

Levin, A., Boruta, M.J., & Vasconcellos, M.T. (1983). Microcomputer-based environments for writing: A writer's assistant. In A.C. Wilkinson (Ed.), Classroom computers and cognitive science. 219-223. New York: Academic Press.

Lewkowicz, N.K. (1980). Phonemic awareness training: What to teach and how to teach it. Journal of Educational Psychology, 72, 686-700.

Lewkowicz, N.K. & Low, L.Y. (1979). Effect of visual aids and word structure on phonemic segmentation. Contemporary Educational Psychology, 4, 238-252.

Liberman, I.Y. (1973). Segmentation of the spoken word. Bulletin of the Orton Society, 23, 65-77.

Liberman, I.Y., Shankweiler, D., Liberman, A.M., Fowler, C., & Fischer, F.W. (1977). Phonetic segmentation and recoding in the beginning reader. In A.S. Reber & D.L. Scarborough (Eds.), Towards a psychology of reading. 207-225. New York: Wiley.

Lie, A. (1991). Effects of a training program for stimulating skills in word analysis in first-grade children. Reading Research Quarterly, 26, 234-250.

Linder, M. & Grissemann, H. (1967). Zürcher Lesetest. Bern: Huber.

Lovegrove, W., Martin, F., & Slaghuis, W. (1986). A theoretical and experimental case for a visual deficit in specific reading disability. Cognitive Neuropsychology, 3, 225-267.

Lovett, M.W., Ransby, M.J., & Barron, R.W. (1988). Treatment, subtype, and word type effect in dyslexic children's response to remediation. Brain & Language, 34, 328-349.

Lundberg, I., Frost, J., & Petersen, O. (1988). Effects of an extensive program for stimulating phonological awareness in preschool children. Reading Research Quarterly, 23, 263-284.

Machemer, P. (1972). Entwicklung eines Übungsprogramms für Eltern zur Behandlung von Legasthenikern nach verhaltenstherapeutischem Modell. Schule und Psychologie, 19, 336-346.

Manis, F.R. & Morrison, F.J. (1985). Reading disability: A deficit in rule learning. In L.S. Siegel & F.J. Morrison (Eds.), Cognitive development in atypical children. 1-26. New York: Springer.

Mannhaupt, G. (1990). Strategieausbildung zur Lautstrukturanalyse mit Hilfe von abstrakten oder konkreten Symbolen während des frühen Schriftspracherwerbs. Ph.D. Dissertation. Universität Bielefeld, Germany.

Meichenbaum, D.H. & Goodman, J. (1969). Training impulsive children to talk to themselves: A means of developing self-control. Journal of Abnormal Psychology, 77, 115-126.

Meis, R. (1970). Diagnostischer Rechtschreibtest für 4. und 5. Klassen (DRT 4 u. 5). Weinheim: Beltz.

Montessori, M. (1913). Selbsttätige Erziehung im frühen Kindesalter. Stuttgart: Julius Hoffmann.

Morais, J., Alegria, J., & Content, A. (1987). The relationships between segmental analysis and alphabetic literacy: An interactive view. Cahiers de Psychologie Cognitive, 7, 415-438.

Morgan, W.P. (1896). A case of congenital word blindness. British Medical Journal, 2, 1378.

Morrison, F.J. & Manis, F.R. (1982). Cognitive processes and reading disability: A critique and proposal. In C.J. Brainerd & M. Pressley (Eds.), Verbal processes in children. 59-93. New York: Springer.

Murphy, J.F., Hern, C.L., Williams, R.L., & McLaughlin, T.F. (1990). The effects of the copy, cover, compare approach in increasing spelling accuracy with learning disabled students. Contemporary Educational Psychology, 15, 378-386.

Neisser, U. (1967). Cognitive psychology. New York: Appleton-Century-Crofts.

Newman, S.P., Karle, H., Wadsworth, J.F., Archer, R., Hockly, R., & P. Rogers (1985). Ocular dominance, reading and spelling: A reassessment of a measure associated with specific reading difficulties. Journal of Research in Reading, 8, 127-138.

Ornstein, P.A. (Ed.)(1978). Memory development in children. Hillsdale, N.J.: Erlbaum.

Ornstein, P.A. & Naus, M.J. (1978). Rehearsal processes in children's memory. In P.A. Ornstein (Ed.), Memory development in children. 69-99. Hillsdale, N.J.: Erlbaum.

Orton, S.T. (1937). Reading, writing and speech problems in children. New York: Norton.

Paivio, A. (1971). Imagery and verbal processes. New York: Holt, Rinehart and Winston.

Pilz, D. & Schubenz, H. (1979). Kindertherapie und Schulversagen. Köln: Pahl-Rugenstein.

Read, C. (1986). Children's creative spelling. London, Boston & Henley: Routledge & Kegan Paul.

Reason, R. (1990). Reconciling different approaches to intervention. In P.D. Pumfrey & C.D. Elliott (Eds.), Children's difficulties in reading, spelling and writing. London: Falmer Press.

Rosner, J. (1971). Phonic analysis training and beginning reading skills. Pittsburgh Learning Research and Development Center Publication Series, No. 9.

Sawyer, D.J. (1988). Studies of the effects of teaching auditory segmenting skills within the reading program. In R.L. Masland & M.W. Masland (Eds.), Preschool prevention of reading failure. 121-142. Parkton, Md.: York Press.

Scheerer-Neumann, G. (1979). Intervention bei Lese-Rechtschreibschwäche. Bochum: Kamp.

Scheerer-Neumann, G. (1981). The utilization of intraword structure in poor readers: Experimental evidence and a training programme. Psychological Research, 43, 155-178.

Scheerer-Neumann, G. (1986). Sprechen, Denken und Rechtschreiben. Grundschule, 18/6, 20-24.

Scheerer-Neumann, G. (1988). Rechtschreibtraining mit rechtschreibschwachen Hauptschülern auf kognitionspsychologischer Grundlage: Eine empirische Untersuchung. Opladen: Westdeutscher Verlag.

Scheerer-Neumann, G. (1989). Lese-Rechtschreibschwäche im Kontext der Entwicklung. In I. Naegele & R. Valtin: LRS in den Klassen 1-10. Weinheim: Beltz.

Schreuder, R. & van Bon, W.H.J. (1989). Phonemic analysis: effect of word properties. Journal of Research in Reading, 12, 59-78.

Seidenberg, M.S. (1987). Sublexical structures in visual word recognition: Access units or orthographic redundancy? In M. Coltheart (Ed.), Attention and performance 12. 245-263. Hillsdale, N.J.: Lawrence Erlbaum.

Seidenberg, M.S. & McClelland, J.L. (1989). A distributed, developmental model of word recognition and naming. Psychological Review, 96, 523-568.

Silberberg, N. & Silberberg, M. (1969). Myths in remedial education. Journal of Learning Disabilities, 2, 209-217.

Skjelfjord, V. (1976). Teaching children to segment spoken words as an aid in learning to read. Journal of Learning Disabilities, 9, 297-306.

Snowling, M. (1991). Developmental reading disorders. Journal of Child Psychology & Psychiatry, 32, 4977.

Spitta, G. (1985). Kinder schreiben eigene Texte, Klasse 1 und 2. Bielefeld: CVK.

Stahl, S.A. & Miller, P.D. (1989). Whole language experience approaches for beginning reading: A quantitative research synthesis. Review of Educational Research, 59, 87-116.

Stein, J.F. & Fowler, S. (1985). Effect of monocular occlusion on visuo-motor perception and reading in dyslexic children. Lancet, July 13. 69-73.

Taft, M. (1979). Lexical access via an orthographic code: The basic orthographic syllable structure (BOSS). Journal of Verbal Learning and Verbal Behavior, 18, 21-39.

Taft, M. (1987). Morphographic processing: The BOSS re-emerges. In M. Coltheart (Ed.), Attention and performance 12. 265-279. Hillsdale, N.J.: Lawrence Erlbaum.

Thomson, M. (1988). Preliminary findings concerning the effects of specialized teaching on dyslexic children. Applied Cognitive Psychology, 2, 19-31.

Thomson, M. (1990). Evaluating teaching programmes for children with specific learning difficulties. In P.D. Pumfrey & C.D. Elliott (Eds.), Children's difficulties in reading, spelling and writing. 155-172. London: Falmer Press.

Torneus, M. (1984). Phonological awareness and reading: A chicken and egg problem? Journal of Educational Psychology, 76, 1346-1358.

Treiman, R. & Baron, J. (1983). Phonemic-analysis training helps children benefit from spelling-sound rules. Memory & Cognition, 11, 382-389.

Vellutino, F.R. & Scanlon, D.M. (1984). Phonological coding, phonological awareness, and reading ability: Evidence from a longitudinal and experimental study. Merrill--Palmer Quarterly, 33, 321-363.

Wagner, R. & Torgeson, J. (1987). The nature of phonological processing and its causal role in the acquisition of reading skills. Psychological Bulletin, 101, 192-212.

Wallach, M.A. & Wallach, L. (1979). Helping disadvantaged children learn to read by teaching them phoneme identification skills. In L.B. Resnick & P.A. Weaver (Eds.), Theory and practice of early reading. Vol. 3, 197-215. Hillsdale, N.J.: Lawrence Erlbaum.

Williams, J. (1979). The ABD's of reading: A program for the learning disabled. In L.B. Resnick & P.A. Weaver (Eds.), Theory and practice of early reading, Vol. 3. 179-195. Hillsdale, N.J.: Lawrence Erlbaum.

Wise, B., Olson, R., & Treiman, R. (1990). Subsyllabic units as aids in beginning readers' word learning: Onset-rime versus post-vowel segmentation. Journal of Experimental Child Psychology, 49, 1-19.

Commentary on Scheerer-Neumann: Organizing the literature on interventions for reading and writing disabilities

Keith E. Stanovich

Gerheid Scheerer-Neumann presents in her paper a most thorough and broad-ranging review of intervention techniques for reading and writing disorders. In less formal terms, let us just say that she deserves a medal for wading through the disparate literatures on drug therapies, ophthalmological interventions, methods related to laterality, psychotherapies, perceptual training, phonics, and structure-linguistics among many others. On a few occasions, I have tried to wade through the training literature in some of these areas and I sometimes have ended up deciding that I would rather go to the dentist. In any case, because Dr. Scheerer-Neumann's review is so wide-ranging, my comments will be fairly unstructured - more free-associations to her paper.

One thing that struck me in reading Scheerer-Neumann's paper was that there was rarely any indication of differential subject responses to any of these treatments. I am specifically referring to indications of whether poor readers with and without IQ-discrepancy (Siegel 1989, in press; Stanovich 1991) respond differently to any of these treatments. In fact, we are simply without good data indicating that discrepancy-defined dyslexics respond differently to various educational treatments than do other poor readers of the same age or than younger nondyslexic children reading at the same level (Pressley/Levin 1987; van der Wissel 1987). This is a rather embarrassing gap in our knowledge base. Differential treatment effects are, in large part, the raison d'etre of special education.

It is of course with great relief that I noted that Scheerer-Neumann's chapter emphasized direct instruction, phonemic awareness and phonics training and de-emphasized such "fringe" training methods as occlusion of an eye, laterality training, or tinted lenses. That Scheerer-Neumann includes many unsubstantiated methods in her review is, I believe, a good thing. Too often, academics are guilty of simply ignoring fringe remedies that are enjoying unopposed publicity in the popular media. Recently, in the U.S. the Irlen colored lens therapy has garnered considerable media attention and was bolstered recently when it was linked on the front page of the *New York Times* with some very legitimate scientific work on visual deficits. Of course, the colored lens idea is backed by no valid empirical research, as Dr. Scheerer-Neumann indicates in her review. And, as those at this conference are aware, visual deficit hypotheses are out of favor among dyslexia researchers at the moment. But it is not enough merely to reiterate this point. The public and the rest of the scientific community deserves a clear statement of why the scientific consensus is what it is - lest we be accused of imposing a Kuhn-type normal-science conspiracy.

Take, for example the work of Lovegrove's group in Australia who have found different spatial frequency functions for dyslexics and nondyslexics (Lovegrove/Martin/Slaghuis 1986). Why is this work less than convincing to most dyslexia researchers? First, most of these studies employ only chronological-age controls and many of the reports appear in the psychophysical literature where it is not as customary to give a detailed description of the subject sample. Thus, the psychometric characteristics of the dyslexic sample are often sparsely reported and inadequate by the standards of accepted practice in the field of learning disabilities - a fact that has impeded the integration of these findings into mainstream theory. But, most importantly, these experiments, as they stand, represent little more than demonstrations. They are the equivalent of the now classic paper by Liberman/Shankweiler/Fischer/Carter (1974) showing the striking developmental trend on the phoneme tapping task that so excited experimental interest. But the Liberman et al. (1974) demonstration was just that - a demonstration. It was left to later work (some of it by the Haskins group itself, of course) to determine the causal and correlative linkages of phonological skills to reading ability - a task that, dozens, if not hundreds of studies later (e.g., Brady/Shankweiler 1991), is still ongoing, as other papers at this conference have revealed.

The tough part always comes later, and is a much more arduous and drawn out procedure because we are a science that depends inordinately on converging evidence. The reason why we are so dependent on converging evidence, rather than critical individual experiments is not hard to discern. Experiments in psychology are usually of fairly low diagnosticity. That is, the data that support a given theory usually only rule out a small set of alternative explanations, leaving many additional theories as viable candidates. As a result, strong conclusions are usually only possible after data from a very large number of studies have been collected and compared. As Horace Judson notes in his book on the history of genetics and molecular biology, *The Eighth Day of Creation*, it took over 10 years of inconclusive experimentation for scientists to change their view about whether genes were made of protein or nucleic acid. We should not be surprised that it took over twice as long to arrive at whatever mild consensus we have on the role of phonological processes in reading. Such a time line suggests that we are in the very early stages indeed of our understanding of the visual processing differences uncovered by the Lovegrove group - a stage in which great caution is in order.

Consider a comparison of the state of the converging evidence vis a vis these alternative theories. The body of converging evidence in the area of phonological processing is basically of four types. Starting with the weakest evidence first: it has been shown that tasks tapping sound sensitivity administered prior to reading instruction predict early reading acquisition (Bradley/Bryant 1983; Fox/Routh 1975; Maclean/Bryant/Bradley 1987; Share/Jorm/Maclean/Matthews 1984; Williams 1984). Additionally, there are some longitudinal studies where cross-lagged correlational methods and/or structural equation modeling have been employed and have led to the conclusion that the development of at least a shallow form of phonological sensitivity leads to superior reading achievement, even when the link from reading to phonological sensitivity is partialed out (Perfetti/Beck/Bell/Hughes 1987; Stanovich 1992). A third class of evidence comes from studies employing the reading-level match design (e.g., Bradley/Bryant 1978; Snowling 1980). Finally, and of course most convincing, are the results of several studies where phonological skills were manipulated via training and resulted in significant experimental group advantages in reading, word recognition, and spelling (e.g., Ball/Blachman 1991; Bradley/Bryant 1983; Cunningham 1990; Lie 1991; Lundberg/Frost/Peterson 1988).

Thus, there are four classes of evidence that have suggested a causal role for phonological sensitivity in early reading acquisition. This converging body of evidence is what has so excited researchers studying individual differences in reading acquisition. There simply is not commensurately strong evidence on causal linkages involving visual processes. Strong claims for visual deficit theories are premature until such evidence is presented. While I am on the issue of visual deficits, let me say a few words about the idea of a visual subtype in dyslexia, because the possibility of such a subtype is often used to justify visual training programs of the type that Scheerer-Neumann covers in her review.

Investigators emphasizing phonological processing theories are often accused of ignoring the possibility of subtypes. I fully agree that we should continue the search for reliably obtainable subgroups of reading disabled children. Let me, however, point to an important asymmetry in the research literature that serves to explain some of the seeming disagreement among reading disabilities researchers on this issue. Most investigators would agree that the following generalization holds pretty well: Those investigators who champion the role of verbal or phonological factors in reading tend not to concern themselves with the subtype issue; whereas investigators supporting the visual deficit hypothesis tend to emphasize the issue of subtypes.

There may be many reasons for this correlation, but I believe that at least part of the reason resides in the fact that the subtypes argument is quite often put forth as an alternative hypothesis to explain null findings in the area of visual processing. The argument - which I have often heard, and it should be noted, do not disagree with - is that in heterogeneous groupings of reading disabled children, the visual processing problems of a small group of children with visual deficits will get swamped when the subgroup is combined with other groups of children with language and phonological deficits. This argument is correct and logical. But we must note a certain asymmetry here. Investigators examining the hypothesis that there is a phonological problem do not have a similar worry. That is, they are not concerned that the speech segmentation performance of the children with phonological problems will be statistically diluted by their being grouped together within a heterogeneous sample including children with visual problems. In short, phonological problems are so large in number that they can be detected even under the most disadvantageous sampling conditions. This, of course, is *not* an argument against the idea of a visual subtype, but it does argue that there must be some restrictive quantitative boundaries on our estimates of this subtype.

This is not a new idea of course. Years ago, Boder (1973) found many more dysphonetics than dyseidetics in her clinical sample and many other theorists have suggested that the visual subtype is considerably smaller than the language/phonological subtypes. But the place of numbers in these disputes is not irrelevant, because therein lies part of the reason why investigators in the various "camps" have had trouble reaching a rapproachment. Phonological deficit theorists - myself, for example - often seem at first to admit that there is a small group of children with visual problems, but then easily slip in their writings into the assumption that they are entirely nonexistent. This understandably raises the ire of the visual deficit theorists. However, the latter are guilty of the same escalation by stealth. Their talk of a small subgroup of children with visual problems often graduates into an argument that large numbers of children are characterized by such a problem or that such children are "typical" - language which teachers quite naturally translate to mean "most common". Thus, an underlying agreement grows into a full fledged controversy because both sides slip into defending their inflated claims. Thus, what is needed is a de-escalation of the rhetoric on both sides.

To return now to Dr. Scheerer-Newmann's review, I should comment that, at times, she paints the state of this literature with a fairly broad brush. But again, I think that this is justified, given the purpose of her review. It is occasionally useful for researchers to step back from their sometimes parochial methodological disputes and to appreciate the scientific progress that has been made in their domain. For example, many of the participants at this conference share certain assumptions about reading that were far from accepted twenty years ago, when cognitive researchers really began to focus on reading. Indeed, an outsider perusing these proceedings is perhaps in the best position to see the magnitude of our progress. To the layperson, our refined disputes about precisely how to fractionate phonological abilities and to trace the causal paths of each component will seem, at best, arcane; whereas the background assumptions that we all share will stand out in bold relief - in contrast, for example, to assumptions held by whole language advocates or socio-constructivist theorists. We must remember this point when communicating current research on phonological processes to educators. They should not mistake our disputes about highly specific issues for disagreements about certain foundational assumptions that we all take for granted.

We have a good example (or perhaps I should say a bad one) in the interminable debate between the Brussels group and the Oxford group (e.g., Bertelson/Morais/Alegria/Content 1985; Bryant/Bradley 1985) regarding whether phonological awareness is a prerequisite for alphabetic reading. I am referring here to the terminology debate and not the real empirical debates in this area (for example, about the role of rhyme in early word learning). This debate reached its "how many angels can stand on the head of a pin" zenith in a 1987 exchange in the *European Bulletin of Cognitive Psychology* when it was finally revealed that everyone basically agreed on the empirical facts - how children perform on which task and when - but no one could agree on what the term phonological awareness meant (see Stanovich 1987, 1992). This is just the sort of attention diverting debate about the meaning of terms that Karl Popper argued was a hindrance to scientific progress. Nothing in this sometimes linguistic debate would change whatever training implications one can derive from our knowledge about the development of phonological sensitivity, defined operationally in terms of performance on particular tasks.

Finally, Scheerer-Neumann cites a study by Kossow (1972) and one by Dummer/Hackethal (1984) in which programs designed to teach the child the movements of the speech organs when pronouncing sounds are described. These programs call to mind the Lindamood auditory conceptualization program (Lindamood/Lindamood 1975) in the U.S. which focuses on what seem to be similar training procedures. Efficacy data is needed on all of these programs, but all of them engender interest in a little-cited study by Montgomery (1981) showing dyslexic children to be extremely bad at choosing which schematic drawing of the articulatory apparatus represented a spoken sound. Thus, in this domain there may be some possibility for reciprocal interaction between training studies like those just mentioned and more basic processing investigations.

These, then, are just a few of my free-associations to Scheerer-Neumann's wide-ranging paper. Training studies are difficult to conduct and the literature on training techniques tends toward extreme fragmentation. Reviews such as Scheerer-Neumann's help to provide organization and coherence to the research literature. And, finally, while reading her review, I was not once tempted to make a dental appointment.

Note

Preparation of this chapter was assisted by a grant from the Social Sciences and Humanities Research Council of Canada.

References

Ball, E.W. & Blachman, B.A. (1991). Does phoneme segmentation training in kindergarten make a difference in early word recognition and developmental spelling. Reading Research Quarterly, 26, 49-66.

Bertelson, P., Morais, J., Alegria, J., & Content, A. (1985). Phonetic analysis capacity and learning to read. Nature, 313, 73-74.

Boder, E. (1973). Developmental dyslexia: A diagnostic approach based on three atypical reading-spelling patterns. Developmental Medicine and Child Neurology, 15, 375-389.

Bradley, L. & Bryant, P.E. (1978). Difficulties in auditory organization as a possible cause of reading backwardness. Nature, 271, 746-747.

Bradley, L. & Bryant, P.E. (1983). Categorizing sounds and learning to read--a causal connection. Nature, 301, 419-421.

Brady, S. & Shankweiler, D. (Eds.) (1991). Phonological processes in literacy. Hillsdale, NJ: Erlbaum.

Bryant, P.E. & Bradley, L. (1985). Reply to Bertelson et al. Nature, 313, 74.

Cunningham, A.E. (1990). Explicit versus implicit instruction in phonemic awareness. Journal of Experimental Child Psychology, 50, 429-444.

Dummer, L. & Hackethal, R. (1984). Handbuch zum Kieler Leseaufbau. Kiel: Veris.

Fox, B. & Routh, D.K. (1975). Analyzing spoken language into words, syllables, and phonemes: A developmental study. Journal of Psycholinguistic Research, 4, 331-342.

Judson, H.F. (1979). The eighth day of creation. New York: Simon and Schuster.

Kossow, H.-J. (1972). Zur Therapie der Lese-Rechtschreibschwäche. Berlin: Deutscher Verlag der Wissenschaften.

Liberman, I.Y., Shankweiler, D., Fischer, F.W., & Carter, B. (1974). Explicit syllable and phoneme segmentation in the young child. Journal of Experimental Child Psychology, 18, 201-212.

Lie, A. (1991). Effects of a training program for stimulating skills in word analysis in first-grade children. Reading Research Quarterly, 26, 234-250.

Lindamood, C.H. & Lindamood, P.C. (1975). Auditory discrimination in depth. Hingham, MA: Teaching Resources Corp.

Lovegrove, W., Martin, F., & Slaghuis, W. (1986). A theoretical and experimental case for a visual deficit in specific reading disability. Cognitive Neuropsychology, 3, 225-267.

Lundberg, I., Frost, J., & Peterson, O. (1988). Effects of an extensive program for stimulating phonological awareness in preschool children. Reading Research Quarterly, 23, 263-284.

Maclean, M., Bryant, P., & Bradley, L. (1987). Rhymes, nursery rhymes, and reading in early childhood. Merrill-Palmer Quarterly, 33, 255-281.

Montgomery, D. (1981). Do dyslexics have difficulty accessing articulatory information? Psychological Research, 43, 235-243.

Perfetti, C.A., Beck, I., Bell, L., & Hughes, C. (1987). Phonemic knowledge and learning to read are reciprocal: A longitudinal study of first grade children. Merrill-Palmer Quarterly, 33, 283-319.

Pressley, M. & Levin, J.R. (1987). Elaborative learning strategies for the inefficient learner. In S.J. Ceci (Ed.), Handbook of cognitive, social, and neuropsychological aspects of learning disabilities (Vol. 2). 175-212. Hillsdale, NJ: Lawrence Erlbaum Associates.

Share, D.L., Jorm, A.F., Maclean, R., & Matthews, R. (1984). Sources of individual differences in reading acquisition. Journal of Educational Psychology, 76, 1309-1324.

Siegel, L.S. (1989). IQ is irrelevant to the definition of learning disabilities. Journal of Learning Disabilities, 22, 469-479.

Siegel, L.S. (in press). Alice in IQ land or why IQ is still irrelevant to learning disabilities. In M. Joshi & C.K. Leong (Eds.), Reading disabilities: Diagnosis and component processes. Dordrecht, The Netherlands: Kluwer Academic.

Snowling, M. (1980). The development of grapheme-phoneme correspondence in normal and dyslexic readers. Journal of Experimental Child Psychology, 29, 294-305.

Stanovich, K.E. (1987). Perspectives on segmental analysis and alphabetic literacy. European Bulletin of Cognitive Psychology, 7, 514-519.

Stanovich, K.E. (1991). Discrepancy definitions of reading disability: Has intelligence led us astray? Reading Research Quarterly, 26, 7-29.

Stanovich, K.E. (1992). Speculations on the causes and consequences of individual differences in early reading acquisition. In P. Gough, L. Ehri, & R. Treiman (Eds.), Reading acquisition. 307-342. Hillsdale, N.J.: Erlbaum Associates.

van der Wissel, A. (1987). IQ profiles of learning disabled and mildly mentally retarded children: A psychometric selection effect. British Journal of Developmental Psychology, 5, 45-51.

Williams, J. (1984). Phonemic analysis and how it relates to reading. Journal of Learning Disabilities, 17, 240-245.

Bei Fragen zur Produktsicherheit wenden Sie sich bitte an:
If you have any questions regarding product safety,
please contact:

Walter de Gruyter GmbH
Genthiner Straße 13
10785 Berlin
productsafety@degruyterbrill.com